Francesco Capasso
Timothy S. Gaginella
Giuliano Grandolini
Angelo A. Izzo

Phytotherapy

A Quick Reference to Herbal Medicine

With 77 Plates, 65 Figures and 57 Tables

Springer

Professor Dr Francesco Capasso
Department of Experimental
Pharmacology
University of Naples "Federico II"
Via D. Montesano 49
80131 Naples, Italy

Professor Dr Giuliano Grandolini
Department of Pharmaceutical
Chemistry and Technology
University of Perugia
Via del Liceo 1
06123 Perugia, Italy

Professor Dr Timothy S. Gaginella
School of Pharmacy
University of Wisconsin
Madison, WI 53706, USA

Professor Dr Angelo A. Izzo
Department of Experimental
Pharmacology
University of Naples "Federico II"
Via D. Montesano 49
80131 Naples, Italy

ISBN 3-540-00052-6 Springer-Verlag Berlin Heidelberg New York

Library of Congress Cataloging-in-Publication Data
Phytotherapy : a quick reference to herbal medicine / Francesco Capasso ...[et al.].
p. cm.
Includes bibliographical references.
ISBN 3-540-00052-6
1. Herbs—Therapeutic use—Handbooks, manuals, etc. 2. Materia medica, Vegetable—Handbooks, manuals, etc. I. Capasso, Francesco.

RM666.H33P497 2003
615'.321—dc21

2003041548

Springer-Verlag Berlin Heidelberg New York
a member of BertelsmannSpringer Science+Business Media GmbH

http://www.springer.de

Printed in Germany

Production Editor: Frank Krabbes, Heidelberg
Typesetting: wiskom e.K., Friedrichshafen
Cover design: design & production GmbH, Heidelberg

SPIN 10869202

Phytotherapy

A Quick Reference to Herbal Medicine

Springer
Berlin
Heidelberg
New York
Hong Kong
London
Milan
Paris
Tokyo

Foreword

It is evident that phytotherapy during the last 20 years has gained significance in drug therapy; in spite of this concerns have been voiced by practitioners of conventional medicine with respect to the use of plant-derived, "herbal" medicines. On balance, most properly cultivated and prepared herbal medicines are usually free of side effects, while synthetic drugs frequently produce undesirable adverse effects. If plant-derived drugs with a low therapeutic index (e.g.foxglove, belladonna) are excluded, most herbs indeed have a low incidence of side effects. Herbal medicines with a high therapeutic index can therefore be considered safe when used for health disturbances and chronic diseases. In this respect phytotherapy must be seen as an integration of pharmacognosy, pharmacology and pathology that enables students, physicians and practitioners to understand why, when and how herbal medicines can be used to treat diseases. It is therefore logical that it would be more efficient to learn pharmacognosy by first reviewing the medicinal plants, then pharmacology and pathophysiology to understand how botanicals may normalise an altered function. It is important to understand how to appropriately use herbal medicines to treat diseases. However, medical practitioners are often confused by the frequently conflicting information available on the safety and efficacy of herbs. In addition, herbal medicines very sometimes co-prescribed without proper attention to adjustment of dosages.

This textbook, unlike many phytotherapy texts, treats the subject of herbal medicines in an integrated fashion relative to pharmacognosy, pharmacology and toxicology. Many tables and figures are included to clarify complex mechanisms and other information. It is hoped that students, physicians and other healthcare practitioners will find this approach not much onerous and useful.

Ludovico Sorrentino MD
Professor of Pharmacology
University of Naples Federico II

Preface

In the last century the sources of natural medicines have expanded to include higher and lower plants, microorganisms, marine organisms, arthropods as well as animals. Nevertheless plants continue to be the major source of biologically active natural products such as teas extracts and tinctures, which may be utilized. The importance of medicinal plants can be realized from their prominence in the market place. Several analysis carried out in recent years have revealed that about 30 % of all prescriptions issued in Europe, USA and Canada contained an herb, a purified extract or an active component (or fraction) derived from herb. In other countries of the world herbs can be present in 70-90 % of the prescriptions. Therefore in spite of the substantial advances that have been made in synthetic chemistry, herbs and their constituents still remain an integral part of modern therapeutics in some countries, while play a role of primary importance in others.

The most frequently documented uses claimed for herbs include constipation and other gastrointestinal disturbances. In the therapy of constipation, especially, herbal laxatives have a leading position. Sleep disturbances and anxiety are other disorders in which herbs are used in the clinical practice. Acute and chronic diseases of the airways and the common cold, but also other disturbances referred to in the present book, are then a domain for herbs in the general medical practice. It's evident that there are controversial opinions with regard to phytotherapy and its efficacy and safety. Those who oppose herbal therapy consider these medicines as placebo while the extreme proponents of phytotherapy consider herbal medicines without side effects, healthful and absolutely safe. Phytotherapy is also an important adjunct to the use of synthetic drugs. However, there is also a political aspect that influences therapy with herbal medicines. For example in some industrialized countries the authorization of herbal medicines occurs on the basis of experimental and clinical studies, while in others the traditional use of herbal medicines is also considered as proof for efficacy and safety.

There are also data of questionable assurance, found in medical journals, books and from internet sources, which frequently do not provide objective information.

This book of phytotherapy is designed to provide phytotherapists with an objective review of the available information on the pharmacognosy and pharmacology of commonly used herbs and approved by Commission E. Clinical and toxicological findings of herbs treated and their dosages are described. A good deal of pathology and therapeutics information is included. A large iconography section can be of some help when the identity of an herbal drug is in doubt. The first part of the book deals with general aspects of herbs, i.e. history, their complexity, efficacy and safety, their preservation, active principles, galenic preparations and specific situations for the use of herbs. An overview of the regulation of herbal medicines concludes the general section. The special section is organized in systems and for each of them there is an introduction of physiopathology, then are treated herbal medicines as follows: botany/key constituents, mode of action, clinical studies, adverse events/contraindications, preparation/dosage.

At the end of the book an Appendix deals with nutraceuticals, herbal medicines and cancer, oriental medicines and a summary of the clinical efficacy of herbal medicines. Finally there is an iconography of the main plants and crude drugs treated in the book. We hope that this book can be useful for a wide variety of students and professionals with various interests.

As documentation throughout the text, we have given preference to review articles, well known book and new original research contributions. We are greatly indebted to colleagues at the Department of Experimental Pharmacology for their help and suggestions. We are also deeply grateful to Dr Emilia Nocerino and Dr Francesca Borrelli for selecting references and plates and for preparing tables.

Naples April 18, 2002

Francesco Capasso
Tymoty S. Gaginella
Giuliano Grandolini
Angelo A. Izzo

Contents

Abbreviations

11-OHSD	11-hydroxysteroid dehydrogenase
5-HT	5-hydroxytryptamine (serotonin)
AC	Adenylate cyclase
ACE	Angiotensin converting enzyme
ACTH	Adrenocorticotrophic hormone
AESGP	Association Européennes des Specialités Grand Publique
AIDS	Acquired immunodeficient syndrome
ALA	Alpha-linolenic acid
AMG	Arzneimittelgesetz
AMM	Authorisation de mise sur marchè
AMP	Adenosine monophosphate
ATP	Adenosine triphosphate
ATPase	Adenosine triphosphatase
BHC	British Herbal Compendium
BHP	British Herbal Pharmacopoeia
BPH	Benign prostatic hyperplasia
cAMP	Cyclic adenosine monophosphate
CAPE	Caffeic acid methyl ester
CE	Cholesterol ester
CHF	Congestive heart failure
CM	Chylomicrons
CRH	Corticotropin-releasing hormone
CNS	Central nervous system
Core-SPCS	Core-Summary of Product Characteristics
COX	Cyclooxygenase
CPMP	Committee for Proprietary Medicinal Products
CRH	Corticotrophin releasing hormone
CSP	Code de la Santè Publique
DGL	Deglycyrrhinized liquorice
DGLA	Dihomoi-gamma-linolenic acid
DHT	Dihydrotestosterone
DNA	Deoxyribonucleic acid
DSHEA	Dietary Supplement Health and Education Act

EEC	European Economic Commission
EEG	Electroencephalograph
EFA	Essential fatty acids
EFPIA	European Federation of Pharmaceutical Industries Association
EGF	Epidermal growth factor
EHPM	European Herbal Products Manufacturers
EMEA	European Medicines Evaluation Agency
ESCOP	European Scientific Cooperatives on Phytotherapy
EU	European Union
FDA	Food and Drug Administration
FSH	Follicle-stimulating hormone
FU	*Farmacopea Ufficiale* (i.e. the Italian Pharmacopoeia)
GABA	Gamma-aminobutyric acid
GAD	Glutamate decarboxylase
GAP	Good Agricultural Practices
GI	Gastrointestinal
GLA	Gamma-linolenic acid
GLC	Gas liquid chromatography
GMP	Good Manufacturing Practices
GnRH	Gonodotrophin realeasing hormone
GRAS	Generally recognized as safe
HCA	Hydroxycitric acid
HDL	High density lipoprotein
HLE	Human leukocyte elestase
HMGCoA	Hydroxymethylglutaryl CoA
HMPWG	Herbal Medicinal Products Working Group
HPLC	High pressure liquid chromatography
HB	Hemoglobin
HR	Herbal remedies
IBS	Irritable bowel syndrome
IDL	Intermediate density lipoprotein
LD_{50}	Lethal $dose_{50}$ = dose which causes death of 50% of treated animals
LDL	Low density lipoprotein
LH	Luteinizing hormone
LHRH	Luteinizing hormone releasing hormone
LOX	Lipoxygenase
LT	Leukotrienes

MAO	Monoamine oxidase
NANC	Non-adrenergic, non-cholinergic
NF	National Formulary
NF-kB	Nuclear factor kB
NO	Nitric oxide
NREM	Non-rapid eye movement
NSAID	Non-steroidal anti-inflammatory drug
NTA	Notice to Applicants
NYHA	New York Heart Association
OTC	Over-the-counter
PAF	Platelet activating factor
PDE	Phosphodiesterase
PDR	Physicians Desk Reference
PG	Prostaglandins
PGE1	1-series prostaglandins
PGE2	2-series prostaglandins
Ph.Eur.	European Pharmacopoeia
PNS	Peripheral nervous system
REM	Rapid eye movement
RNA	Ribonucleic acid
SCFA	Short-chain fatty acids
SHBG	Sex hormone binding globulin
SOD	Superoxide dismutase
TG	Triglycerides
TLC	Thin layer chromatography
TM	Tincture Mothers
TMC	Traditional Chinese Medicine
TNF	Tumor necrosis factor
TRH	Thyroxin releasing hormone
TTO	Tea tree oil
UDA	Urtica dioica agglutin
USP	United States Pharmacopoeia
VLDL	Very low density lipoprotein
WHO	World Health Organization

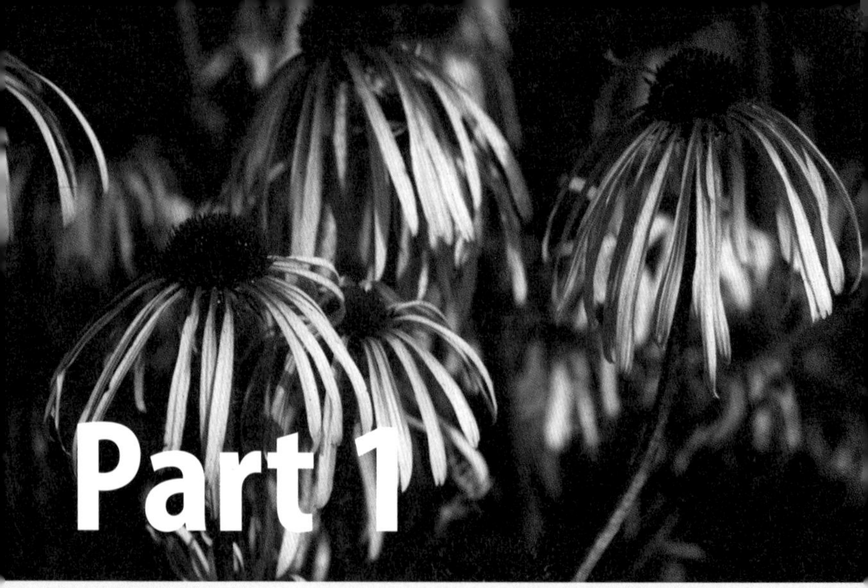

Part 1

Chapter 1
Introduction

For centuries plants have provided mankind with useful, sometimes life-saving, drugs. Even as the world entered the 20th century about 100 years ago, "modern" pharmaceutical manufacturers were primarily involved in extracting, developing and marketing the active constituents present in medicinal plants. In cases where correlations between chemical structure and biological activity were noted, "empirical" science began to give way to "rational" drug design. This emerging approach by newly formed pharmaceutical companies to identify, test and develop potential new drugs was largely successful due to the intellectual cooperation of chemistry (i.e. "medicinal chemistry"), pharmacognosy (which can be thought of as "medicinal botany") and pharmacology. Initially the focus was on the synthesis of analogous or homologous molecules but with advances in knowledge and technology emphasis shifted more towards the synthesis of new chemical entities (Figure 1.1, p. 4). Along with the advent of synthetic drugs medicinal plants began to rapidly disappear from use in most industrialized countries including the United States, Canada, Australia and England; in other countries such as Austria, Germany, Italy and France plant-derived (herbal) remedies continued to be used but generally in a minor role compared to more highly purified synthetic drugs produced for modern medicine.

Today there is a renewed interest in the consumption of herbs even though there is a decline in some of them (Table 1.1, p. 5). This return to things more "natural", which would seem to be in contrast to the trend of modern medical science, has been recognized by the World Health Organisation (WHO), which has campaigned to promote more research on and the better use of medicinal plants. However, this growing trend to use medicinal plants to treat a wide range of problems from insomnia, anxiety, obesity, eczema, arthritis to immunodeficiency syndrome, has been facilitated by the realization by patients that modern medicine cannot always resolve symptoms of medical disorders or prevent the progression of disease. Patients have increasingly begun to recognize that physicians are indeed limited in their ability to "heal". Time constraints

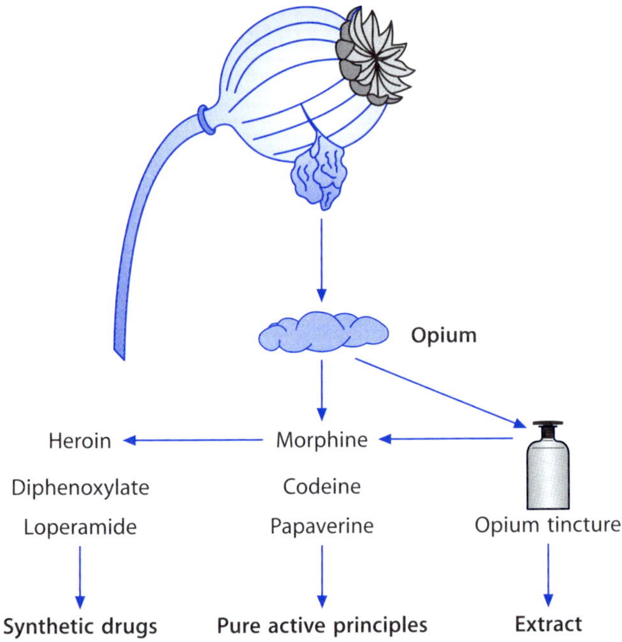

Figure 1-1 ▲ **Examples of crude drug (opium), extract, active principles, and synthetic drugs**

(and even "quotas") imposed on physicians working within the "managed care model", in operation in many countries around the world, has added to patient discontent. The often less than satisfying experience of a trip to one's doctor in the 21st century, along with increased awareness that even sophisticated synthetic pharmaceuticals have undesirable side effects, has led to greater consumer demand for herbal drugs. And, the idea that "natural can only be good" has been bolstered by ecological movements throughout the world over the last 20 years.

Herbal medicines originated from the ancient use of wild plants. Depending on the locality and conditions under which the plant was grown, the content of active components can vary. Today, with the possibility of carefully controlling the cultivation of medicinal plants and even improving them genetically, it is possible to develop and market a wide variety and quantity of herbal drugs of consistent chemical com-

Table 1.1
Sales of herbal medicinal products in the USA (Herbal Gram 2002; 55: 60)

Herbal medicine Common name	Herbal medicine Latin name	Condition frequently treated	Retail sales (US $) in 2001	% Change (compared to 2000)
Ginkgo	*Ginkgo biloba*	Cognitive deficit, tinnitus, intermittent claudication	46,115,692	−35.3
Echinacea	*Echinacea spp.*	Respiratory tract infections (cold)	39,700,408	−20.2
Garlic	*Allium sativum*	Hypercholesterolemia, prevention of arteriosclerosis	34,834,928	−17.3
Ginseng	*Panax ginseng*	Stress states, lack of stamina	30,964,420	−32.8
Soy	*Glycine max*	Menopausal complaints	27,625,944	−3.6
Saw palmetto	*Serenoa repens*	Prostatic hyperplasia	24,616,420	−13.5
St John's wort	*Hypericum perforatum*	Mild-to-moderate depression	24,132,972	−40.5
Valerian	*Valeriana officinalis*	Insomnia	11,777,825	−13.3
Cranberry	*Vaccinium macrocarpon*	Urinary tract infections	10,279,853	+6.9
Black cohosh	*Cimicifuga racemosa*	Premenstrual syndrome	9,639,506	+105.8
Kava kava	*Piper methysticum*	Anxiety	9,316,924	−16.3
Milk thistle	*Silybum marianum*	Liver diseases	7,044,696	+12.8
Evening primrose	*Oenothera biennis*	Inflammatory states, menopausal complaints, psoriasis, atopic eczema	5,760,010	−11.5
Grape seeds	*Vitis vinifera*	Prevention of cancer and arteriosclerotic diseases	4,002,785	−15.1
Bilberry	*Vaccinium myrtillus*	Chronic venous insufficiency, cancer prevention, diarrhea, mouth inflammation	3,521,756	−10.5
Yohimbe	*Pausinystalia yohimbe*	Erectile dysfunction	2,013,491	−2.8
Green tea	*Thea sinensis*	Cancer prevention	1,717,237	−13.2
French maritime pine	*Pinus pinaster*	Chronic venous insufficiency	1,448,488	−27.5
Ginger	*Zingiber officinale*	Nausea, vomiting	1,211,835	−21.1
Feverfew	*Tanacetum parthenium*	Headache, fevers	667,353	−23.9
Multi herbs			**6,355,926**	**+68.8**
All other herbs			**34,688,456**	**−26.9**
Total herbs			**337,431,200**	**+21.0**

position and excellent quality (Table 1.2, p. 6). Apart from these advantages, important progress has been made in processing and preserving the raw material of medicinal plants through modern methods of freezing, stabilization, dehydration through drying in vacuum, and lyophili-

Table 1.2
Advantages of cultivation of medicinal plants vs. wild flora

	Wild flora	Cultivation
Availability	Decreasing	Increasing
Fluctuation of supply	Unstable	More controlled
Quality control	Poor	High
Botanical identification	Sometimes not reliable	Not questionable
Genetic improvement	No	Yes
Chemical constituents	Unstable	Consistent and constant
Agronomic manipulation	No	Yes
Post-harvest handling	Poor	Usually good
Adulteration	Likely	Relatively safe

zation, making it possible to store raw material for long periods of time. Therefore, today it is possible to find on the market herbal medicines of high quality, with well-defined chemical composition and pharmacological activity.

Herbal medicines offer the advantages of relative safety, lack of significant side effects and generally lower cost compared to conventional medicines. The use of herbs also has application as adjuncts to complement traditional pharmacotherapy. For example, echinacea may be used to ameliorate cold and flu symptoms, possibly reducing the improper use of antibiotics in such conditions, thus minimizing the possibility of developing resistant strains of microorganisms and side effects (e.g. diarrhea). Regarding costs, it has been demonstrated that migraine headache prophylaxis with feverfew costs less than (US) $0.25/day compared with propanolol or methysergide from $2.5 to $8/day. Hypercholesterolemia may benefit from garlic at a cost of about $0.15/day compared with cholestyramine at $54/day; benign prostatic hyperplasia is treatable both with saw palmetto at $0.4/day and finasteride at a cost of about $2/day. Finally, "Mother Nature" seems to "do her best" as evidenced by the fact that often times plants possess medicinal effects that are not found with isolated components, making the whole greater than the sum of the parts. Therefore, while it is possible to extract biologically active plant constituents and to perform structural modifications, this approach is unlikely to lead intentionally to the discovery of completely new drugs. The plant kingdom seems to be an inexhaustible source of medicaments and herbal medicine must be regarded as "one active ingredient in its entirety, whether or not the constituents with therapeutic activity are known".

Chapter 2
Definitions

"Medicinal plants" contain chemicals with pharmacological activity in humans and/or animals. This definition excludes those plants used in surgery (*Gossypium herbaceum*, *Hevea brasiliensis*). Likewise such a definition does not consider those plants used to extract substances in the synthesis of compounds with known pharmacological activity, a good example being the *Dioscorea* species which contains diosgenin, a substance used to synthesize progesterone. Excluded from this definition are also those plants used as parasite repellents (e.g. *Derris elliptica*, *Chrysanthemum cinerariaefolium*) or agents poisonous to animals such as *Antiaris toxicaria*, *Alstonia scholaris*, *Barringtonia racemosa*. There are, then, a limited number of plants that qualify either as drugs, foods or both (e.g. *Allium sativum*), depending on their specific use. Medicinal plants are, therefore, those used for medicinal purposes and must be considered to be drugs.

Another term commonly encountered is "herbal medicine" or "botanical medicine", as preferred by the Food and Drug Administration (FDA). This definition refers to the use of plants or plant substances as medicinal agents, as does the term "herb", "herbal drug" and "herbal remedy". However, herbal remedy is not synonymous for homeopathic remedy, as frequently stated by people and practitioners. Both entities employ plants, but herbal remedies contain active principles which exert a pharmacological effect, while homeopathic remedies contain herbal and active principles in amounts so low to be immeasurable (a sufficient molecular memory exerts a therapeutic effect). The "crude drugs", called "simples" in the Middle Ages, represent the dried or fresh herbs or the starting material from which chemically pure compounds can be isolated. "Phytopharmaceutical" is a term used for those medicinal preparations made by extracting botanical products with appropriate solvents to yield extracts, tinctures, or the like. Ideally, such preparations have been standardized to a chemical marker or pharmacologically active constituents, named "active principles". "Phytomedicine" is another term proposed by the European

Union (EU) and the European Scientific Cooperative for Phytotherapy (ESCOP) to indicate phytopharmaceuticals.

The discussion about the most appropriate term is old and will probably continue in future. To avoid confusion we prefer to use the expression **herbal medicine** to also indicate complex preparations from medicinal plants, which, with rare exceptions, have a large therapeutic index. "Phytotherapy", which is based upon herbal medicines, is the bridge between herbal folklore (i.e. traditional) and allopathic (conventional) medicine. The term phytotherapy was coined by Henri Leclerc, a French physician (1870-1955), who summarized his lifetime in a work entitled "*Precis de Phytotherapie*". Phytotherapy describes the efficacy and limitation of herbal medicines in the treatment of human diseases: it covers everything, from herbal medicines with powerful actions (foxglove, belladonna, etc.) to those with "very gentle" (or mite) action (chamomile, mint, etc.). The herbs with gentle action must not be considered ineffective, but rather that one would not expect these herbs to produce instant and powerful effects like foxglove or have appreciable toxic effect, and may be safely taken over a long period of time. Between gentle and powerful herbal medicines there are the majority of herbal medicines, liquorice, senna, echinacea, St. John's wort and ginkgo to mention just a few. This branch of herbal medicine is practiced by physicians trained in herbalism. Other branches of herbal medicine are "phytochemistry" (studies the chemicals in the plants) and "phytopharmacy" (dealing with the preparation of vegetable medicines). The botanical study of the medicinal plants is another scientific branch of herbal medicine. Crude drugs, botanical medicines, phytomedicines and phytopharmaceuticals, like conventional medicines should be included in every country's Pharmacopoeia, an official book which lists all the medicines and the characteristics that those must posses in order to go on sale. In contrast to these products, "nutraceuticals" are food-derived nutrients which, at doses sometimes exceeding their minimal daily requirement, have beneficial pharmacological effects. Nutraceuticals support human health or return one to relative health from a disease or medical disorder. Vitamins and minerals, but also plant-derived antioxidants such as flavonoids, isoflavones and proanthocyanidins, can be considered common nutraceuticals (see Appendix).

Chapter 3
History

The healing properties of plants were discovered by chance, no doubt by early mankind in the quest for daily food. The observation that animals favored certain plants when they were injured or ill may have helped to guide primitive man in the search of cures for his ailments. Knowledge of the medicinal value of these plants was initially passed on verbally. Eventually, with the development of society and written language, records on the use of medicinal plants were preserved in writing.

The first documented use of medicinal plants can be found in the early Egyptian and Asian cultures. The Egyptians had extensive knowledge of plants derived from their technique of embalming. The Ebers Papyrus (about 1550 BC) presents a large number of crude drugs that are still of great importance (castor seed, gum arabic, aloe, etc.). Knowledge of the virtues of medicinal plants later spread to Greece and other countries of the ancient Western World. Many authors of antiquity described plants that could be used as drugs. Among them were Hippocrates (460–370 BC), Theophrastus (370–287 BC), Pliny the Elder (AD 23–79), Dioscorides (AD 40–80) and Galen (AD 130–210). The Greek Dioscorides rigorously collected information about 600 plants and remedies and collected them in his seminal *Materia Medica*, a term used to define the knowledge of drugs for many hundreds of years. If Discorides was "The Father of Medicine", Galen was "The Father of Pharmacy". Regarded as the pivotal Graeco-Roman authority in medicinal plants, he wrote extensively about the subject and also proposing a research agenda for establishing the powers of a remedy. In the Middle Ages medicinal plants began to be catalogued according to their therapeutic action, and medical schools such as the one in Salerno, Italy, published the book *Ortus Sanitatis*. In the 15th century several so-called herbals were published containing information, with pictures, on medicinal plants. During the 16th and 17th centuries medicinal plants continued to play a primary function in medicine. In the 18th century, Linnaeus made an important contribution to the development of plant science through the introduction of the new system for naming and classifying plants.

During the 18th and 19th century plants and crude drugs were still being used as powders, extracts or tinctures. However, during this period began the isolation and chemical identification of pharmacologically active compounds from crude drugs. For example, morphine was isolated in 1803, strychnine in 1817, quinine and caffeine in 1820, nicotine in 1828, atropine in 1833, cocaine in 1855 and foxglove glycosides in 1868. The 20th century is characterized by the development of synthetic chemistry, which began generating a stream of pure new drugs which could be standardized and for which quality could be easily controlled. Today the constituents of the main herbal drugs have been isolated and their structure determined. The last century has also witnessed the discovery of hormones and vitamins from the animal Kingdom, although in amounts too small to permit isolation of enough quantities for use as drugs. Some of these are today prepared from plant-derived compounds while others are obtained by biotechnological methods. In any case, since 1980 there has been a gradual increasing appearance of herbal medicines and their galenical preparations from medical practice and pharmacy shelves.

Chapter 4

The Complexity of Herbal Medicines

The quality of a herbal medicine is believed to be directly related to its active principles. These constituents have been referred to as "secondary" plant substances. However, herbal medicines contain other substances, often neglected and poorly understood, which render the ingredients "active" as medicinal agents. Thus, it is often difficult to reproduce the effect of the herbal drugs by isolating its individual constituents and recombining them in the laboratory. They are generally inactive substances (cellulose, lignin, etc.) but also substances of minimal pharmacological interest, such as the bitter or aromatic substances that stimulate the gastric and intestinal secretions thus making the dissolution, and consequently the absorption of the active principle possible or more complete. The tannins and saponins, very common in the vegetable kingdom, as the salts of organic acids may facilitate intestinal absorption of active plant principles through effects on intestinal motility or bile secretion. Like the mucilages and peptic substances, vitamins can also modify the functions of the intestine mucous membrane and consequently the absorption.

There is also the possibility of interactions between plant constituents. These agents may be closely related both chemically and therapeutically to the main constituents responsible for the pharmacological activity. Foxglove, for example, contains about 30 different closely related glycosides. These cardiotonic agents, with small structural differences, have different rates of onset of action and different durations of their effects (digitoxin, given orally, has an onset of action of 1–4 hours with peak activity at 8–14 hours; digoxin has an onset of action of 1/2–2 hours and reaches a peak activity level in 2–6 hours). For these reasons foxglove preparations provide an activity of short onset and long duration but they are very seldom used because it is difficult to standardize. In some cases a herbal medicine may contain a variety of pharmacologically active agents that are not related chemically or therapeutically. In most cases, therefore, herbal medicines represent a synergic complex of active principles whose actions and applications can be difficult to reproduce. Contrary of conventional drugs, herbal medicine must be seen as a complex pharmaceutical preparation (Figure 4.1) and as such should preferably be administered in the form of an extract.

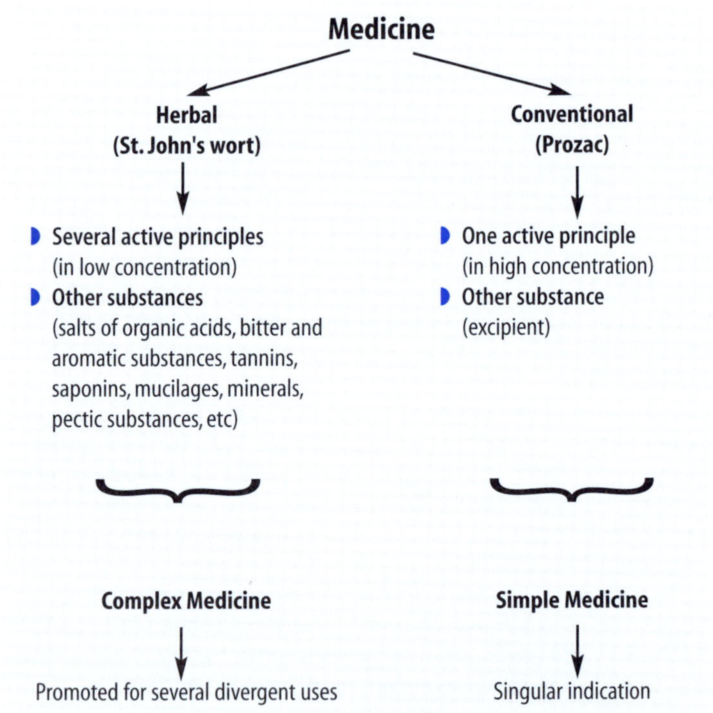

Figure 4-1 ▲ **Differences between herbal and conventional medicines**

Chapter 5

Are the Herbal Medicines Safe?

Medical opinion is that any medicine has the potential to do harm and adverse reactions are a cost of medical therapy. It is not possible to eliminate the adverse reactions because these are part of the normal, pharmacological actions of all medicines or represent an indirect consequence of the principal action of the medicine. Such reactions, being pharmacologically predictable and dose-dependent, can be anticipated and also reduced by dose reduction but never eliminated. Therefore, the statement that medicines are safe and effective is very relative. On the other hand, there is a native view that what is "natural" can only be good and the belief that herbal medicines are completely innocuous in contrast to conventional medicines. The use of herbal medicines by millions of people since prehistory is an aspect emphasized by herbalists. Another point, for the safety reputation of herbs, is that herbal medicines promote healing responses rather than obstacle pathologies and this is because herbs have a complex chemical composition. It is also deduced that herbal medicines are free from adverse reactions, probably because they are not effective like conventional medicines. It is not easy to give satisfactory answers to these discrepancies and for the absence of serious information about adverse reactions and toxicity of herbs.

Many herbal medicines widely available today have not been properly evaluated for untoward effects in clinical studies. Certainly there is substantial evidence for adverse reactions to herbal medicines (Table 5.1, p. 14). The situation is complicated in several ways: the sources of herbal material are diverse; the active (and toxic) components vary as a result of climate, soil quality, genetic factors and exposure to chemicals; quality control is lacking so that problems such as contaminations with heavy metals or microorganisms and adulteration with botanicals and/or chemicals may arise during preparation, storage or shipping; several common herbal medicines contain a mixture of herbal drugs and in

Table 5.1
Some herbal medicines associated with adverse reactions

Herbal Medicine	Indication/use	Adverse effect
Aloe gel	Wound healing	Allergic reactions
Artichoke	Liver and gallbladder complaints, cholesterol-lowering	Allergic reactions
Chaparral	Expectorant, anti-inflammatory	*Liver damage
Comfrey	Blunt injuries	*Liver damage
Dandelion	Dyspeptic complaints	Allergic reactions
Feverfew	Headache migraine	Allergic reactions
Garlic	Cholesterol-lowering, antihypertensive, arteriosclerosis	Allergic reaction, abdominal discomfort
Ginseng	Stimulant, tonic	Mastalgia
Goldenseal	Digestive disorders	Excitatory states, constipation
Guar gum	Obesity	*Obstruction of the GI tract
Liquorice	Gastritis, cough/bronchitis	*Hypokalemia, hypertension, arrhythmias, edema
Ma huang	Stimulant, asthma	GI, cardiovascular and CNS effects
Pennyroyal	Digestive disorders	*Liver damage
Saw palmetto	Prostatic complaints, irritable bladder	Stomach complaints

* adverse effects frequently reported; GI, gastrointestinal; CNS, central nervous system

some cases are self-prescribed. Other risks that may contribute to the toxicity of herbal medicine are listed in Table 5.2. (p. 15) In the United States and other countries, herbal drugs are sold as dietary supplements, without intervention or advice by a pharmacist or other healthcare professional. Standardization would seem to be a step forward, but this makes little sense when (i) most herbal medicines have yet to yield identity of their pharmacological active principle(s), (ii) attempts at standardization are confounded by the complex composition of herbs, (iii) active principles (antagonists as well agonists) may coexist. The desired effect may require concerned action of some or all components of the particular herb. For this reason too, differences in desired/undesired activities, and potency differences may be noted when comparing whole herb, infusion and extract. The problem is to determine the active component upon which standardization will be based. Just recently it has been recognized that echinacea and St. John's wort appear to be improperly standardized for therapeutic activity by their levels of echinacosides and hypericin, respectively.

It is also important to consider that some of the many herbs available to treat diseases may interact with prescribed drugs to produce unde-

Table 5.2
Risks contributing to the toxicity of herbal medicines

- Presence of potentially toxic constituents (apiole, asarone, estragole, safrole, pyrrolizidine alkaloids, lectins, cyanogenetic glycosides, sesquiterpene lactones, etc.) in medicinal plants
- Use of herbal medicines in addition to conventional drugs
- Herbal medicine contains numerous plants
- Automedication
- Misidentification of the plant
- Inadequate preparation and storage
- Presence of contaminants (microorganisms, heavy metals, microbial toxins, pesticides, fumigation agents, radioactivity, synthetic and animal drug substances)
- Adulteration during conditioning
- Mislabelling of the final product

sirable effects (Table 5.3, p. 16). Clearly more research into all aspects of herbal therapy is warranted. The resurgence of interest in herbal medicines presents a challenge: identify and characterizing the constituents of herbal medicines, standardizing products in a manner appropriate to the intended use, discourage misuse and concurrent ingestion of multiple drugs. Until better control of herbal medicines is gained on several levels, it seems prudent to follow the suggestion of De Smet and apply "pharmacovigilance" in the marketing and use of herbal medicines. Finally, the safety of herbal medicines depend on their correct use. Table 5.4 (p. 18) lists the conditions that can establish the "powers" of a herbal medicine. A herbal medicine, like any medicine, is a double-edged word. Therefore, both patients and physicians must be able to make the risk/benefit assessment, before using any herbal medicine (Figure 5.1, p. 18). It is also important to have in mind the fundamental principles of toxicology proposed by Parcelsus (1493–1541): *sola dosis facet venenum.*

5.1 Standardization of Herbal Medicines

We have just stated that one of the main problems of phytotherapy is the standardization of herbal preparations. If a preparation of a given herb is shown to be effective, this does not necessarily mean that another preparation of the same drug is similarly effective. The use of preparations inadequately standardized involves a considerable risk of distortion and produces a false negative overall result. To carry out reliable clinical trials the herbal medicines must be of standardized quality. The standardization, in the case of a herbal drug, is not simply an analytical

Table 5.3

Clinical reports of suspected interaction between herbal medicines and prescribed drugs. (Data from Fugh-Berman and Ernst, 2001 and Izzo and Ernst, 2001)

Type of herbal remedy	Use of herbal remedy	Interaction with	Clinical effect	Possible mechanism	Causality
Danshen	Chinese herb with various uses	warfarin	over – anticoagulation	danshew has anti-platelet activity	very likely
Dong quai	pre-menstrual symptoms	warfarin	over – anticoagulation	not known	possible
Garlic	to lower cholesterol	warfarin	over – anticoagulation	garlic has anti-platelet activity	possible
Gum guar	to reduce body weight	digoxin	reduced absorption	Gum guar reduces absorption since it reduces gastric emptying	very likely
Papaya extract	indigestion	warfarin	over – anticoagulation	not known	possible
Ginkgo	to enhance memory and circulation	warfarin	over – anticoagulation	ginkgo biloba has anti-platelet activity	possible
Ginkgo	to enhance memory and circulation	aspirin	over – anticoagulation	ginkgo biloba has anti-platelet activity	possible
Ginkgo	to enhance memory and *circulation*	thiazide diuretics	hypertension	not known	possible
Devil's claw	arthritis	warfarin	over – anticoagulation	not known	possible
Green tea	prevention of cancer	warfarin	decreased antico-agulant effect	Green tea contain vitamin K, which antagonise the effect of warfarin	likely
Ginseng	various indications	phenelzine	mania, headache, hallu-cinations, insomnia	not known	likely
Kava	anxiolytic	alprazolam	coma	synergism of action	likely

Continued on next page

Table 5.3

Clinical reports of suspected interaction between herbal medicines and prescribed drugs. (Data from Fugh-Berman and Ernst, 2001 and Izzo and Ernst, 2001) (*continued*)

Type of herbal remedy	Use of herbal remedy	Interaction with	Clinical effect	Possible mechanism	Causality
St. John's wort	anti-depressant	theophyllin, cyclosporine, warfarin, ethinyloestradiol, indinavir, digoxin, simvastatin	decreased plasma levels of concomitantly administered drugs	hepatic enzyme induction and/or induction of P-glycoprotein	very likely
St. John's wort	anti-depressant	loperamide	delirium	potentiation of MAO inhibition	possible
St. John's wort	anti-depressant	paroxetine,seraltine, nefazodone	serotonin syndrome: dizzeness, weakness, confusion, nausea/ vomiting	synergistic serotonin uptake inhibition	likely
Shankhapushpi	Ayurvedic remedy with various indication	phenytoin	loss of seizure control	not known	possible
Evening primrose oil	eczema, pre-menstrual syndrome	phenytoin	loss of seizure control	not known	possible
Ispaghula	laxative	lithium salt	none	lowering of lithium level due to reduced intestinal absorption	possible
Betelnut	various indications	procylidine	extrapyramidal syndrome	antagonism on acetylcholine receptors	possible
Liquorice	antiulcer, hepatoprotective	anti-hypertensive drugs	hypokalemia	aldosterone effect	very likely

Table 5.4

A research agenda of establishing the powers of a herbal medicine

- The remedy must be of good unadulterated quality
- The illness must be simple, not complex
- The illness must be appropriate to the action of the remedy
- The remedy must be more powerful than the illness
- One should make careful note of the course of illness and treatment
- One must ensure that the effect of the remedy is the same for everybody at all times
- One must see that the effect of the remedy is specific for human beings (in an animal it can have another effect)
- One must distinguish between the effect of botanical medicines (working by their quality) from foods (working by their substance)

evaluation, i.e. the identification and assay of active principles or of a marker. It means "the body of information and controls that are necessary to guarantee the constancy of composition, and consequently the constancy of activity, of an herbal medicine".

We must take into account that the vegetable material to be examined has a complex and inconstant chemical composition. The composition of herbal medicines is inevitably inconstant, depending on a variety of

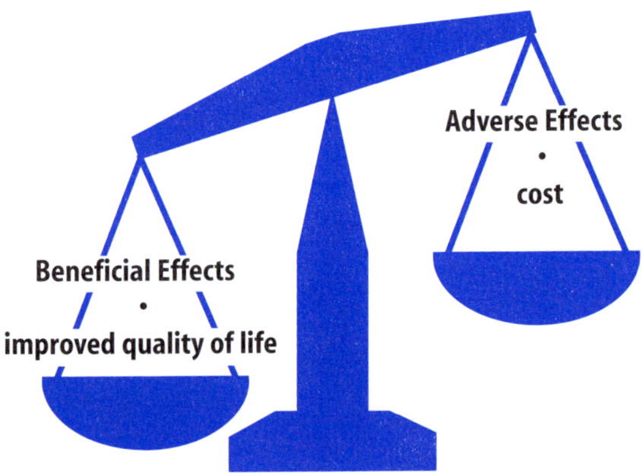

Figure 5-1 ▲ **Risk/benefit ratio. The beneficial effects of a herbal medicine can outweigh the adverse effects**

factors: age and origin, harvesting period (Table 5.5), the specific parts of the plant to be processed, the extraction methods employed, the drying and storage, etc. The use of cultivated rather than wild plants may reduce some causes of inconstancy of chemical composition. In fact, cultivated plants grow in homogeneous climatic conditions, are harvested quickly at the right time and dried in a controlled time and temperature. Correct drying is the most important phase in the whole process of production. Besides, because of the complex composition of herbal medicine the process of production of botanical preparation (extract, etc.) must be kept constant; only in this way it is possible to obtain from a standard herb a standardized herbal preparation. With regard to the definition of chemical composition, chromatographic techniques (TLC, GLC, HPLC) yield good results and are considered the most suitable. However, in the absence of a specific chromatographic method, other methods have to be used: spectrophotometry, colorimetry, gravimetric determinations, etc.

Table 5.5

Optimal harvesting period of whole herb and its organs

Material*	Time
Root, rhizome and bulb	From Autumn (end of the vegetation period) to Spring (before germination) They must be washed free of adhering soil and sand
Wood	In the Winter (before formation of buds)
Bark	In the Spring (when the parenchymatous cells are not yet differentiated)
Leaf and herb	In the Spring (the flowering stage)
Flower	From Spring to Easter (when fully developed)
Fruit and seed	From Easter to Autumn (when fully ripe)

* The material is collected when the organ in question has reached its optimal state of development

An important aspect of standardization is the need to use a homogeneous nomenclature for herbal preparations. This aids to compare pharmacological and clinical results carried out in different laboratories, permits the physicians to compare herbal preparations containing the same active principles and excludes mistakes in dosage. Therefore in the case of a crude drug, the name of the drug should be followed by the drug/extract ratio, by the solvent used for extraction and by the physical form (for example: *Rhamnus purshiana* bark, 1:1, 20% hydroalcoholic extract). In the case of purified extract the name of the herbal drug (i.e. latin name of the plant followed by the part of the plant used) should be followed by the content of active principles (for example: *Atropa belladonna* leaves, 90% total alkaloids calculated as hyoscyamine). However, where possible, it is better to define a fingerprint of the herbal medicine.

Chapter 6

The Herbal Medicines and the Importance of the Scientific Research

Herbal medicines, before appearing in the pharmacy's as a medicine, should be required to undergo pharmacological and toxicological testing on animals and clinical trials in humans. Unfortunately, this is not usually the case. The cost of such an endeavour, especially for products that will not have patent protection, is perhaps the major reason for the lack of research on herbal medicines. Although approximately 13,000 plants are used therapeutically around the world, few have been studied in a systematic way. The situation may be improving. In the United States, where most herbal medicines are sold as dietary supplements without a physician's prescription, companies themselves are beginning to conduct research on their products in order to regulate quality to avoid governmental regulation.

6.1 Toxicity Studies

Ideally a botanical product should eliminate symptoms of or cure medical disorders and alleviate suffering. Therapeutic dosages should not provoke untoward effects such as gastro-intestinal disturbances, blood pressure changes or cutaneous reactions, nor alter enzymatic reactions. Today, ascertaining the safety of a drug is perhaps more important than ascertaining its effectiveness. Acute toxicity should be assessed in animals by determining the maximal tolerated dose. Chronic toxicity can be determined after repeated exposure to the product (3–10 days subacute toxicity, 15–30 days subchronic toxicity, 1 month to 2 years for chronic toxicity). Prolonged toxicity is determined on the basis of data supplied by daily or periodic observation of some parameters: weight curve, daily food consumption, the animal's general state (appearance, condition of its coat, behavior, muscular tone, pupil diameter, quantity, appearance and consistency of urine and feces), metabolic constants (leukocyte count, hematocrit, Hb, etc.), blood chemistry, and macro- and microscopic examination of the main organs at the end of the treatment period. Toxicity tests also include *teratogenic*, and *carcinogenic* potential and *tolerability* tests. As herbal medicines may sometimes interfere with sexual function, giving rise to impotence or infertility, tests for these functions should be included in the safety evaluation of any botanical product.

6.2 Efficacy Studies (see also appendix D)

The effectiveness and therapeutic application of herbal medicine is the other requirement to be taken into consideration. This requires specific biological tests for every pharmacological action on laboratory animals. In practice this means studying the effects of the drug on tissues and organs in experimental models of the disease or disorder for which the product is intended. Preliminary estimates of the therapeutic dose may also be determined in these studies. However, the evaluation of herbal drugs for medicinal properties is complicated by the presence of multiple components in addition to the active principle(s). As a consequence, it is much more difficult to extend the experimental results in animals with botanicals to humans than with conventional drugs. The chemical complexity of herbal medicines causes multiple effects in humans which must be tested only throughout clinical trials. When evaluating human studies, additional considerations come into play. It is essential to rule out a placebo effect. This can be accomplished through thoughtful experimental design, specifically using a double-blind, cross-over method. This makes it possible to minimize the influence of the expectations of patients and physicians. Anyway, even rigorous randomized clinical trials do not always agree in their conclusions. An example may be the use of feverfew in patients with headache. Some randomized clinical trials suggest that feverfew is more efficacious than placebo in alleviating headache, while other trials show no significant effect. In these cases the matter can be achieved by conducting systematic reviews (which provide a summary of the clinical evidence by assessing individual clinical studies) and meta-analysis. Meta-analysis represents a subspecies of systematic reviews which give data from individual trials and calculate a new overall effect size of a particular outcome measure. Meta-analysis is a useful, albeit not infallible, approach to assess the efficacy of herbal medicines. Germany has a strong tradition in phytotherapy and hence controls are more stringent. The **German Commission E** (*Kommission E*), a special committee of the *Bundesgesundheitsamt* (Federal Department of Health), is a consulting body appointed by the German equivalent of the U.S. Food and Drug Administration (FDA). The German Commission E prepares monographs using historic information, chemical, pharmacological, clinical and toxicological studies, case reports, epidemiological data and unpublished manufacturer's data.

Chapter 7

Parts of the Plant to be used, Nomenclature, Drug Acquisition and Preservation

Herbal medicines are obtained from either wild or cultivated plants with economic factors usually determining the choice. It may be more advisable to obtain the drug from wild plants which are particularly common, therefore limiting the costs; however, scarcity and consequently high costs of wild plants make cultivation a valid alternative. Dioscorea (*Dioscorea mexicana*) and cascara (*Rhamnus purshiana*) are almost exclusively obtained from wild plants in Mexico and the United States, while in Europe foxglove (*Digitalis purpurea*) is obtained from cultivated plants. Marshmallow (*Althea officinalis*) is obtained from both wild and cultivated plants in Europe. Without doubt cultivation offers many advantages: the main is the possibility to have plants with a constant chemical composition.

7.1 Parts of the Plant used for Therapeutic Ends

Botanical medicines may take many forms. They may contain crude drug in the form of powdered material from the part of the plant determined to have biological activity, or as various aqueous, alcoholic or other extracts. It is essential to identify the part of the plant used in the preparation. In order to minimize expense, many herbal medicines tend to be marketed in the form of powder or cut up into small pieces. **Roots** are the underground parts of the plant and serve to anchor it. They are free of buds, leaves, knots and interknots. In dried state they are of a cylindrical or conical form, with a wrinkled surface, free of knots or lichen traces. **Rhizomes** are cylindrical-shaped underground stems, more or less swollen and fleshy, with small scales from which leaf, root and bud systems are developed. In dried state they have an elongated, cylindrical form with marks and scarring from leaves, roots and shoots. **Tubers** are fusiform or spheroidal form underground organs (stems, rhizomes, roots and leaves). In dried state they have a spheroidal form showing the marks of shoots and roots. **Bulbs** are spheroidal underground organs with short stems at the center, which are covered by numerous and rather fleshy leaves (scales). The isolated scales (which are in the form of lamellae) or the whole bulb with roots or remains of these can be used for the drug. The **cortex** is the external part of the stems, branches and roots. When dried it is in flat pieces, rugose and rough, cylindrical or grooved. The **wood** is the part of the stem between (and including) the cambium and medulla. When dried it is hard with a stratified structure.

Herbs are drugs which are composed of the entire herbaceous plant. The dried parts used are the caulis, leaves and flowers. **Flowering tops** are the terminal flowers. When dried the parts used are the leaves and at times the fruit. The **leaves** are appendices and extensions of stems and have a respiratory function. They are composed of a main stem (petiole) and a leaf (lamina). Those without a main stem are called sessiles. Dried leaves are distinguished from one another by the form of the lamina (oval, lanceolate etc.), by the form of the lamina margin (serrated, crenated etc.), by the form of the nervature (single or parallel veins etc.) and by the presence or lack of a main stem. **Flowers** are the reproductive organs. They can be with or without a peduncle, in the latter case sessile; they can be isolated flowers or in a clump (raceme, spike, corymb, etc.). In dried state the latter are distinguished by the easiness with which they are crushed. **Fruits** are ovary transformations after fertilization and following ripening. Their function is to propagate the species. In dried state the parts that can be used are the skin or epicarp, the fleshy part or mesocarp, the peduncle or main stem or the whole fruit. The **seeds** are transformed ovules after fertilization. Each seed consists of a husk and a kernel. In dried state they are hard, of different shapes, coloured and in some cases covered with fine hair. They can be used with or without the husk removed (for example, ricinus seeds). **Sprouts** are undifferentiated lower plant bodies (thallophytes), not as cormophytes, roots, stems, and leaves, etc. Their cellular tissue is always morphologically homogeneous. In dried state they are filiform or membraneous branches (algae, lichen) or spungy bodies differing in volume and appearance (fungus). **Galls** (cecids) are caused by parasites which establish themselves in a plant organ stimulating abnormal development. These pathological formations are constant in form, thus permitting description. When dried they are globular bodies, hard, heavy with a small base main stem and with roundish surface projections.

7.2 Nomenclature

The names of the plant drugs are most appropriately expressed in pharmaceutical Latin. The Latin names generally indicate the genus and/or species of the plant, followed by the Latin name of the part of the plant from which the drug derives. So when referring to the whole plant, the botanical name is followed by the Latin name **herba** (*Malva sylvestris herba*). When referring to the root, rhizome, bulb, tuber, caulis, wood, bark or leaf, these names are followed by **radix** *(Glycirrhiza glabra radix)*, **rhizome** *(Rheum palmatum rhizome)*, **bulbus** *(Urginea maritima bulbus)*, **tuber** *(Colchicum autumnale tuber)*, **caulis** *(Equisetum arvense caulis)*, **lignum** *(Quassia amara lignum)*, **cortex** *(Cinchona succirubra cortex)*, **folium** *(Digitalis purpurea folium)*. When referring to the fruit the term used is **fructus** *(Vaccinium vitis fructus)*, **epicarpum** *(Citrus aurantium epicarpum)*, or **pulpa** *(Tamarindus indica pulpa)*. For seeds the term **semen** *(Linum usitatissimum semen)* and for sprouts the term **thallus** *(Cetraria islandica thallus)* is used.

7.3 Acquisition of Crude Drugs

The crude drugs sold in industrialised countries are mostly imported from Eastern Europe and developing countries. In these countries the personnel employed in the plant picking and drug separation processes may lack proper qualifications. This and the fact that local names are used, not scientific ones, create confusion among the same personnel. Consequently there is the risk of finding one drug instead of another on the market; this is the case of echinacea (*Echinacea angustifolia*) confused with parthenium (*Parthenium integrifolium*), gentian (*Gentiana lutea*) confused with tormentilla (*Potentilla erecta*), burdock (*Arctium majus*) for belladonna (*Atropa belladonna*) and for many other drugs. For this reason, plus the fact that today drugs are sold in rather small pieces or even in powder form, it is absolutely necessary to issue the following information in order to guarantee the soundness and quality of any botanical drug:

(i) The place of origin of the plant which provides the drug (economic and environmental factors influencing the drug active principle content).
(ii) The nature of the plant itself, wild or cultivated (exogenous, endogenous and biotic factors significantly modifying the drug active principle content).
(iii) The date of plant picking and drug preparation (the activity of many drugs ceases after a few months, while others are still usable after 8—12 months, such as some anthraquinone drugs).
(iv) The absence or presence of contaminants indicated in percentages (moulds, microorganisms, pesticides, heavy metals, radionuclides, preservatives, foreign vegetable substances).
(v) The processing method used (dehydration, stabilization). It should never be forgotten that a homogenous and correct drying is often the most delicate and essential phase in the whole process of production of a vegetable drug preparation (extracts, tinctures, etc.).
(vi) The active principle strength.
(vii) The botanical name of the plant, therapeutic information and possible disadvantages (side effects, etc.).
(viii) Information on drug preservation.
(ix) Information about the drug producer.

7.4 Crude Drug Preservation

It is essential that crude drugs be well preserved and protected from external and internal agents which could influence their shelf-life, not only the quality of the storage conditions but also the stability of active principles. Among the most important factors having a harmful effect on drugs are: physical (light and heat); chemical (atmospheric oxygen and humidity); biological (moulds, insects). Among the internal agents are enzymes, although in some cases enzymatic activity is useful because it stimulates the formation of therapeutically useful substances. Crude drugs sensitive to light should therefore be stored in containers, which prevent the infiltration of light rays (terra-cotta, clay and wood containers, etc.). Crude drugs sensitive to humidity should be stored in hermetically sealed containers. This is valid, for example, for marshmallow, mullein and opium poppy. Crude drugs sensitive to atmospheric oxygen should be stored in hermetically sealed containers thus preventing any contact with air. Crude drugs sensitive to heat, which encourages mould and bacteria growth, should be stored away from heat sources such as radiators and stoves, etc. Storage places should be kept cool, dry and well aerated. Hygroscopic substances (drying agents) should be placed both in the containers and storage places in order to keep local humidity low. If these rules are respected the risk of drug alteration – changes in color, taste, smell and consistency – and the presence of mould, all of which can be detrimental to the drug, can be avoided.

Color change is caused by exposure to direct or indirect light and humidity. Direct or indirect light mainly alters the leaves and flowers causing rapid discoloration and yellowing, giving the crude drug the appearance of a decidedly inferior quality. Light also affects other types of crude drugs such as the stigmas of *Crocus sativus* (saffarin) and the bark of *Cinnamomum zeylanicum* (cinnamon), producing reddish marks in the latter. Photodecomposition also occurs with santonin (the active principle of aormseed) which become black, and powdered rhubarb that change from yellow to a more reddish color. The smell caused by humidity and heat can become unpleasant as in the case of *Althaea officinalis* (marshmallow), ammoniacal as *Claviceps purpura* (ergot), or not to mention the characteristic smell of mould due to the presence of mycetes. These and other microorganisms are responsible for the change in taste. Humidity affects drug consistency – roots, tubers, wood, rhizomes, bark, seeds and bulbs are easily softened if not stored in a completely dry environment.

Woodworm is caused by the presence of insects inside the storage containers. Roots, leaves and tubers etc. appear perforated and partly eroded, while a deposit of powered drug and organic insect waste is found on the bottom of the container. Periodic control is essential to check the preservation state and thus enabling immediate removal of the affected parts. Such checks reduce the risk of losing whole quantities of the plant drug and above all of using affected parts which could be harmful to the patient. Even if stored correctly, a drug progressively loses its strength with the passing of time. At the moment of picking a drug contains a large quantity of water, very many enzymes and chemical substances, apart from pharmacologically active substances, and their activity continues despite the dehydration process. The most important of these activities is hydrolysis, which can change or weaken the active components. Thus careful preservation does not avoid but only delays this inevitable ageing process and progressive drug inactivation. For these reasons batches of botanical drugs should undergo periodic evaluation for the presence of microorganisms and potency of the active component(s).

Chapter 8
Active Principles

The term "active principle" refers to *the intrinsic chemical substance which induces pharmacological activity*. Plant organisms, though different in form, organization and environmental adaptability, use a rather limited number of substances for their biochemical processes (carbohydrates, lipids, proteins, nucleic acids, co-enzymes and vitamins). Plants are often capable of synthesizing a large variety of organic compounds, the significance of which is clear only in some cases - essential oils of the *Coniferae* are useful in that their resin solvents function as a protective for wounds. The biosynthesis of these compounds comes about through metabolic processes which use intermediary products of the primary metabolism. Through this process certain biochemicals accumulate in plant cells. The metabolic conversions that take place vary from one plant species to another, and depend on environmental and genetic factors. The active principles are mainly formed during the period of plant growth when metabolic transformation is at its greatest. The active principle may be represented by primary cellular constituents (proteins, lipids, polysaccharides), by intermediary metabolites (organic acids) and by secondary cellular constituents (alkaloids, glycosides, flavonoids, saponins, tannins, essences, etc.). It is the latter which contains the most interesting active principles from a pharmacological point of view. The study of active principle biosynthesis is very important because it permits clarification of: a) the mechanism which leads to active principle formation, b) the relationship between their formation and that of normal cellular metabolites, c) the physiological meaning of active principles. Figure 8.1 (p. 32) illustrates the main biosynthetic pathways. Box 8.1, a–f (p. 33) illustrates chemical structures of the main active ingredients.

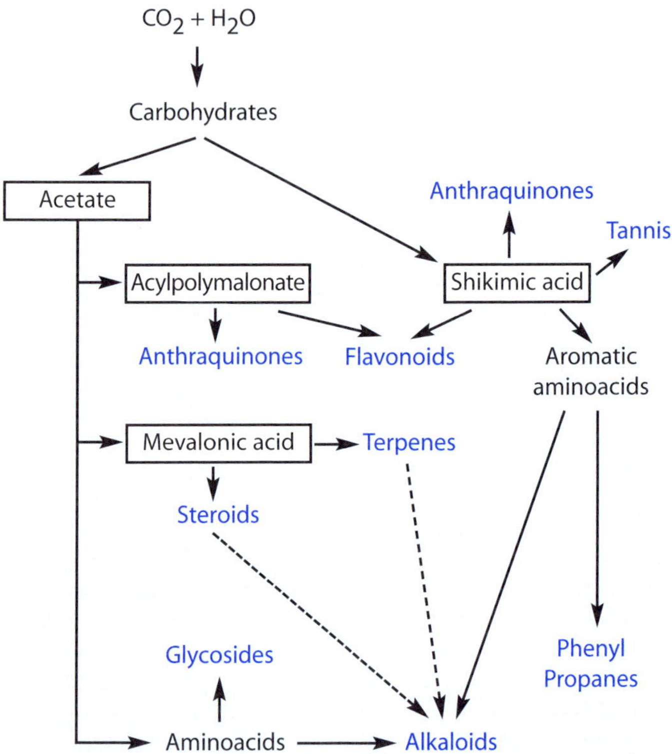

Figure 8-1 ▲ **General biosynthetic pathways**

8.1 Alkaloids

Alkaloids form a very large family of nitrogen-containing substances present in the plant kingdom. They are highly heterogeneous from a chemical point of view (Box 8-1a) as well as for the pharmacological action they possess. It can generally be said that these basic molecules, apart from nitrogen, contain carbon and oxygen. Oxygenated alkaloids are solid, crystallizable and not very volatile. Those without oxygen can take the form of liquid, oily liquid or crystallizable solids. Most of these are colorless, little soluble in water but soluble in organic solvents. Of course, salts are more soluble in alcohol and water. Natural alkaloids are levorotatory but addition of sodium or prolonged heating may induce variations in their sense of deviation from fine polarized light until they become optically inactive (racemization). They are generally present in low amounts in the plant of origin. As a plant nearly always produces more than one type of alkaloid, these should be extracted and separated using suitable techniques which exploit their various physicochemical characteristics. The alkaloids are synthesized mainly from amino acids and have been hypothesized to be useful as a defence mechanism to protect the plant from insects and other animals. Recent research, however, has disproved this hypothesis, showing that alkaloids probably act as intermediaries in the synthesis of other products. Considering the heterogeneity of alkaloids, various criteria for classification are possible:

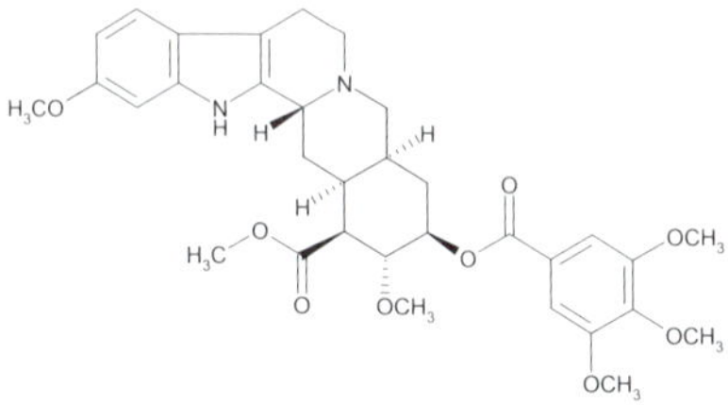

Reserpine

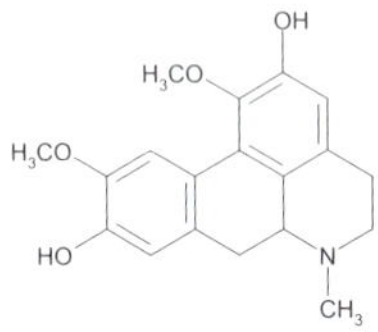

Boldine

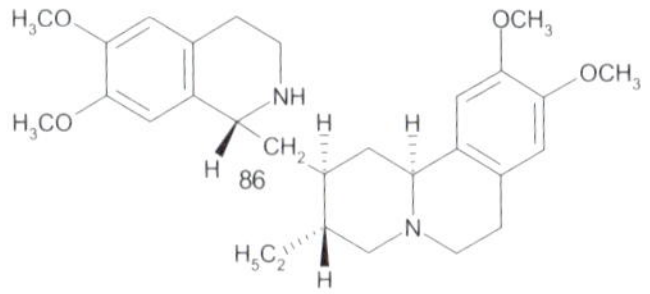

Emetine

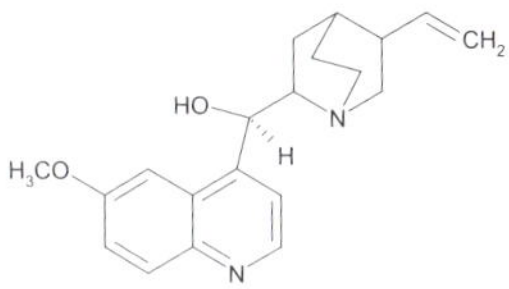

Chinine

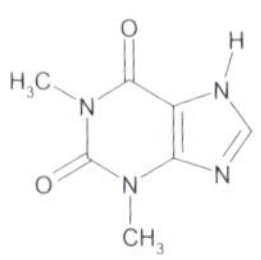

Theophylline

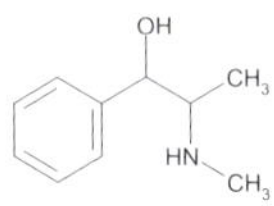

Ephedrine

Box 8-1a ▲ **Alkaloids**

a. Botanical - according to plant species.
b. Pharmacological - based on therapeutic activity and/or toxicity.
c. Chemotaxonomical - based on botanical, morphological or chemical criteria.
d. Chemical - depending on the nucleus, whether it is heterocyclic or carbocyclic nitric at the base of the structure. In some cases the nitrogen is esocyclic and therefore there exists a class of alkaloids called amminics, which do not show the classic nitrogen-containing ring.

Observing the various types of heterocycles it is possible to follow the course of alkaloid biosynthesis (e.g. those with a tropane nucleus probably derive from glutamic acid; the indoles and chinilinic from tryptophane, the pyridotine acid, the isochinolinic from phenylalanine and the imidazole-containing from histidine) or to specify how the fusion of some rings gives rise to the formation of more complex alkaloids (e.g. pyrrolidine and piperidine generate the tropanic nucleus, pyrimidine and imidazole generate the purine nucleus). These structures contain one or more asymmetric carbon atoms and therefore, as said previously, the alkaloids are optically active; the dextro- or levorotatory forms show different levels of pharmacological activity. It is not possible to specify a structure-activity relationships between alkaloids of a given chemical class. Indeed, there are alkaloids with different activities within the same chemical class, as exemplified by antineoplastics, hallucinogenes, some neuroleptics, sympatholytics, parasympathomimetics and analeptics, even though all of these alkaloids contain an indole nucleus. It is therefore difficult to propose a systematic classification of alkaloids, the most acceptable rational method until now being to group alkaloid drugs according to their therapeutic use.

8.2 Glycosides

These are complex organic substances mainly present in the plant world. They consist of two parts, of which one is a sugar (saccharide) molecule and the other an aglycone. The sugar moiety can be joined to the aglycone in various ways. The most common bridging atom is oxygen (O-glycoside), but it can also be sulphur (S-glycoside), nitrogen (N-glycoside) or carbon (C-glycoside). They are usually solid, sufficiently soluble in water and alcohol but little soluble in ether. The glycosidic link is resistant to alkaline hydrolysis but is easily separated by enzymatic action of glycosidases or by dilute mineral acids. To extract the

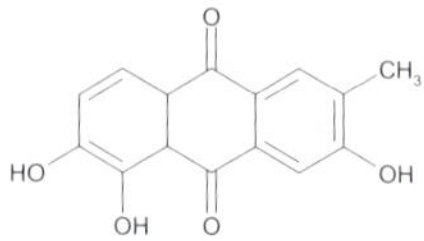

Chrysarone

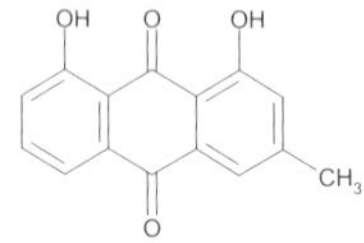

Crysophanol

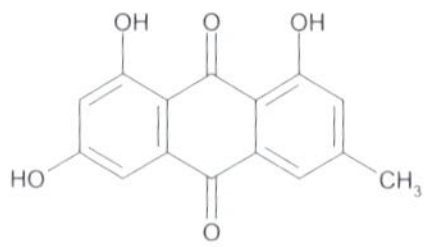

Frangula-emodin

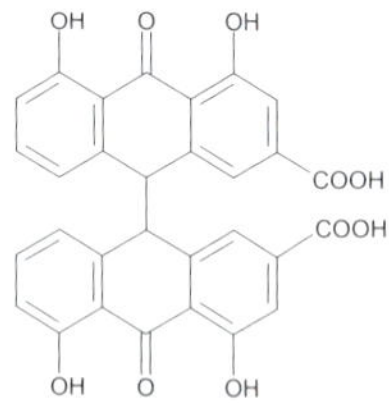

Sennidin

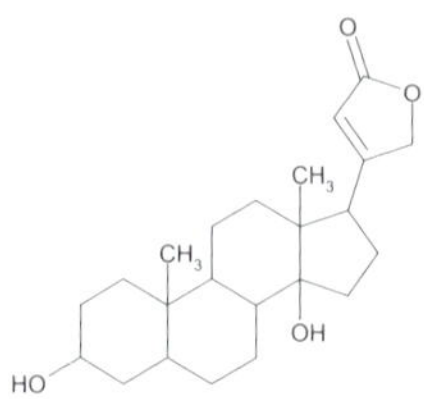

Digitoxigenin

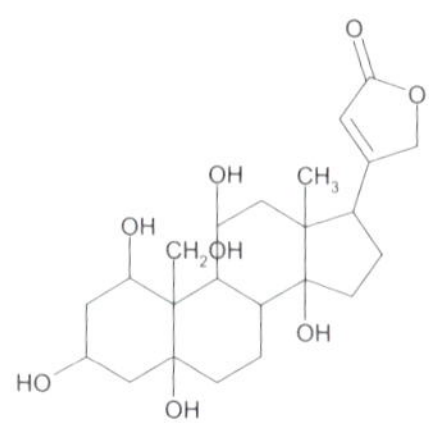

Diabegenin

Box 8-1b ▲ **Aglycones of glycosides**

glycosides, the glycosidases must be inactivated or made insoluble by suitable treatment. From a pharmacological point of view glycosides are a heterogeneous family. The aglycone portion of the molecule is responsible for the pharmacological action while the sugar component influences the absorption, distribution, metabolism and excretion. Because of the chemical or pharmacological heterogeneity of this large family of compounds, both criteria should be borne in mind when making a rational classification.

8.3 Flavonoids

Flavonoids are yellow compounds, very common in nature. Citrus fruits, such as *Citrus medica* (lemons), *Citrus aurantium* (oranges) in their bitter and sweet varieties, and some wild fruits like *Rosa canina* are very rich in these flavonoids. Chemically they are derivatives of flavone (2-

phenyl-benzo-γ-pyrone) (Box 8-1c) and some (named isoflavonoids) from isoflavone (3-phenyl-benzo-γ-pyrone); they are usually soluble in water and boiling alcohol. Many flavonoids constitute the aglycone of natural glycosides which are formed by the link of one or more sugars in position 7 or in position 3. Due to their wide availability and intense coloring, flavonoids were widely used as industrial dyes before the advent of synthetic dyes. Flavonoids reduce permeability and capillary fragility. They also possess anticoagulant and antihepatotoxic properties. Many flavonoids also possess anti-inflammatory, antioxidant, antibacterial and spasmolytic properties. However, several of these actions have not been completely and unequivocally proved to be demonstrated in man. It should be remembered that isoflavone derivatives (also named **phytoestrogens**) show a considerable estrogenic action linked to the stilbene structure. This is very important in that isoflavones are present in many animal foods, particularly soy products. The isoflavones not only have antioxidant and hormonal activities but, because of their estrogenic activity they appear to promote retention of calcium in bones. For this reason, numerous isoflavone products are now available in the United States to prevent or treat osteoporosis.

Chemically related to flavonoids are flavonolignans, anthocyanins and proanthocyanidins. **Flavonolignans** (or flavolignans) are hybrid lignans derived from the flavonoid taxifolin (2,3-dihydroquercetin) and coniferyl alcohol. Silybin is a flavonolignan isolated from the fruit of *Sylibum marianum* (milk thistle). **Anthocyanins** are pigments responsible for the red, pink, mauve, purple, blue, or violet color of most flowers and fruits. These pigments occur as glycosides (the anthocyanins), and their aglycones (the *anthocyanidins*) are derived from the 2-phenylbenzopyrylium cation, more commonly referred to as the flavylium cation. Anthocyanins decrease capillary permeability and fragility, act like radical scavengers and possess antiedema activity. These pharmacological actions lead to the use of anthocyanin-containing herbal medicines [e.g. bilberry (*Vaccinium myrtillus*), grape seeds (*Vitis vinifera*)] in the symptomatic treatment of venous insufficiency and capillary fragility. **Proanthocyanidins** (condensed tannins) are complex polymers, whose chemistry is only partly known. Their building blocks include catechins and flavonoids (see paragraph 8.5). Chief proanthocyanidin-containing drugs include witch hazel (*Hamamelis virginiana*), oak (*Quercus* spp.) and bilberry (*Vaccinium myrtillus*). Proanthocyanidins possess the typical pharmacological activity of tannins (i.e. astringency and antioxidant activity).

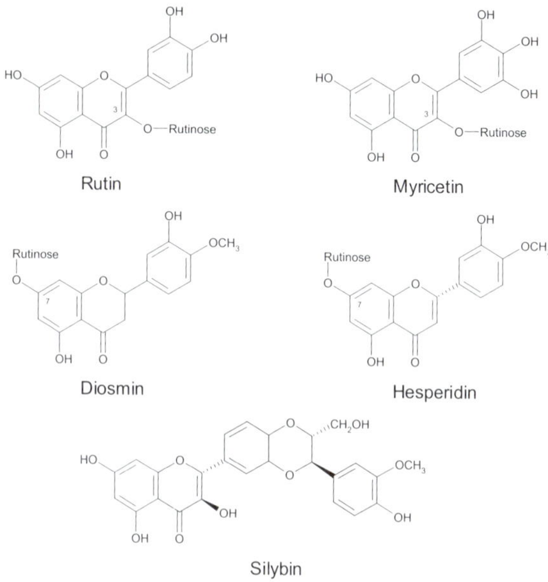

Box 8-1c ▲ **Flavonoids**

8.4 Saponins

These is a group of natural glycosides forming colloidal solutions with water which foam when shaken - thus their name. Sugars and aglycones (Box 8-1d) (which are separated into steroids and terpenes according to chemical structure) are released of these glycosides by acid hydrolysis. They are devoid of nitrogen, usually odorless and with a bitter taste (excluding glycyrrhizin). Pharmacologically, saponins possess expectorant and antitussive action. When administered in small doses saponins stimulate the secretion of fluid mucus thus facilitating expectoration. This effect is due to gastric mucus irritation which by reflex action causes an increase in bronchial secretion. After administration saponins come into contact with mucus, and their ability to reduce superficial tension makes the mucus more fluid and easy to eliminate. This irritant effect is in some cases exploited to aid the absorption of other medicines (synergic effect). If administered in higher doses saponins may induce purgative effects. In the cosmetics industry they are employed as emulsifying agents in the preparation of foam.

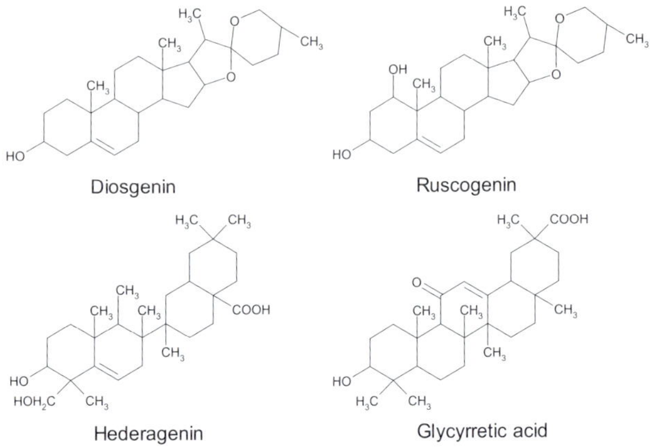

Box 8-1d ▲ **Aglycones of saponins**

8.5 Tannins

Tannins are polyphenolic organic compounds (Box 8.1e) with a strong bitter taste and astringent effects. Gallic acid is a building block of many tannins. Tannins are able to transform leather skins, precipitating proteins and forming insoluble compounds with them. Low concentrations of tannic substances, if applied locally, induce a significant reduction in vascular permeability. When applied in high concentrations they can have a caustic effect causing profound modifications of protein structure. In therapy tannins are used externally (mouth washes and gargling products) as astringents and hemostatics. They are also employed for their astringency on rectal blood vessels, making them useful for the treatment of hemorroids. In the past tannins were employed as antiseptics while today they are sometimes employed in antiseborrheic and antidandruff lotions. Plant drugs which are used most as sources of tannins are the leaves of *Hamanelis virginiana* (witch hazel), roots of *Krameria triandra* (rathany), rhizomes of *Potentilla erecta* (tormentilla), seeds of *Aesculus hippocastanum* (horse chestnut), leaves and husk of *Juglans regia* (walnut), bark of *Quercus robur* (oak). In plants tannins are found in complex form – tannoids – and sometimes in combination with sugars – tannosides. Tannins can be divided into two groups: *hydrolysable tannins*, which are split into simpler molecules on treatment with acids or enzymes, and *condensed tannins* (catechin tannins, also named **proanthocyanidins**) which give complex insoluble products on similar treatment (see paragraph 8.3). *Procyanidins* are compounds which can be formed by treating proanthocyanidins with acid at high temperature. They are also referred to as dimeric proanthocyanidins (i.e. proanthocyanidins consisting of two units).

8.6 Essences (Essential or Volatile Oils)

Essences or essential oils consist of a complex mixture of volatile organic substances with varying chemical constitution (Box 8.1f). They are contained in particular tissues of different plants, and are usually obtained by distillation in steam currents or extraction with solvents or suitable mechanical procedures. The chemical constituents of essences are very heterogeneous: hydrocarbons, aromatics, open and closed chain terpenes, sesquiterpenes, alcohols (aromatic or terpenic), acids (aliphatic or aromatic), aldehydes and ketones (esters and ethers), phenols, various cyclic ethers, nitrogen and sulfate. Essences can be subdivided into several types. Preformed essences are the most numerous and are found in various parts of the plant. Non-preformed essences are more complex substances which are separated by hydrolysis on distillation or maceration. For example, during maceration in water of *Prunus*

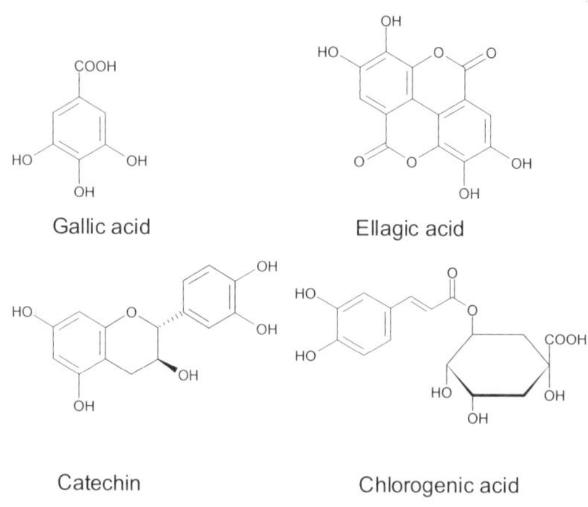

Box 8-1e ▲ **Tannins**

laurocerasus leaves, enzymes hydrolyse amagdalin glucoside, releasing glucose, benzoic aldehyde and cyanic acid, the drug's volatile principle. Essences are lipophilic, generally liquid, not very soluble in water but soluble in organic solvents. They refract light and are optically active, some showing a characteristic color and degree of fluorescence when exposed to ultraviolet light. They usually have the smell of the plant from which they are obtained and after extraction often have to be purified. Essences used in perfumes are converted to diterpenes to increase their smell. The elimination of terpenoid hydrocarbons with little smell, makes it possible to obtain an essence with 30–70% increased odor strength. These are typically more soluble in alcohol, with greater antiseptic properties and greater stability.

Essential oils are present in nearly all plants, though in different quantities. The botanical families most rich in these are: *Asteraceae, Lauraceae, Apiaceae, Rutaceae, Liliaceae, Magnoliaceae, Cupressaceae* and *Pinaceae.* The pharmacological action of essence-containing drugs depends on their capacity to irritate tissue or simply by their smell and taste. Some of these essences have been found to have an important action on central nervous system or the uterine musculature.

The pharmacological action of the volatile oils can be summarized as follows:

1. Antiseptic action (eucalyptus, thyme) in the lungs and kidneys.
2. Counter-irritant action. This action is taken advantage of in ointments and lotions used to treat muscular aches and pains. When applied to the skin certain volatile oils, particularly those from camphor and arnica, irritate receptors in the skin causing a warming, mildly irritating sensation which tends to lessen perception of the underlying muscle pain. When inhaled, camphor has an expectorant effect; taken orally aniseed, fennel and cinnamon have carminative effects on the gastrointestinal tract.
3. Central nervous system action (oxygenated compounds). Camphor seems to have a direct stimulatory effect on the respiratory and vasomotor centers, others act as stimulants on the motor cortex (e.g. wormwood, thuja) and can induce convulsions.
4. Antihelminthic action (wormseed).
5. Uterine stimulant action, inducing abortion in case of intoxication. Examples are rue, wormwood, savin, thuja.

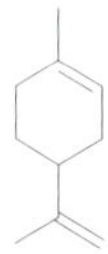

Limonene

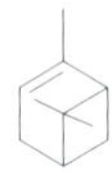

α-Pinene

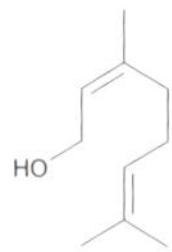

Geraniol

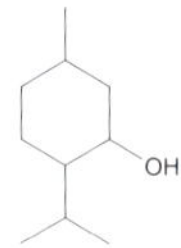

Menthol

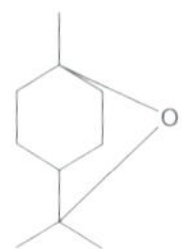

Eucalyptol

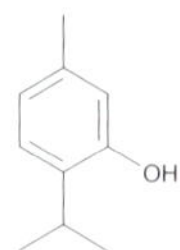

Thymol

Box 8-1f ▲ **Some constituents of essential oils**

8.7 Bitters

Bitter compounds come from different phytochemical classes like monoterpenes, sesquiterpenes, diterpenes, flavonoids and triterpenes. The other bitter compounds include alkaloids and substances with a steroid skeleton. However, the most notable bitter compounds are the monoterpene secoiridoid glycosides of gentian (amarogentin), centaury (gentiopicroside) and bog bean (foliamenthin), and sesquiterpene lactone dimers of wormwood (absinthin). When bitter agents are introduced into the mouth, they stimulate (i) the bitter receptors located at the base of the tongue and (ii) gastric secretion; the result is an increase of the flow of secretions. Gastrin stimulates the upper digestive function and the secretion of bile and pancreatic juice.

The main indications for bitters are dyspepsia and anorexia. However, patients' responses to bitter herbs depend on their upper digestive function. In fact the ability of the digestive system to produce low molecular weight compounds (more active) from the natural polymers (less active) existent in herbal drugs is essential for the efficacy of bitters. Bitters may be classified as pure bitters [gentian, (*Gentiana lutea*), bog bean (*Menyanthes trifoliata*), etc.], aromatic bitters [calamus (*Acorus calamus*), angelica (*Angelica archangelica),* blessed thistle (*Cnicus benedictus*), yarrow (*Achillea millefolium*), etc.], acrid (pungent) bitters [ginger (*Zingiber officinale*), galangal (*Alpinia officinarum*), etc.] alkaloidic bitters [quinine (*Chincona pubescens*)]and mucilaginous bitters [iceland moss (*Cetraria islandica*), colombo (*Jatrorhiza palmata*), etc.]. Gentian has the highest bittering power followed by centaury and bog bean. Aromatic bitters also contain volatile oils, and therefore can develop spasmolitic, carminative or cholagogue action. Acrid bitters also contain acrid compounds and, therefore must be used cautiously in children and elderly patients. All bitters are contraindicated in gastric and duondenal ulcers because an increase of stomach secretion with higher acid secretion is not desirable in these patients.

8.8 Gums

These are heterogeneous polysaccharides of high molecular weight which on prolonged boiling with acids are hydrolyzed into pentoses (arabinose, xylose) and hexoses (glucose, galactose), and glucuronic and galacturonic acids. They form adhesive substances with hot water which are subdivided into: solubles (arabic gum) when they give colloidal solutions, insolubles (tragacanth gum) when they swell in water producing a jelly, and semisolubles which behave as insolubles becoming solutions when a further quantity of water is added. Natural gum formation is believed to be a pathological process in the plant of origin, caused by the bacterial transformation of starch and cellulose following trauma. It is thought that the purpose of gum production is to cover wounds in the plant to limit water evaporation. This notion is reinforced by the fact that gum production increases if the plant is cut and most gum producing plants are found in tropical regions where the process of evaporation is intense. The pharmacological uses of gums are very varied. They are used as excipient and emulsifying agents, and to treat constipation. Gum obtained from *Astragalus gummifer*, for example, is used as a mild laxative.

8.9 Mucilages

These are amorphous substances composed of heterogenous polysaccharides, which produce viscous non-adhesive colloidal solutions with water. They have not yet been chemically defined with precision but it would seem that they are derived from the transformation of endocellular amide and cellulose membranes. They are very diffuse in nature and are extracted from the plant with hot or boiling water. True mucilages are those obtained from marshmallow, marigold, flax, mallow, aloe vera and psyllium, but they are also found in lichens, mushrooms and algae. The drugs are usually sold as such and not the extracted mucilages, which are difficult to preserve. Their pharmacological action is linked to their capacity to swell in water, producing a plastic mass or viscous dispersions. When swallowed they have a laxative action, caused by softening of the intestinal contents, increased pressure on the intestinal wall and increased peristaltic activity. Used in dressings on inflamed or damaged skin and mucus, their action is protective. (See Chapter 18 for the use of mucilages in cough).

8.10 Other Phytochemicals

Several other compounds are recognized in plants. Some of them are toxic and could be considered poisons (e.g. cyanogenic glycosides, pyrrolizidine alkaloids), but many others may be of some therapeutic interest (Table 8.1).

Table 8.1

Some chemical constituents found in plants (other constituents, i.e. alkaloids, glycosides, flavonoids, saponins, tannins, essences, bitters, gums and mucilages are described in the text of this chapter)

Class	Chemistry	Source (example)	Component (example)	Pharmacological activity of the component
Coumarins	5,6-benzo-2-pyrone derivatives	Tonka bean (*Dipteryx odorata*) Sweet clover (*Melilotus officinalis*) Bishop's weed (*Ammi visnaga*)	Coumarin, dicoumarol	Anticoagulant
Enzymes	Proteins able to catalyze biochemical reactions	Pineapple (*Ananas comosus*)	Bromelain	Anti-inflammatory
Fats (Triglycerides)	Esters of long-chain fatty acids. The alcohol component is glycerol	Castor oil (*Ricinus communis*)	Ricinolein	Laxative

continued on next page

Table 8.1
Some chemical constituents found in plants (other constituents, i.e. alkaloids, glycosides, flavonoids, saponins, tannins, essences, bitters, gums and mucilages are described in the text of this chapter) (*continued*)

Class	Chemistry	Source (example)	Component (example)	Pharmacological activity of the component
Fatty acids (Fatty oils)	Carboxylic acids with a long chain	Borage oil (*Borago officinalis*) Evening primrose (*Oenothera* spp.) Blackcurrant oil (*Ribes nigrum*)	γ-Linolenic acid	Anti-inflammatory
Glucosinolates	Glycosides containing nitrogenous and sulfur. Isothiochyanates are products of glucosinolates hydrolysis	Shepherd's purse (*Capsella bursa-pastoris*) White mustard (*Sinapis alba*)	Sinigrin	Antitumoral, anti-inflammatory
Iridoids	Compounds containing a cyclopentanotetrahydropyran ring system	Valerian (*Valeriana officinalis*)	Valtrate	Hypnotic
Lectins	Protein which is not an antibody or an enzyme, but which has the ability to attach itself to specific sugars	European mistletoe (*Viscum album*)	Viscumin	Anticancer
Lignans	Cinnamyl alcohol dimers	Schizandra (*Schizandra chinensis*)	Schizandrine A-C	Hepato-protective
Pectins	Amylase-resistant polysaccharides	Banana (*Musa paradisiaca*)	Dextrin, α-glucans	Antidiarrheal
Phloroglucinol derivatives	Compounds containing phloroglucin (1,3,5-Trihydroxybenzene)	St John's wort (*Hypericum perforatum*)	Hyperforin	Antidepressant
Poly-saccharides	Macromolecules containing a large number of monosaccharides (sugars formed by one unit, e.g. glucose and fructose)	Echinacea (*Echinacea* spp.) Aloe gel (*Aloe* spp.)	Echinacin Acemannan	Immunostimulant
Purines	Methylxanthines	Tea (*Thea sinensis*) Maté (*Ilex paraguariensis*) Guarana (*Paullinia cupana*)	Caffeine	Central stimulant

Chapter 9

Therapeutic Overview of Galenical Preparations

Over the centuries, after much trial and error, many techniques have been developed for the preparation of herbal medicines. Today it is well known that herbal medicines must be used in a specific type of formulation (dosage form) in order to achieve the desired results. Knowing the composition and physicochemical characteristics of active principles allow us to establish the best or most appropriate method of extraction, and therefore administration in order to obtain the desired effect. Herbal medicines and their active ingredients possess various beneficial properties which can be used in the treatment of different illnesses (Figure 9.1, p. 46). As will be shown later, appropriate drug mixtures or their derivatives are used to obtain a particular synergistic effect. Many drugs turn out to be equally effective for a particular disease, but as people react differently it is important to be aware of the alternatives (Table 9.1). This topic is dealt with in a separate section of this book.

Table 9.1
Indications and contraindications of herbal medicine

Indications	Contraindications
When herbal medicines are the treatment of choice, e.g. constipation, toxic liver disease, etc.	When herbal medicines are not efficacious
When herbal medicines can be an alternative to synthetic drugs, e.g. dyspepsia, skin disorders, urinary infections, etc.	When herbal medicines protract a rational therapy with synthetic drugs
When herbal medicines can be used in combination with synthetic drugs, e.g. respiratory diseases	When herbal medicines impede a rational therapy with synthetic drugs

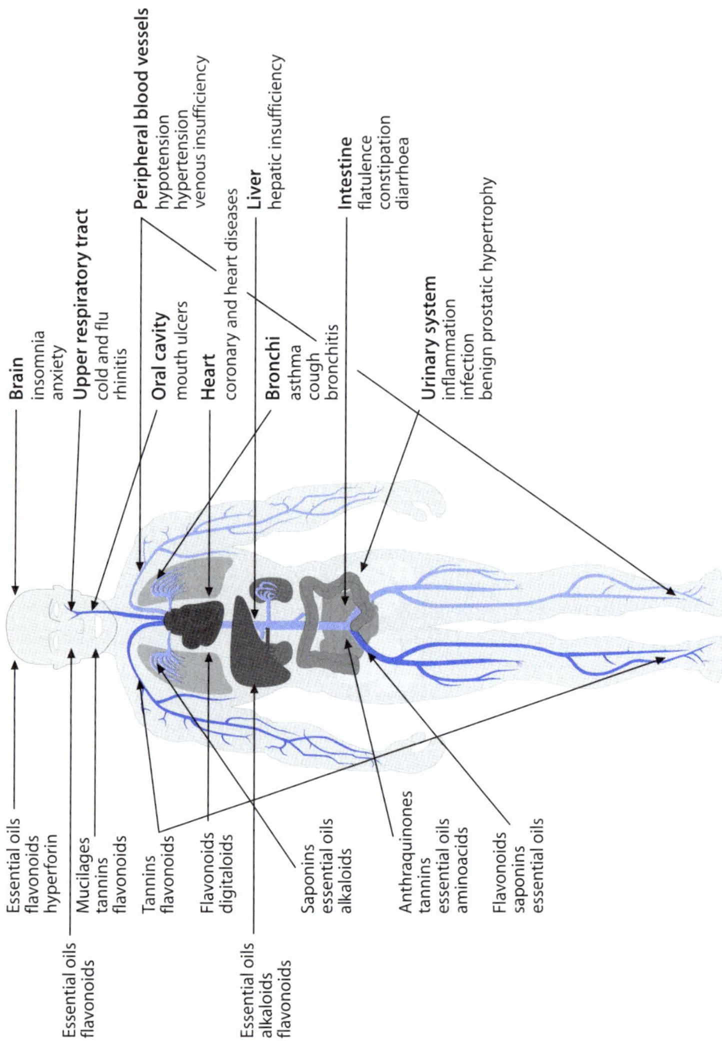

Figure 9-1 ▲ **Active principles, organs and related disturbances**

9.1 General Therapeutic Principles

The ailments that most frequently require the use of drugs of botanical origin are those involving the gastrointestinal system. The wide variety of "natural" medicines used today for gastric acidity, constipation and diarrhea is evidence of this. Many herbal medicines are able to stimulate the appetite, reduce or increase digestive secretions and intestinal motor functions. Herbal medicines that can lower or increase arterial pressure are often used to treat disorders of the vascular system. In practice the botanicals most exploited are those that reduce blood pressure. These same drugs often induce diuresis, which is also helpful in hypertension. Various respiratory conditions can be improved with vegetable drugs. Coughs, mucus obstruction of the respiratory system and constriction of bronchial smooth musculature can be treated with botanical products. Other botanicals are used for diseases such as urogenital conditions, and diabetes mellitus. Remedies for skin and mucous membrane disorders, as a consequence of trauma, inflammation or irritation, are derived from the mucilages and tannin-containing materials. Anxiety states and insomnia can also be improved with infusions prepared from medicinal herbs. Other uses will be considered in subsequent chapters. However, care should be taken in assuming that serious pathologies such as most cardiac disorders, liver or kidney disease can be cured with botanical drugs by themselves. Natural drugs should not be relied upon to treat malaria and cancer. Before using botanical drugs as "mono-therapy" or in combination with other pharmaceuticals, one must accurately diagnose the patient's illness. It may be most appropriate to combine herbal medicines with conventional drugs to improve the benefits to the patient. Such combinations may permit the use of a lower dose of the synthetic drug, thus reducing side effects and minimising the potential for iatrogenic illness. Another indirect "benefit" from the use of plant-derived drugs is their value as a source of nutrients (vitamins, protein, fiber, enzyme content).

9.2 Galenic Formulations

Herbal medicines can be administered in the form of powders manufactured in capsule or tablet form, or various extracts can be prepared. These are classified as teas, infusions, decoctions and tinctures. Apart from these traditional pharmaceutical extracts, prepared with water, ethanol or water/alcohol mixtures, today many extracts are made with glycerine or combinations of glycerine with other solvents. The purpose

Absorption of the active principle	Drug formulation	Comment
Fast	**Liquid form** Tea Extract Tincture Syrup	Active principle is present in a soluble form and then easily absorbed
↓ Slow	**Solid form** Capsule Coated capsule	Disintegration and dissolution of the preparation slow active principle absorption

The oral ingestion is most convenient, economical and usually safer

Figure 9-2 ▲ **Oral drug formulation and bioavailability**

of the therapy must be borne in mind when choosing the form of preparation in that different forms of the same drug can induce very different pharmacological effects. For example, if a relaxant effect on the intestine is desired from chamomile it is necessary to prepare it as an infusion. In general the simpler the pharmaceutical form, the more quickly the active principle is absorbed by the target tissue (Figure 9.2). Many substances are added to extracts to facilitate or improve galenic preparations. These include agglutinating agents, absorbents, lubricants and diluents. To improve taste aromatic flavours and natural sweeteners may be added; to increase stability and preservation, antimicrobials or antioxidants can be added. For dried extracts intended for encapsulation or use in tablets, lactose is often used as a diluent (as opposed to calcium sulphate) to increase active principle bioavailability. Apart from the pharmaceutical factors there are physiopathological factors to be taken into consideration (gastric motility, pH at the absorption site, area of absorbing surface, blood flow, presystemic elimination, ingestion with or without food, etc.), which can also alter active principle bioavailability. Figure 9.3 (p. 49) shows some factors that may determine a variability in response to herbal medicines.

Prescription	Factors determining herb effect
Dosage prescribed ↓	
	patient compliance
Dosage administered ↓	rate of absorption distribution in body fluids binding in plasma and tissue rate of excretion
Hematic concentration ↓	physiopathological conditions genetic factors herb/drug interactions development of tolerance
	herb-receptor interaction placebo effects
Intensity of effect	

Figure 9-3 ▲ **Factors that may determine a variability in response to herbal medicines**

9.2.1 Fresh and Dried Botanical Drugs

Plant-derived drugs can be used either in fresh or dry states. The section *Vegetable Drugs and Preparations* of the Italian Pharmacopoeia (FU) states that unless a limit is fixed, dried drugs should not contain more than 10% humidity. The use of fresh drugs, theoretically the ideal, causes practical problems in the manufacturing process. There are cases in which enzymatic transformation is necessary before the drug can be used, as is the case for frangola and belladonna. Fresh drugs are used for

Mother tinctures; they are preferable in the preparation of pulps, juices and especially essential oils. Dried drugs are used in the preparation of powders, infusions, decoctions, extracts and tinctures. They offer advantages such as ease of availability throughout the year, ease of transport and preservation, better stabilization and preservation. Dried drugs are also referred to as "raw drugs" which means that the drug has only been dried and stabilized. The fresh drugs in greatest demand today are hamamelis, angelica, burdock, birch, hawthorn, marion thistle, echinacea, ginkgo and tormentilla.

9.2.2 Botanical Drug Preparation

Every botanical drug should be accompanied by a technical index card with the name of the plant and producer, the picking, packing and expiry dates, the strength of the active principles and certification of the absence of contaminants. Any drug, before being used, must be identified and checked for the possible presence of moulds, insects and other plants and suitably cleaned to reduce pieces of a suitable powdered form. It is obvious that the drug must be well preserved so as not to alter its active principle content. The dried drug used in extractive and tincture preparations must be moistened before use with the extractive solvent, the so-called "menstrum", and left to soften for a period varying from half an hour to several days according to the nature of the drug, the solvent employed and the type of preparation. "Softening" (*maceration*) is an extractive process carried out at room temperature (when carried out in gentle heat it is called "digestion"), permitting the solvent to penetrate the plant cellular structure and solubilize the active principles.

Steeping is carried out in glass, enamel-coated iron or china containers, provided with a suitable lid and stirred from time to time. After filtration the resulting extract can be drunk either cold or warm. This preparation is suitable for mucilages and when one wishes to avoid the extraction of useless substances, toxic substances such as viscotoxin, gentian pectin, or thermolabile active principles (e.g. devil's claw iridoids). Steeping is almost never exhaustive, usually constituting a preliminary operation followed by percolation leading to drug depletion. The whole extraction process depends on the degree of drug fragmentation being facilitated and is more thorough if solvent action is not hindered by cellular walls. The choice of extractive solvent is therefore of paramount importance to provide efficient extraction of the active principle(s) and elimination of the unwanted components, without compromising the intended pharmacological activity. The extractive processes and the solvents which obtain the best results for most botanical drugs are now well known. When extraction is carried out with water, it can be more convenient to remove fatty substances and waxes by preliminary washing with hexane, petroleum ether or dichloromethane; when using water as a menstrum, the addition of a preservative is necessary to reduce bacterial contamination and prevent mould formation.

9.2.3 Powders

These are the oldest form of botanical drug administration. They are obtained by trituration of the dried drug, the size varying, depending on the method used. The powder is sieved to obtain homogeneous granules and is graded depending on the sieves used from very coarse, coarse, semi-fine, fine and very fine (micronized powder). Powders are classified as simple (consisting of only one drug), or compound when mixed with powders from other drugs. Powders from the whole plant can be administered suspended or dissolved in water or another liquid, mixed with honey, as a tablet, pill or capsule form. Hard gelatin capsules are preferable when the powder has an unpleasant taste or smell, or when the preparation is mucilaginous. The bitter taste is thought by some to be important to stimulate biliary secretion, release insulin and gastric hormones. Such a preparation is therefore useful in the treatment of digestive and liver disorders, diabetes, and even other ailments.

In France a pulverizing technique has been perfected called cryofractionation, to obtain a product as similar as possible to the composition of the medicinal plant. This technique works by injecting liquid nitrogen at -196°C into the pulverizer. The plant material becomes fragile and breaks down without an increase in temperature, which might otherwise destroy thermolabile products. Grains of about 125 microns are separated by sifting and are incapsulated. This size permits an easy transfer of active principles. This technique is interesting but it has the disadvantage of the drug drying out which can always lead to some alteration. Thus another fresh plant cryofractionation procedure has been perfected to eliminate this problem and obtain uniform suspension (discussed below). Capsules are easy to use and can be made gastric acid-resistant with coating substances as modified cellulose. Insoluble in the acidic milieu of the stomach the coated capsules dissolve when the pH rises above 7. Capsules are made commercially in eight sizes indicated by numbers from 000 to 5, with a capacity from 1.37

to 0.13 ml (from 10 to 0.8 grains; 1 gr = 0.0648 g). The sizes 0 and 1 are usually used for botanical drugs. Excipients are generally added to the powdered drug to reach the appropriate capsule mixture volume. Other excipients are added to improve absorption, stabilization and to facilitate mechanical filling. Moistened powdered drugs can be incorporated with the usual excipients into ointments for external application.

9.2.4 Infusions and Decoctions

Unlike other galenic formulations these are extemporaneous preparations obtained from previously prepared drugs. Infusions are liquid preparations obtained by pouring warm or boiling water over the plant material. This is the manner in which medicinal and non-medicinal "tea" is also prepared (see below); flavors and any nutrients or pharmacological agents are thus extracted prior to ingestion. The extent of extraction usually depends upon the length of time the material is exposed to the extraction fluid. After cooling the resulting solution can be filtered through cotton wool or gauze and the eluent is then brought up to the prescribed weight by adding hot water (the residue and filter should be washed to recover as much drug as possible). In some cases it may be necessary to add small quantities of acid or alkaline substances to the solvent to facilitate active principle extraction. Generally 1–10 parts of drug are needed for the preparation of 100 parts of infusion.

Infusion is used when the drug is composed of tender or delicate tissues such as leaves and flowers and other upper parts of the plant. Often the infusion technique does not permit the extraction of substances with little solubility in water. For example, only 10–15% of chamomile oil passes into the infusion even after prolonged extraction time. Clearly the preparation of a pleasant infusion like tea to be drunk with friends or during a work break is one thing and a therapeutic infusion is another. In the latter case it is necessary to define the quantity of drug relative to water (usually 3–5 parts for 100 parts infusion), the duration of infusion, and the appropriate extraction containers (for example aluminium containers should be avoided). In many cases, however, therapeutic effectiveness (and therefore potential drug toxicity) is modest; this, plus the fact that active principles are rather diluted does not permit precise control of dosage. Information concerning the quantity of infusion to be taken daily is given in another section of this book.

Decoctions are liquid preparations obtained extemporaneously by boiling in water the suitably pulverised drug from which the active principles are to be obtained. This operation is never applied to volatile active principle drugs. Usually 5 parts of drug are used to prepare 100 parts of decoction; in the case of drugs containing alkaloids, water is added to promote extraction. A quantity of diluted citric acid corresponding approximately to the total alkaloid content of the drug may be added to improve extraction. Decoction is used when drugs are composed of not very permeable compact tissues which release active principles with difficulty (e.g. wood, bark, roots, seeds, etc.) and is often preceded by steeping in cold water for some hours. Boiling varies from 15–45 minutes depending on the physical characteristics of the material to be extracted. There are of course exceptions as in the case of lichen or barley where the drug is first boiled and then the liquid is substituted before undergoing the final decoction. Decoctions are never used when drugs to be extracted are known to be thermolabile (e.g. foxglove). Decoctions are often cloudy due to the presence of mucilages which can be extracted by boiling, and precipitate upon cooling. Few decoctions are used today because the protracted boiling inactivates alkaloid or heterocyclic molecules, causing loss of activity or conversion to substances with undesirable effects.

9.2.5 Herbal Teas

Teas are watery preparations obtained extemporaneously from one or more herbal drugs and are administered orally for therapeutic purposes (medicinal teas), or are consumed for pleasure (non-medicinal teas) or used as a vehicle for other medicines. They can be sweetened or flavoured and should be consumed immediately. Herbal drugs should be carefully chosen and cleaned and are used whole or in pieces of a suitable size. Three kinds of tea are generally sold as ready-to-use products: tea-bag teas, species (blended teas) and soluble teas. For the species any drug, after the removal of foreign elements, is reduced to a suitable volume to facilitate mixing and to limit possible drug mixture separation. Usually plant materials are sieved after initially being reduced in size. Sieves are classified by a number indicating mesh width (μm), the choice depending on the drug type; sieve n° 5600 is used for leaves, flowers and grasses; n° 4000 for leaves, flowers and grasses of a particular consistency or thickness exceeding 300 μm; sieve n° 4000 is also used for roots, rhizomes, bark, woody parts, fruits and seeds. Small dimension drugs can be used whole, while essence containing fruits and seeds are cut up just before mixing. The mixture must be as homogeneous as possible and if different components separate easily, homogeneity must be restored in a suitable manner before use. Usually 10–20 g of plant material is needed to produce one liter of tea. Teas are prepared by steeping, digestion, infusion or decoction, using tap water and are decanted or filtered through cotton wool or gauze before use. Preferably they are prepared by infusion. Compared to infusions and decoctions they are more diluted and can therefore be administered in greater quantities even habitually, without unpleasant side effects. The teas quoted in the Italian Pharmacopoeia are all prepared by infusion for immediate use: one spoonful of drug of species (about 5 g) for one cup (about 250 g). A therapeutic action (laxative) has only been reported for tisanes prepared from senna.

The preparation of drugs for teas follow precise methods. Other substances (potentiating agents, etc.) are sometimes mixed with the base remedy drugs. The species (tea mixtures) referred to in Italian Pharmacopoeia are all composed of 4–5 drugs. Worthy of note is the tea express, a fashionable tisane today. The drug, in very small pieces is filtered through the coffee machine as when making coffee, but great care must be taken to use water and drug in the correct proportions. Today, teas can be prepared simply and quickly with greater dosage accuracy, permitting fluid extracts to absorb inert and easily water-soluble excipients such as sucrose, lactose or maltodextrin. The advantages of these teas are that they can be prepared instantly by dissolving them in hot water and that they can be preserved over a long period, the active principles being dry. Recently liquid preparations, composed of dry extracts in a water solution to be diluted in hot water before consumption, have been commercialized on a large scale. Another preparation which is easy for a patient to prepare is "simple syrup", composed of sugar and water. Sugar (about 180 g to 100 ml of tisane) is added to the tisane and heated gently until dissolved. After filtering through a strainer it is administered by spoon. Syrups are preferable to tisanes when it is necessary to administer drugs with an expectorant or antitussive action. They can be prepared by infusion and also by adding flavors to the simple syrup. The slogan "drink tea, wait and see" is with good reason correct because these simple formulations can mainly reduce the anxiety and stress of patients who are constantly worried about their own health. Thus, medicinal teas are today widely used, being a recommended, effective therapy without toxicological risk.

9.2.6 Extracts and Tinctures

These are pharmaceutical preparations obtained from dry or fresh drugs using a suitable extractive process. Extracts may be liquids or solids or of a soft consistency obtained from usually dry primary plant material. Extracts are classified according to the solvents: aqueous, hydroalcoholic, alcoholic or ethereal. Other solvents may be used (vinegar, glycerine, propylene glycol, etc.). After chopping the plant material into small pieces, if required, lipids can be removed and/or enzymes can be inactivated.

Extracts are usually prepared in two phases. The first phase involves getting the active principles into solution followed by partial or total evaporation of the liquid obtained in order to concentrate the product. **Fluid extracts** are prepared so that one part by weight corresponds to one part by weight of the dried drug. They are first steeped and then percolated. The percolation technique used is to pass the solvent through a glass or enamel tube filled with the drug to be extracted. The menstrum is collected drop by drop until 85% of the final volume is obtained; the remaining 15% is obtained by draining the solvent-saturated plant material and concentrating the liquid obtained. According to the pharmacopoeias, fluid extracts can also be obtained by dissolving a soft or dry drug extract in alcohol of appropriate strength followed by filtering if necessary. Whatever the preparation method, fluid extracts must have identical composition. The most commonly used fluid extracts are hydroalcoholic (prepared by draining the drug with alcohol at 60–70%) and alcoholic (alcohol at 95%). Alcohol, apart from possessing greater solvent capacity than water also acts as a preservative. Fluid extracts can be used in drop form directly but are usually used in the preparation of syrups or other dosage forms. Fluid extraction can sometimes be improved by the addition of fruit juice. For example, prune juice improves the therapeutic action of a laxative, pear juice may act as a cholagogue, and black cherry juice enhances the effect of diuretics.

Soft and dry solid extracts are prepared by concentrating hydroalcoholic or alcoholic fluid extracts at reduced pressure and at a temperature below 50°C. **Soft solid extracts** are obtained if the evaporation process of the extractive solution is interrupted when the residue begins to stick on the paper. Other methods for **dry solid extract** preparation are nebulization (drying the liquid reduced to minute drops with hot air) or lyophilization (cryodesiccation). These techniques produce excellent results and are applied especially to drugs containing thermolabile or easily degraded active principles. Other techniques may be used, such as thin-layer evaporation. The presence of active principles in terms of percentage is obviously higher in soft or dry solid extracts than in that of the initial drug; in dry solid extracts the proportion between extract and drug is the same or higher than 1:4. Dry drugs are brought up to prescribed strength by means of appropriate inert substances. Soft extracts are used in the preparation of pills, poultices, and suppositories, while dry extracts are sold in capsules as they are extremely hygroscopic. They should be stored in dry places and away from light.

Tinctures are liquid preparations obtained by treating usually dried primary vegetable or animal material (drugs) or their extracts with an appropriate strength alcohol. Tinctures may also be prepared exceptionally from fresh drugs although this should be stated in the instructions. The instructions for each tincture must indicate the name of the drug or extract and any solvent other than alcohol to be used. Thus tinctures can be prepared either by direct treatment of the drugs subdivided by percolation with alcohol and steeped from 2–8 days or by diluting the fluid extracts. Tinctures are always more diluted than fluid extracts and the proportion between drug and tincture weight is typically 1:5 (1:10 when requiring a high dosage). Thus tinctures are five or ten times less potent as compared to an equal amount of fluid extract. Tinctures are called simple if only one drug is used in their preparation and compound if there are more than one drug included. Simple tinctures containing very active drugs are prepared with 70% alcohol; aconite tinctures with 90% alcohol; those of nux vomica and poppy are prepared by diluting the relative fluid extract with 60% alcohol. Tinctures are not usually diluted with water (those mentioned in the Italian FU use 60% alcohol) because this can cause precipitation of non-active and active substances; even the mixing of different tinctures can cause turbidity. Today fluid extracts with tannins removed (to avoid precipitation of alkaloids and glycosides) are commercially available. Tinctures are sometimes used in drop form but more commonly they are used in the preparation of syrups and various preparations (e.g. "laudanum oral drops", Sydenham laudanum). Mild laudanum (0.05% morphine) is obtained by dilution of laudanum oral drops (morphine 1%) with 30% alcohol. The preparation is steeped in a well-sealed glass vessel for seven days before being strained and filtered.

Liquors are pharmaceutical forms obtained by steeping the fresh drugs in alcohol. 95% ethyl alcohol is usually used because the fresh plant contains large quantities of water which dilutes the alcohol. Liquors are prepared from plants that would lose all or part of their active principles when dried. They are used as aids to digestion when prepared with the bark of some citrus plants (lemon, sweet orange and mandarin). Some types of liquors are considered **Tincture Mothers (TM)**, their name deriving from the fact that they are used as basic material for homeopathic preparations but today are also used in phytotherapy. They are prepared using fresh wild drugs picked in warm weather (exceptionally dried drugs). Steeping is carried out after the water content has been removed by drying at 105°C, using appropriate strength alcohol (established by the French Pharmacopoeia – usually 80–90°). The quantity of solvent used is such that a TM of 10 parts to 1 part of dry plant material is produced. After steeping for precisely three weeks the fluid is decanted, filtered and the residue expressed from the wet solids. The well-known German method of TM preparation consists of diluting the plant juice with an equal weight of 86% alcohol at which point the TM obtained has an alcoholic grade of 43% and active principle concentration of 50%. The TM alcoholic grade (from 45–60°) is lower than that in dry drug tinctures. The length of preservation is also different: TM are valid for five years while the others are valid for only two years. TM have superior therapeutic activity compared to traditional tinctures in that they are richer in active principles, either because they are obtained from the untreated whole plant or because of the longer steeping period.

At this point we must distinguish between **stabilized alcoholic liquors**, which are prepared by extraction with boiling alcohol (e.g. valerian and horse chestnut liquors), and **alcoholic distilled liquors**, which are rich in volatile substances (essential oils). **Medicinal wines** are particular types of tincture obtained by using wine as an extractive solvent. They are also known as vinous tinctures obtained by steeping the dry drug from 10–15 days. Red wines are used to obtain an astringent action. White wines are used to prepare extractive from alkaloid plants and which would precipitate with red wine tannins. Wine liquors such as Marsala are used for the extraction of plants with high resin content. Today they are no longer used as they cannot be preserved for long.

Medicated oils (oleates) are extractive preparations obtained either by digestion of prepared drug in a vegetable oil (olive oil) or by displacement; in other words by first extracting the liposoluble substances with a petroleum ether or other suitable solvent, and then evaporating the solution and dissolving the residue in oil, the remaining solvent traces are evaporated in a water bath. However, this pharmaceutical form is also little used today due to its instability. Oleates are also prepared from monkshood, chamomile, marigold, mullein and St John's wort.

9.2.7 Other Types of Fresh Plant Preparations

Plant Juices

Some freshly harvested plants yield fresh juices that may have therapeutic application and are used chiefly for self-medication. This is an ancient method of administering medicinal agents in which there is renewed interest due to modern methods of preservation. Dissolved or suspended substances in the juice content include carbohydrates, organic acids, mineral salts, amino acids, proteins and metabolites which represent the plant active principles (e.g. alkaloids, flavonoids). Since everything contained in the plant passes into the juice, this is much more complete than the extracts obtained by solvents. Owing to the preparation method (squeezing and compression) of freshly expressed juice, there is no possibility for loss of active constituents if it is consumed immediately. Today excellent, inexpensive products are available, without added preservatives or coloring. Commercial preparations of such juices as those from carrots, watercress, nettle, garlic, juniper and artichoke can be prepared at home with a liquidizer.

Integral Fresh Plant Suspension

This modern pharmaceutical form is prepared by treating the fresh plant (within 6–12 hours after picking) with liquid nitrogen thus blocking all enzymatic activity. The frozen plant is crushed into a homogeneous paste and then combined with alcohol to a final concentration of 30% (w/v). The resulting solution suspension is then subjected to "molecular ultrapression", which transforms it into a stable microsuspension. Analytical tests have proved that this technique yields a preparation of identical composition to that of the medicinal plant. Such preparations are stable and can be preserved for at least three years. They are taken in doses of 5 ml diluted in a little water during meals.

These juices are sold with a certificate of analysis certifying the presence of a known amount of active principle and the absence of heavy metals and pesticides. Because of greater cost this method is only used for delicate plants with poorly soluble or highly unstable active principles. Only 15 of such products have been commercialized to date: hawthorn, artichoke, burdock, horse chestnut, horsetail, eucalyptus, kelp, sweet clover, nettle, passion flower, blackcurrant, dandelion and valeriana.

Steeped Glycerites (Bud Derivatives)

These are important preparations fundamental to bud therapy. They originated from the work of the Belgian doctor Paul Henry, who in his treatise on phytoembryology, published in 1958, foresaw the therapeutic use of plant buds. He pioneered the use of immature plant material believing that these tissues contain particularly active components which on growth lose this desired activity. The most important components in this regard are plant hormones. Gemma-derivatives were mentioned in the French Pharmacopoeia until 1965 and which explained their preparation. The method is simple: the material consisting of buds, young shoots and roots etc. is cleaned and dried in such a way that the water content is established, allowing successive treatments to be carried out with reference to dry weight. The material is then steeped for three weeks in a mixture of glycerine and alcohol in equal parts. The resulting liquid is diluted with glycerine, alcohol and water (in proportion 9:3:2), to obtain 10 parts of steeped material to 100 parts of solution. It is usually sold in dark glass dropper bottles. The dosage is 30–50 drops three times daily, diluted in a little water and held in the mouth so that it can be first absorbed under the tongue before swallowing - generally on an empty stomach.

9.3 Preparation, Flavoring and Preservation

The presence of bitter and unpleasant tasting substances in the drug make flavoring necessary for oral use preparations. This is done by adding at least 10–15% of an aromatic drug to the material to be extracted. Herbal medicines often used for this purpose are: *Mentha piperita* leaves (peppermint), *Glycirrhiza glabra* roots (liquorice), *Citrus sinensis* peel (sweet orange), *Pimpinella anisum* fruits (anice), *Verbena officinalis* flowering plant (vervain), *Phoeniculum vulgare* fruits (fennel) and *Citrus lemon* peel (lemon). Natural colours, e.g. hibiscus (*Hibiscus sab-*

dariffa) or corn poppies (*Papaver rhoeas*) for red and marigold (*Calendula officinalis*) for yellow, can be added to improve the appearance. Natural sweeteners (honey, cane sugar, molasses, malt and maple syrup), or synthetic sweeteners can be added to improve taste. For diabetic patients synthetic or polyalcoholic sweeteners are preferable. These preparations remain "fresh" for only 24 hours at room temperature, and 3–4 days if kept in a refrigerator. The Italian FU advises the addition of suitable preservatives for syrups. Since muddying and precipitation are easily manifested in compound preparations, it is advisable to reduce to the minimum drug or extract combinations. In the case of insufficient active principle solubility, co-solvents (glycerine, glycols, sorbitol, etc.) or emulsifiers (polysorbates, polyhexylene glycols, etc.) or organic acids (citric, tartaric, lactic) can be added during extraction. Varying the pH content of the latter facilitates alkaloid solubility.

In conclusion it is always necessary to protect all phytotherapeutic preparations from external agents (light, heat), chemical agents (air, humidity) and microbiological agents. Care must be taken to store them in a dry and aerated place and in suitable well-sealed containers (dark glass).

9.4 Dosage

The dosages stated throughout this text is for adults aged 18–65 and a weight of 70 kg. For **unweaned** babies up to 10 kg in weight the dosage should be 1/6–1/10 of that for an adult; for children up to 20 kg in weight the dosage should be 1/3, and up to 40–50 kg must be 3/4 of the adult dosage. If taking age as a parameter the adult dose should be reduced by 1/10–1/15 up to 2 years of age; 1/8–1/6 up to 4 years of age; 1/4 up to 9 years of age; 1/2 up to 14 years of age; 2/3 up to 18 years of age and 3/4 over 65 years of age.

▸ *See Part II, Chapters 13–23 for special plant dosages*

Chapter 10

Uses of Herbal Medicines in Specific Situations

The use of plant-derived drugs in pregnancy and in the mother who is breast feeding requires particular care. Caution is also required for the very young or old patients and for those suffering from hepatic or renal insufficiency

10.1 Pregnancy

Since the 1960s, following the tragic teratogenic consequences of using thalidomide in pregnant women, the use of natural or synthetic medicines during the first phase of pregnancy should in general be avoided. Unfortunately, in practice this recommendation has not always helped to resolve the problem of mutagenicity because by the time the patient is aware of the pregnancy (usually 5–6 weeks after conception) she may have been exposed to the mutagen/teratogen for quite some time. Generally speaking it is accepted that the toxic effects of medicines are more pronounced during cellular differentiation. Thus the risk is highest if the medicine is administered during the period of blastogenesis (from the moment of conception to the 14th day of pregnancy) and embryogenesis (from the second week to the end of the third month of pregnancy): in the former there is the death of the embryo (blastogenesis) and in the latter malformation of the limbs or organs (embryogenesis). Although the possible teratogenic effects of a medicine prescribed in the first three months of pregnancy are known to everyone, very few are aware of the risk of collateral effects in the fetal period. When the mother receives a medicine it may reach the fetus in a concentration great enough to produce a toxic effect. In addition, the mother may be at risk of abortion or hemorrhage during birth (this has been shown with the prolonged use of salicylates). If it is necessary to resort to medicines during pregnancy, as in diabetes, epilepsy, cardiopathy, hypertension, infection, or the threat of abortion, those medicines suspected of affecting the fetus obviously need to be avoided. This is equally valid for botanical drugs and especially for drugs which may affect uterine motility. Table 10.1 lists some herbal medicinal products which potentially can cause health problems during pregnancy. Clinical data on the possible risk associated to pregnant women and their babies are shown in Table 10.2.

10.2 Nursing

Maternal milk is without doubt the most suitable nutrient for a child in the first months of life. The yield of carbohydrates, mineral salts, fats and proteins is the ideal. Maternal milk also contains antibodies able to protect the infant from microorganisms and infections. Thus, in cases of insufficient milk secretion lactation-stimulating substances are sometimes administered, even if there are doubts as to their safety. Milk can transmit chemical or substances of alimentary origin which cause allergies in the newborn such as nettle-rash, diarrhea (from aloe) or sleepiness from sedatives for anxiety or narcotics (e.g. opiates) for pain. The nursing mother, therefore, should always be advised to avoid or reduce the intake of medicines, including herbal medicines containing laxatives, xanthines such as caffeine, tranquillizers, contraceptives and anticoagulants.

10.3 Pediatric Age Group

Children, because of their immaturity, are often more susceptible than adults to the effects of drugs. Some medications can adversely affect normal development in children. In newborn babies hepatic microsomial and non-microsomial enzyme systems involved in the transformation of medicines are not fully functional, the blood-brain barrier is not completely developed and the excretory system (in particular the kidneys) is immature. This clearly makes the newborn particularly vulnerable to drug-induced toxicity, especially to the liver and kidneys. Therefore, the use of botanical drugs in this age group must be carefully evaluated.

Table 10.1

Herbal medicinal products and potential adverse effects during pregnancy

Common Name	Latin Name	Relevant Adverse Effect
Alfalfa	*Medicago sativa*	May cause uterine stimulation
Aloe	*Aloe spp.*	Stimulation of uterine muscle activity
Angelica	*Angelica archangelica*	Emmenagogue effects
Asafoetida	*Ferula asafoetida*	Emmenagogue effects
Ashwagandha	*Withania somnifera*	Abortifacient properties
Barberry	*Berberis vulgaris*	Uterine stimulant
Basil	*Ocimum basilicum*	Emmenagogue, abortifacient, mutagenic
Bearberry	*Arctostaphylos uva ursi*	Oxytocic action
Bitter melon	*Momordica charantia*	Emmenagogue and abortifacient effects
Black cohosh	*Cimicifuga racemosa*	Oestrogenic activity, suppresses endogenous luteinising hormone secretion (in rats) and binds uterine oestrogen receptors,reduces circulating luteising hormone levels. Emmenagogue effects
Blood root	*Sanguinaria canadensis*	Emmenagogue and uterine stimulant
Blue cohosh	*Caulophyllum thalictroides*	Gastrointestinal symptoms, stimulates contraction of uterine muscle, causes arterial constriction, inhibits embryo implantation (in rats), alleged to induce menstruation and promote abortion.
Boneset	*Eupatorium perfoliatum*	Abortifacient effects
Borage	*Borago officinalis*	Mutagenic (contains pyrrolizidine alkaloids)
Buckthorn	*Rhamnus catharticus*	Abortifacient, mutagenic, genotoxic effects
Bugleweed	*Lycopus virginicus*	Antigonatotrophic and antithyrotropic activity
Burdock	*Arctium lappa*	Oxitocic and uterine stimulant action
Butterbur	*Petasites hybridus*	Emmenagogue, hepatotoxic, genotoxic and carcinogenic effects
Buttercup	*Ranunculus acris*	Uterine stimulant
Calamus	*Acorus calamus*	Emmenagogue and genotoxic effects
Camphor	*Cinnamomum camphora*	Emmenagogue and uterine effects
Cascara sagrada	*Rhamnus purshiana*	Abortifacient, mutagenic and genotoxic action
Cassia cinnamon	*Cinnamomum aromaticum*	Emmenagogue and abortifacient effects
Castor bean	*Ricinus communis*	Emmenagogue and abortifacient effects
Catnip	*Nepeta cataria*	Emmenagogue and abortifacient effects
Celandine	*Chelidonium majus*	Uterine stimulant
Celery	*Apium graveolens*	Uterine stimulant, abortifacient and emmenagogue action
Chamomile (Roman)	*Chamaemelum nobile*	Emmenagogue and abortifacient effects
Chasteberry	*Vitex agnus castus*	Emmenagogue effects
Chicory	*Cichorium intybus*	Emmenagogue and abortifacient effects

Continued next page

Table 10.1

Herbal medicinal products and potential adverse effects during pregnancy (*continued*)

Common Name	Latin Name	Relevant Adverse Effect
Cinchona	*Cinchona spp.*	Abortifacient, uterine stimulant, oxytocic, teratogenic effects
Cinnamon	*Cinnamomium verum*	Emmenagogue effects
Cola	*Cola nitida*	Low birthweight, birth defects, premature birth
Coltsfoot	*Tussilago farfara*	Contains hepatotoxic pyrrolidizine alkaloids, risk of fatal hepatic veno-occlusive disease, abortifacient effects
Comfrey	*Symphytum officinale*	Contains hepatotoxic pyrrolidizine alkaloids, risk of foetal hepatic veno-occlusive disease, hepatotoxic and carcinogenic in animals
Echinacea	*E. angustifolia or E. purpurea or E. pallida*	Weak oxytocic effects
Ephedra	*Ephedra spp.*	Contains ephedrine and related alkaloids, increases blood pressure, heart rate and causes CNS activity, stimulates uterine muscle
Fennel	*Foeniculum vulgare*	Emmenagogue effects
Feverfew	*Tanacetum parthenium*	May promote menstruation and induces abortion
Flax	*Linum usitatissimum*	Emmenagogue effects
Frangula	*Rhamnus frangula*	Endometrial stimulation, mutagenic and genotoxic effects
Garlic	*Allium sativum*	Emmenagogue effects
Ginger	*Zingiber officinale*	Abortifacient, emmenagogue and mutagenic effects
Goldenseal	*Hydrastis canadensis*	Uterine stimulant
Gotu kola	*Centella asiatica*	Emmenagogue effects
Guarana	*Paullinia cupana*	Low birthweight, birth defects, premature birth
Hemp agrimony	*Eupatorium cannabinum*	Emmenagogue and abortifacient effects
Hibiscus	*Hibiscus rosa sinensis*	Emmenagogue effects
Horehound	*Marrubium vulgare*	Emmenagogue and abortifacient effects
Horseradish	*Armoracia rusticana*	Abortifacient effects
Hyssop	*Hyssopus officinalis*	Emmenagogue and abortifacient effects
Ipecac	*Cephaelis ipecacuanha*	Uterine stimulant
Joe-pye weed	*Eupatorium purpureum*	Abortifacient effects
Juniper	*Juniperus communis*	Allergenic, cathartic in large doses, diuretic, increases uterine tone; possible anti-amplantation, abortifacient and emmenagogue effects
Kava	*Piper methysticum*	Loss of uterin tone
Khella	*Ammi visnaga*	Emmenagogue and abortifacient effects
Knot grass	*Polygonum aviculare*	Abortifacient effects
Lavender	*Lavandula angustifolia*	Emmenagogue effects
Leptandra	*Veronicastrum virginicum*	Teratogenic effects
Liquorice	*Glycyrrhiza glabra*	Emmenagogue effects
Life root	*Senecio aureus*	Emmenagogue and teratogenic effects

Continued next page

Table 10.1
Herbal medicinal products and potential adverse effects during pregnancy (*continued*)

Common Name	Latin Name	Relevant Adverse Effect
Lobelia	*Lobelia inflata*	Loss of uterine tone
Lovage	*Levisticum officinale*	Emmenagogue effects
Madagascar periwinkle	*Vinca rosa*	Abortifacient effects
Madder	*Rubia tinctorium*	Genotoxic and emmenagogue effects
Male fern	*Dryopteris filix-mas*	Abortifacient effects
Marigold	*Calendula officinalis*	Emmenagogue and abortifacient effects
Marsh tea	*Ledum palustre*	Abortifacient effects
Masterwood	*Heracleum lanatum*	Emmenagogue effects
Mate	*Ilex paraguariensis*	Low birthweight, birth defects, premature birth
Mistletoe	*Viscum album*	Uterine stimulant
Motherwort	*Leonurus cardiaca*	Emmenagogue effects
Mugwort	*Artemisia vulgaris*	Emmenagogue and abortifacient effects
Myrrh	*Commiphora myrrha*	Emmenagogue and abortifacient effects
Nutmeg	*Myristica fragrans*	Abortifacient and mutagenic effects
Papain	*Carica papaya*	Emmenagogue and abortifacient effects
Pareira	*Chondrodendron tomentosum*	Emmenagogue and abortifacient effects
Parsley	*Petroselinum sativum*	Emmenagogue and abortifacient effects
Passion flower	*Passiflora incarnata*	Uterine stimulant
Peach pit	*Prunus persica*	Emmenagogue and abortifacient effects
Pennyroyal	*Hedeoma pulegioides* or *Mentha pulegium*	Traditionally used an abortifacient, hepatotoxic and neurotoxic
Paeony	*Paeonia officinalis*	Emmenagogue effects
Peppermint	*Mentha piperita*	Emmenagogue effects
Pine	*Pinus spp.*	Abortifacient effects
Pleurisy root	*Asclepias tuberosa*	Uterine stimulant
Pomegranate	*Punica granatum*	Emmenagogue and abortifacient effects
Prickly ash	*Zanthoxylum americanum*	Emmenagogue effects
Pulsatilla	*Anemone pulsatilla*	Uterine stimulant
Queen anne's lace	*Dancus carota*	Emmenagogue and abortifacient effects
Raspberry	*Rubus idaeus*	Stimulates contraction in strips of pregnant human uterus, antigonatrophic activity
Rhubarb	*Rheum palmatum*	Uterine stimulant, mutagenic, genotoxic effects
Rosemary	*Rosmarinus officinalis*	Emmenagogue and abortifacient effects
Rue	*Ruta graveolens*	Emmenagogue and abortifacient effects
Safflower	*Carthamus tinctorius*	Emmenagogue and abortifacient effects
Saffron	*Crocus sativus*	Emmenagogue and abortifacient effects
Sage	*Salvia officinalis*	Emmenagogue and abortifacient effects
Sandalwood	*Antalkum album*	Abortifacient effects
Sassafras	*Sassafras officinale*	Emmenagogue effects
Savin	*Juniperus sabina*	Abortifacient effects
Scotch broom	*Cytisus scoparius*	Abortifacient effects

Continued next page

Table 10.1
Herbal medicinal products and potential adverse effects during pregnancy (*continued*)

Common Name	Latin Name	Relevant Adverse Effect
Scullcap	*Scutellaria laterifolia*	May inhibit pituitary and chorionic gonadotropins, as well as prolactin, liver damage in humans
Senna	*Cassia acutifolia, angustifolia*	Endometrial stimulation, mutagenic and genotoxic effects
Shepherd's purse	*Capsella bursa-pastoris*	Emmenagogue and abortifacient effects
Snakeroot	*Polygala senega*	Emmenagogue and uterine stimulant effects
St.John's wort	*Hypericum perforatum*	Emmenagogue and abortifacient effects
Stinging nettle	*Urtica dioica*	Emmenagogue and abortifacient effects
Sweet marjoram	*Origanum majorana*	Emmenagogue effects
Tansy	*Tanacetum vulgare*	Emmenagogue and abortifacient effects
Thyme	*Thymus vulgaris*	Emmenagogue effects
Turmeric	*Curcuma longa*	Emmenagogue and abortifacient effects
Valerian	*Valeriana officinalis*	Stimulates uterine contraction
Watercress	*Nasturtium officinale*	Emmenagogue and abortifacient effects
Wild cherry	*Prunus serotina*	Emmenagogue effects
Wild ginger	*Asarum canadense*	Emmenagogue and abortifacient effects
Wild marjoram	*Origanum vulgare*	Emmenagogue and abortifacient effects
Wood sorrel	*Oxalis acetosella*	Emmenagogue effects
Worm seed	*Chenopodium ambrosoides*	Emmenagogue and abortifacient effects
Wormwood	*Artemisia absinthium*	Emmenagogue and abortifacient effects
Yellow cedar	Thuja occidentalis	Emmenagogue and abortifacient effects

data from Ernst E (2002); BJOG 109:227–235 (modified); CNS = central nervous system

10.4 Geriatric Age Group

It has been estimated that for people over 65 years of age undesirable effects are double those of young people. In the elderly, side effects are more probable due to impaired absorption, biotransformation and elimination. An additional consideration is the fact that the elderly often have medical conditions that further compromise the ability of their body to handle drugs. Furthermore, for therapeutic intervention to be effective it is essential to take into consideration the patient's capacity to follow instructions. This may be impaired in the older patient due to cerebral insufficiency and social isolation. For these reasons pharmacological therapy should be simplified as far as possible (in oral form), not only for the patients but for those who are involved in their care. Because of the perceived safety and "gentle" action of many herbal medicines, in recent years there has been an increase in the use of these-products in geriatric patients.

Table 10.2

Clinical reports of adverse events (in mother and their neonates) associated to herbal use during pregnancy

Herbal medicine (Common and latin name)	Promoted use	Adverse effect	Possible mechanism	Source of information
Chasteberry (*Vitex agnus castus*)	Premenstrual syndrome, menopausal complaints	Derangement of gonadotrophin and ovarian hormone levels	Chasteberry may lead to ovarian hyperstimulation and may increase the risk of miscarriage	Case report
Blue cohosh (*Caulophyllum thalictroides*)	Gynecological disorders	Myocardial infarction and cardiovascular shock in the neonate. Kidney damage, seizure and need for mechanical ventilation in the neonate	Cardiotoxic alkaloids (e.g. caulosaponin) in blue cohosh may cause constriction of coronary blood vessels and causes myocardial toxic reactions	2 case reports
Dong quai (*Angelica sinensis*)	Gynecological disorders; circulatory disorders	Postpartum acute headache, weakness, vomiting and high blood pressure; high blood pressure in the neonate	Not known	Case report
Ginseng (*Panax ginseng*)	Stress states, lack of stamina	Black pubic hear, hear over the entire forehead, swollen and red nipples in the neonate	Androgenization may be caused by hormonal effects of ginseng	Case report
Solomon's seal (*Polygonatum multiflorum*)	Inflammatory states; respiratory and lung disorders	Symptom of hepatitis	Hepatotoxity of the herbal product	Case report
Thunder god vine (*Tripterygium wilfordii*)	Rheumatoid arthritis	Occipital meningoencephalocele and cerebellar agenesis in the neonate	Not known	Case report
Castor oil (*Ricinus communis*)	Constipation	Pregnancy complicated by fetal meconium passage. Caesarean section more frequent	Not known Zoapatle possess oxytocin-like effects	Retrospective surveys (n = 8)

continued next page

Table 10.2
Clinical reports of adverse events (in mother and their neonates) associated to herbal use during pregnancy (*continued*)

Herbal medicine (Common and latin name)	Promoted use	Adverse effect	Possible mechanism	Source of information
Zoapatle (*Montanoa tomentosa*)	Contraception, induction of labour, treatment of post-partum bleeding	Cardiorespiratory depression in the neonate		Case series (n = 8)
Evening primrose oil (*Oenothera biennis*)	Dermatological conditions, rheumatoid arthritis, premenstrual syndrome, menopausal complaints	Increase in the incidence of prolonged rupture of membranes, oxytocin augmentation, arrest of descent and an increased frequency of vacuum extraction	Gamma-linolenic acid (a component in Evening primrose) can be converted to prostaglandins which could modify the course of childbirth	Clinical trial (n = 108)

data extracted from Ernst E (2002); BJOG 109:227-235

10.5 Precautions

The risks from herbal medicines, and indeed all drugs, are greatly reduced if some precautionary norms are followed:

- Patients over 65 years of age should begin treatment with low doses of herbal medicines
- Pregnant and breast-feeding mothers should not take herbal medicines
- Herbal medicines should not be used in children under two years old
- Chronically ill patients should bear in mind that plant-derived drugs may interact with conventional drugs taken concurrently
- Do not ignore toxic symptoms of any kind
- Essential oils should be used with caution (they are highly concentrated and small quantities which seem innocuous may cause serious harm)
- Herbal medicines should be taken only at the prescribed dose and for limited periods of time

Chapter 11

Sources of Herbal Medicine Information

It is obvious that physicians need objective and concise information on herbal medicines (Table 11.1, p. 72). Textbooks of pharmacognosy and phytotherapy, leading scientific journals, meetings and seminars are the main sources available. Although this multiplicity of information is available, most phytotherapists are unable to collect appropriate information required for the practice of rational phytotherapy. In general pharmacognosy textbooks provide basic principles and detailed descriptions of herbal drugs organized by chemical classes of active components. Phytotherapy textbooks include information on the therapeutic use of herbal medicines. They certainly are books of medicine but often superficially. Both cannot contain information about new herbal drugs.

Another source of information is the Physicians Desk References (PDR) for Herbal Medicines. This book, supported by manufacturers, includes for each herbal medicine indications supported by the German Commission E (German Regulatory Authorities – a herbal watchdog agency) and by the Food and Drug Administration. The United States Pharmacopoeia (USP) and National Formulary (NF) are two official compendia, which list therapeutic agents used in medical practice for their proven efficacy. Then there are journals that specifically refer on the medicinal properties of herbal drugs (e.g. Phytomedicine, Journal of Ethnopharmacology, Phytotherapy Research, Fitoterapia, Alternative Medicinal Review, Journal of Alternative and Complementary Medicine).

There are a variety of on-line databases that contain valuable information on the biological and chemical properties of herbal medicines. MEDLINE is the most complete and useful source of information on medical sciences, including experimental and clinical studies of herbal medicines; it provides information in the form of abstracts. Database

Table 11.1
Information pertaining to herbal medicine

Ethnomedical use (ancient and recent)
Pharmacological assessment of the herbal medicine and its preparations
Clinical studies and meta-analysis
Amount of active principles in the herbal medicine and its preparations
Pharmacological assessment of active principle
Quality control data
The disease for which herbal medicine is safe and effective

specialized in phytotherapy include NAPRALERT, CISCOM, AMED and PHYTOBASE. Another on-line database is THE COCHRAINE LIBRARY which includes all clinical studies, including those using herbal medicines.

Chapter 12
Herbal Product Regulations

Officinal plants and their products have great social and economic consequences, and today they are used in four principal sectors: food, cosmetics, health and medicine. In 2001 sales of herbal products exceeded US $ 337 millions. The medicinal use of the herbal drugs, Phytotherapy, is differently controlled in different countries, but with only marginal differences because phytotherapeutic products must possess quality, safety and efficacy. The use of herbs as health foods, as well as food supplements, complicates the formulation of regulations by countries throughout the world. The increasing supply of herbal products to international markets makes it necessary for international organizations, such as the World Health Organization (WHO) to develop standards relative to their commercialization throughout the world.

12.1 WHO Guidelines for Herbal Medicines

During the last decades, WHO has played a fundamental role in the promotion and the development of the international regulation of medicinal plants. The activity of WHO to promote the investigation of medicinal plants used in traditional medicine is directed towards rational and scientific use of herbal drugs and standardization of their preparations.

In 1979, WHO instituted the "Programme on Traditional Medicines" devoted to the study of the cultivation, identification, preparation, and the use of plants in traditional medicine. In October 1978, the "Committee for the Selection and Specification of the Medicinal Plants" was founded. The committee, besides defining the therapeutic importance of medicinal plants and their preparation all over the world, prepared a list of 230 plants considered to be used most in the world, among 12,000 inventoried by WHO. The documents of greater interest defined the task of the WHO centers. These are "Guidelines for the Assessment of Herbal Medicines", München, June 1991 and "Research Guidelines for Evaluation of the Safety and Efficacy of Herbal Medicines", published by the Regional Office for the Western Pacific, Manila 1993. The guidelines of 1993, for the evaluation of the safety and efficacy of herbal medicines, consist of detailed criteria to establish the specification of quality of the herbal material and the information related to the pharmaceutical forms used. They also established tests for the determination of the toxicity of the plants and have emphasized the importance of conducting pharmacological, pharmacodynamic and clinical studies.

12.2 The European Regulation

In an attempt to coordinate the marketing and distribution of herb-based medicinal products, marketing authorization in the EU for drugs of herbal origin began with the promulgation of the directives EEC 65/65 and 75/318 and with the publication of the European Pharmacopoeia (Ph. Eur.). The basic directive 65/65 EEC, art. 1 gives definitions of medicine, medicinal specialty and substance, including drugs of herbal origin. Subsequently, directive 75/318 authorized diversified standards for the drugs of botanical origin. The application of such directive, however, would have caused the elimination from the market of many herbal medicines, because of the practical impossibility to apply the procedures required for the marketing of complex herbal mixtures. In fact, it is known that the herbal medicines, because of the complexity and variability of their chemical composition, introduce problems of standardization and reproducibility of their biological effects. The process to harmonize the procedures of authorization of the medicines has been effected fully with the institution as of January 1, 1995 by the European Medicines Evaluation Agency (EMEA); it also guarantees the uniformity and quality of the currently marketed medicines in the 15 Countries of the EU. Within the framework of the European Community there has been an increasing interest in herbal medicines, not withstanding the fact that coordination of legal issues on herbal medicines within the EU is very complex.

In 1977, in Bruxelles, the Committee for Proprietary Medicinal Products (CPMP) adopted the term "herbal remedies" (HR) for all the medicinal products containing herbal drugs and/or preparations as active ingredients. The group proposed the application of simplified standards to the majority of herbal products and the application of the standards required by the directive 75/318 EEC only for products with remarkable biological activity. In the same period the CPMP also proposed to admit provisionally products that do not contain dangerous herbal substances and are intended to be used (without a physician's prescription) for the symptomatic treatment of the minor pathologies. The necessity of a specific and complete norm for the herbal remedies was indicated by the European Parliament, with the resolution of October 16th, 1987 (GUCE n. C 305 of 16-10-1987). The resolution recommended university training of those working with scientifically documented natural medicines, as well as the formulation of a special list of medicinal plants which would be excluded from the most rigid regulatory requirements.

In 1989, the Commission of the European Communities, in the document *The Rules Governing Medicinal Products in the European Community, vol. III, Guidelines on the Quality, Safety an Efficacy of Medicinal Products for Human Use*, established the definitions of vegetable drugs, herbal remedies or herbal medicines, and vegetable drug preparations. They defined the formalities of application of the part 1 of the directive 75/318/CEE, regarding the quality of the starting material and the final products of vegetable origin. The guidelines set forth required qualitative and quantitative control of the components, the description of the methods of preparation, the control of intermediate product and of the final product and the tests of stability for herbal products. It also required disclosure of the origin of the plant or vegetable drug, the possible presence of contaminants and, if the substances responsible for therapeutic activity are unknown, a guarantee of quality based upon production according to "Good Manufacturing Practices" (GMP). In the same year, directive 89/341/CEE set the application of the same standards of quality, safety and efficacy provided by directives 65/65/CEE and 75/318/CEE for galenicals and all medicines of natural origin. These standards also related to the European Court of Justice's recommendations that herbal products with preventive activity or therapeutic use must be considered a medicinal product, even if it is generally used as a food or if therapeutic effects have yet to be shown.

In 1996, the European Commission announced a competition for a contract to study the marketing of medicines of vegetable origin relative to production, distribution and retail sale. In this regard the Ph. Eur. monographs on vegetable drugs and preparations has been very important. Also important was the "European Scientific Cooperatives on Phytotherapy" (ESCOP). Constituted in 1989, ESCOP is an association to which the most important national associations of the different European countries that take an interest in medicinal plants and phytotherapy. ESCOP promotes studies in the field of the phytomedicines which it defined as "medicinal products containing as active principle only plants, parts of plants or vegetable materials and their combinations in either the raw or refined state". This definition has been adopted by other national and international organizations. To promote the unification of the criteria for evaluation of vegetable medicines, ESCOP organized an international symposium on the theme "European Harmony in Phytotherapy".

In the January 1997, the EU published the *Notice to Applicants* (NTA), guidelines for the use of phytomedicines. In this document were also the requirements for herbal drugs as to synthesis, but not as to geographical origin, macroscopic and microscopic description, toxicity and/or adulteration. It has become more and more evident that a revision of the document on the procedures of authorization of the vegetable medicines was necessary. In 1997, within the EMEA, the "EMEA's ad hoc Working Group on Herbal Medicinal Products" (HMPWG) was founded, composed by experts and representatives of the most important community organizations of the sector, as the ESCOP, the *European Federation of Pharmaceutical Industries Association* (EFPIA), the *Association Européenne des Specialités Grand Publique* (AESGP), the *European Herbal Products Manufacturers* (EHPM), as well as of the European Parliament and of the European Pharmacopoeia. The group committed itself to revise and to elaborate new guidelines addressed both to the manufacturing firms and the licensing authorities, respectively, - to require and to grant the authorization for "*Herbal Medicinal Products*" and to establish specific criteria as to the quality, safety and efficacy of phytomedicines.

The HMPWG, which might evolve into a permanent committee, has issued the "Report from the *ad hoc* Working Group on Herbal Medicinal Products 1997/1998". Perhaps the most important document of the HMPWG is the revision of the guidelines *Manufacture of Herbal Medicinal Products.* In order to ensure that vegetable drugs have reproducible characteristics of quality and efficacy, herbal substances need to follow the norms on the *Good Agricultural Practices* (GAP) of the European Herb Growers and Producers Association. Another very interesting point of the work is represented by the proposal of guideline "Non Clinical Testing of Herbal Drug Preparations with Long-term Experience – Guidance to Facilitate Mutual Recognition and Use of Bibliographical Data". It discusses the lack of need to tightly regulate herbal ingredients or whole herbs for which exhaustive bibliographical data exist; it is not necessary to introduce the results of new toxicological and clinical studies unless the scientific literature is insufficient. HMPWG has to establish the general criteria to evaluate the efficacy and the safety of the phytotherapy, elaborated in the monographs known as *Core - Summary of Product Characteristics* (Core-SPCS). Such monographs are and will be based on those of ESCOP, WHO, the experience of the Commission E in Germany and the current original research. The document was revised in regard to GMP in l989. This change concerns the declaration of the composition, description of the method of preparation and the control of the starting material, the description of the procedure of preparation and its validation as Drug Master File, according to *European Drug Master Files Procedure for Active Substances.*

In conclusion, the EU is preparing a community directive that, according to the recommendations of WHO, will favour the rational use of herbal drugs. According to art. 3 of the draft, state members of the EU can authorize the products for traditional use with an alternative procedure to those established from the previous directives. Article 5 defines the requirement that a product has to possess to be authorized as a traditional medicine: it should not be dangerous; it has to be suitable only for minor pathologies, recommending specific dosage and only be a way of administration. Article 6, moreover, establishes that the "simple preparations" (drugs to prepare tea, infusion, tisanes, etc.) can be authorized with the presentation of a simplified dossier. Thus in some countries of the EU, the new directives on the traditional medicines will require only some changes to the existing regulations, while in other countries, including Italy, it will be necessary to make major alterations in the general EU directives.

12.3 Laws and Regulations in some European Countries

France

In France, according to the art. L 601 of the *Code de la Santè Publique* (CSP), all the medicines of vegetable origin must get the *Autorisation de mise sur marchè* (AMM), based on conformity with the dispositions of the articles R 512–R 5136 of the CSP. For herbal medicines, whose use is well known, the presentation of a shortened dossier is enough (art. 5133 of the CSP); it is not necessary to attach the pharmacological and clinical documentation to the application. Since 1990 the *Ministere des*

Affaires Sociales et de là Solidaritè published a "Notice to the Manufacturers", a wide guide that allowed the simplified authorization for medicines obtained by 174 vegetable drugs of consolidated traditional use. In France, therefore, it has been possible, following the above procedure, to maintain in commerce traditionally used medicines for which a suitable scientific documentation was not available. New drugs based on already known drugs always require the presentation of a complete dossier, in line with the EU general directives on medicines. In 1998, the *Ministère de l'emploi et de la Solidarité-Agence du Médicament* published the volume *Les Médicaments à Base de Plantes*. The volume is divided in five chapters and four enclosures. Chapter I gives the definitions and the characteristics of herbal drugs of well known use, with the relative preparations, therapeutic indications, and required specifications for the AMM. Chapter II, divided in four parts, specifies the necessary documentation for the preparation of the dossier. Chapter III covers information on vegetable drugs which are considered rational in France. The fourth chapter is about the vegetable laxatives. It brings a classification of the laxative drugs and their possible associations, dosage and conditions of employment. Chapter V defines therapeutic categories and gives a list of words related to therapeutic indications, according to the traditional use.

Germany

Germany, together with France, is a leader in the regulation of phytotherapy, because of the long-time traditional use of herbal medicines in these countries. The *Arzneimittelgesetz* (AMG) was instituted in 1976 and the regulation of herbal medicines has been enforced since January 1, 1978. A 12-year extension was granted for products already in commerce, but because many products could not meet the new requirements in Germany they disappeared from the market. In consideration of the EU directives of January 1, 1990, the Office of Health in Germany founded the *Kommission E* (German Commission E). This commission was constituted of 24 experts (naturalists, doctors, chemists and pharmacologists) who were given the task of collecting and evaluating existing documentation on phytotherapeutic products. The German Commission E elaborated 300 monographs, each devoted to a single drug. The reports include information on constitution, pharmacology, pharmacokinetics, toxicology, indications, contraindications, adverse effects, interactions with other substances, dosage and uses of plant-derived medicinal substances. The monographs were first published in provisional layout in specialized journals and, after three months, with some revisions, in the *Bundesanzeiger* (Federal Official Gazette), in order to establish legality. The monographs, continually brought up-to-date, represent a useful tool for doctors and other healthcare professionals interested in phytotherapy. The monographs of drugs, whose therapeutic indications have not been sufficiently documented, brought about the saying "not having shown the activity of the drug for the proposed indications, we cannot sustain the therapeutic use of it". These drugs are included in a negative list of drugs and their use is not recommended, even if not forbidden. The monographs of plants and vegetable drugs with well defined qualitative and quantitative standards, approved by the German Commission E, have been inserted in the German Pharmacopoeia. Simple and composed formulations, and preparations based on vegetable drugs that can be prepared both in the pharmacy and in industry as officinal galenic, have been inserted in the German national formulary. The opinion of the German Commission E is compulsory for the Farmacopoeia and the National Formulary. The monographs elaborated by the German Commission E have been of fundamental importance in the revision of the medicines in commerce in Germany: around 148,000 products, of which half are herbal remedies (HR). In 1991, only 115 HR were authorized as medicinal specialties, while about 25,000 products were exempted from authorization from the *Bundesgesundheitsamt* (the Office of Health) and, conforming to art. 4 of the directive EEC 65/65/CEE, could be authorized on the base of the monographs of the Kommission E. In August 1994, the *Federal Authorities* emanated a new AMG that established criteria more specific about the active ingredients. Currently, the herbal substances considered to be without any human health risk and conforming to the requirements provided for by the monographs of the Kommission E, can be authorized for sale. These products have to be labeled with the statement "used traditionally" but they are not necessarily subject to quality control.

Great Britain

Herbal products in the United Kingdom are available to the public in varied ways: in pharmacies, health/natural food shops and supermarkets. Some products are simply dried herbs sold alone, or combinations for internal and external use. The greatest part of the vegetable-based products is used for alimentary problems. They have been submitted to regulation by the *Ministry of Agriculture, Fisheries and Foods*. Different vegetable drugs and their derived products are recorded as medicinal specialties. The norms regulating authorization in the market of the vegetable medicines are the same as those for synthetic medicines. Some plants and drugs can be sold only by the chemist, and others distributed by the chemist with medical prescription only. After the 1968 *Medicines Act* the HR were regulated as other medicines, but from September 1971 provisional authorization was granted (*Product Licence of Right*) to the products already in the market. The *Medicines Act* allowed the "Herbal Practitioners" to practice their activity even within the national health service. With some important documents (MO 1977 SI 2130; MO 1983 SI 1212; MO 1984 SI 796), the practitioners established some restrictions to the sale and the supply of the HR.

In 1991, as a consequences of the revision of the HR, 600 HR were approved according to the directive 75/318; their efficacy and safety were recognized based on the existing bibliography. The authorities agreed to accept the efficacy based on existing herbal and/or the pharmacological literature. These HR had to be labeled as "a traditional vegetable remedy to assuage the symptoms of..." and "if the symptoms persist do consult the physician." As of January 1995, Rule 1994 SI 3144 (according to the European legislation), introduced new procedures for approval of herbal medicines, including the requirement for more detailed labeling. Currently, before marketing, all the new herbal products authorized as medicinal, are evaluated by the Medicines Control Agency for safety, quality and efficacy according to the British and European legislation.

In the United Kingdom the *British Herbal Pharmacopoeia* (BHP) exists. It was revised and published in 1990 and in 1992, and was integrated by the *British Herbal Compendium* (BHC), republished in 1997. It is a manual that furnishes detailed technical information on the medicinal plants for which the standards of quality are defined in the BHP. The BHC was published and edited by the *British Herbal Medicine Association*, founded in 1964 to promote the study and the use of the medicinal plants in the United Kingdom. The BHC is particularly interesting because every monograph, beside providing scientific information on the drug (composition chemistry and pharmacological aspects), gives *Regulatory Status* in the UK as well as in the United States and the EU. Every monograph has references to the other pharmacopoeias including the "Regulatory Guidelines from other EC Countries."

Italy

The plants or drugs with medicinal properties must be submitted to the same procedures for all the medicines in order to get authorization, such as for DL vo 178/91, modified by the DL vo 44/97. It is not possible to effect simplified procedures and a specific norm does not exist as in other European countries. A proposal of law in Parliament called *Discipline of the Phytotherapy* exists which sets out a simplified procedure for approval of medicinal substances of vegetable origin. The vegetable drugs for general and customary use are anchored to old laws (law January 6th 1931, n 99, RD November 19th 1931, n 1793, and May 26 1932, n 722), without changes in about 20 years. In the current 14th legislature there are also some additional proposals relative to herbal preparations.

Austria

The vegetable products can be commercialized only after notification to the Office of Health and concession of authorization.

Belgium

There is a positive list of plants that can be commercialized after notification and approval from the Office of Health.

Ireland

All the products that contain vegetable substances are considered to be medicines and so can be commercialized only if authorized by the Irish Medicinal Board.

Holland

There is, in progress of elaboration, a new norm based on a negative list of substances that can be sold only as medicines and on a positive list of plants saleable as foods.

Denmark

Recording is necessary for the most part of the vegetable products, with a dossier on the starting materials, on the toxicology, etc. Some plants that are considered to be safe can be sold as foods, with the condition that they do not have therapeutic properties.

Sweden

In this country the authorization for vegetable products is necessary. But an intermediary category of products exists, called a *Grey Area*, placed between the medicines and the foods.

Finland

Some vegetable products are commercialized as foods but they are not therapeutic products. Other products (excluded those of the negative list) can be authorized with a simplified procedure.

Spain

Some 23 plants can be commercialized as foods. All the other vegetable products require the authorization from the Office of Health.

Portugal

All the medicinal plants and the vegetable products must be authorized for marketing. The medicinal plants and their derivatives must be authorized and the presentation of a detailed dossier is required.

12.4 Regulations in Non-European Countries

United States

In the United States, as in the EU, during the last decades there has been an increasing interest in the natural products of vegetable origin. Much of the legislation in the United States for the products of vegetable origin is inadequate. From 1962, subsequent to the *Drug Amendments to Federal Food, Drug and Cosmetic Act* (1938), safety and efficacy had to be shown for all the medicines commercialized in USA. Thus the *Food and Drug Administration* (FDA), helped by the *Division of Medical Sciences of the National Academy of Sciences*, started a huge work of revision of all the medicines in commerce. In 1990 the results of a study conducted by the FDA on the over-the-counter medicines (OTC) were published, in which many HR were examined. The results were rather disappointing. For the greatest part of the HR and the vegetable drugs traditionally employed, it was not possible to document therapeutic activity adequately. Like the European authorities, the FDA had to confront the problem of dealing with currently marketed products in terms of the concept known as "grandfathering". In addition, the pharmaceutical industry had little interest in carrying out expensive clinical studies on old products based on vegetable drugs, which could not be patented. The FDA has maintained for a certain time a list of substances "Generally Recognized as Safe" better known as GRAS list. This list contains about 250 plants mainly used as additives in the food industry. Herbal medicines can be sold in pharmacies, health food stores and supermarkets. On the container, in the package leaflet or in the information accompanying the product, no declaration of therapeutic activity may appear. The labeling of the product with only the common name introduces some serious drawbacks, together with the lack of information on the use of the product. The popular names of the plants are numerous and often inaccurate.

Since 1994, after publication of the *Dietary Supplement Health and Education Act* (DSHEA), for the most part HR have been purchased as dietary supplements in health food stores. The intention of the DSHEA was to make natural/herbal products readily available to consumers. On January 6th, 2000, the FDA published the final edition of the rule that introduces some changes to the 1994 DSHEA. Among the new norms there is the exact list of the allowed and forbidden indications for the dietary supplements.

Canada

In 1984 the *Health Protection Branch* appointed a committee for the study of the classification of the vegetable products and in 1986 it codified a new class of remedies called "Folklores Medicines". This class includes safe herbal medicines, whose efficacy must be shown, although not necessarily with the same methods required for the other standardized medicines. The *Health Protection Branch* established that for the authorization of herbal products, it is necessary to introduce references of scientific works and information reported in the Pharmacopoeia. The labeling follows the general norm on the medicines to inform the consumer of the therapeutic use of the product and of the dosage. In 1993, however, there was a regression with the closing of the Natural Products Section of the Bureau of Drug Research, Health and Welfare.

Further Reading

Books

Balick MJ, Cox PA (1996) Plants, People, and Culture. The Science of Ethnobotany. Scientific American Library, New York

Blumenthal M (1998) The complete German Commission E monographs. Therapeutic guide to herbal medicines. American Botanical Council, Austin, Texas, USA

Bruneton J (1999) Pharmacognosy. Phytochemistry. Medicinal Plants. 2nd edn. Lavoisier Pub, Paris

Capasso F, Grandolini G (1999) Fitofarmacia. Impiego razionale delle droghe vegetali, 2nd edn. Springer Verlag Italia, Milan

Capasso F, De Pasquale R, Grandolini G, Mascolo N (2000) Farmacognosia. Farmaci naturali, loro preparazioni ed impiego terapeutico. Springer Verlag Italy, Milan

Dewick PM (1997) Medicinal natural products. John Wiley & Sons, Baffins Lane

Ernst E (2000) Herbal Medicine. A Concise Overview for Professionals. Butterworth Heinemann, Oxford

Ernst E (2001) The desktop guide to complementary and alternative medicine. An evidence-based approach. Mosby (Harcourt Publishers limited), Edinburgh

Gruenwald J, Brendler T, Jaenicke C (2000) PDR for Herbal medicines. Medicinal Economics Company, Montvale, New Jersey

Johnes Cupp J (2000) Toxicology and clinical pharmacology of herbal product. Humana Press, Totowa, New Jersey

McKenna DJ, Hughes K, Jones K (2001) The natural dietary supplement desktop reference, 2nd edn. Haworth Press, Binghamton, New York

Newall CA, Anderson LA, Phillipson JD (1996) Herbal medinines. A guide for health-care professional. The Pharmaceutical Press, London

Robbers JE, Tyler VE (1998). Herbs of Choice. The Therapeutic Use of Phytomedicinals. The Haworth Press Inc, New York

Samuelsson S (2001). Drugs of natural Origin. A textbook of pharmacognosy. Swedish Pharmaceutical Press, Stockholm

Schulz W, Hänsel R, Tyler VE (2000) Rational Phytotherapy. A Physician's Guide to Herbal Medicine, 2nd edn. Springer Verlag, Berlin Heidelberg New York

Williamson EM, Okpako DT, Evans FJ (1996) Selection, preparation and pharmacological evaluation of plant material. John Wiley & Sons, Chichester

Articles

Ang-Lee MK, Moss J, Yuan C-S (2001) Herbal medicines and perioperative care. JAMA 286:208–216

Barrett B, Kiefer D, Rabago D (1999) Assessing the risks and benefitss of herbal medicine: an overview of scientific evidence. Altern Ther Health Med 5:40–49

Boullata JI, Nace AM (2000) Safety issues with herbal medicine. Pharmacotherapy 20:257–269
Calixto JB (2000) Efficacy, safety, quality control, marketing and regulatory guidelines for herbal medicines (phytotherapeutic agents) Braz J Med Biol Res 33:179–189
Capasso R, Izzo AA, Pinto L, Bifulco T, Vitobello C, Mascolo N (2000) Phytotherapy and quality of herbal medicines. Fitoterapia 71 (suppl 1):S58–S65
Clepser TB, Klepser ME (1999) Unsafe and potentially safe herbal medicines. Am J Health Syst Pharm 26:125–138
Conover EA (2002) Over-the-counter products: nonprescription medications, nutraceuticals, and herbal agents. Clin Obstet Gynecol 45:89–98
De Smet PAGM (2002) Herbal remedies. N Engl J Med 347:2046–2056
Ernst E (2000). Herbal medicines: where is the evidence? Br Med Journal 321:395–396
Ernst E (2002) Toxic heavy metals and undeclared drugs in Asian herbal medicines. Trends Pharmacol Sci 23:136–139
Ernst E. (2002) Herbal medicinal products during pregnancy: are they safe? BJOG 109:227–235
Forte JS, Raman A (2000) Regulatory issues relating to herbal products. J Medicinal Food 3:23–39
Hahn MJ (1998) Is it a food or a dietary supplement? J Medicinal Food 1:264–267
Izzo AA, Ernst E (2001) Interaction between herbal medicines and prescribed drugs. Drugs 61:2163–2175
Kabelitz L (1998) Heavy metals in herbal drugs. Eur J Herb Med 4:25–29
Kiefer D, Shah S, Gardiner P, Wechkin H (2001) Finding information on herbal therapy: a guide to useful sources for clinicians. Altern Ther Health Med 7:74–78
Linde K, Riet G., Hondras M, Vickers A, Saller R, Melchart D (2001) Systematic reviews of complementary therapies. An annotated bibliography. Part 2: Herbal medicine. Compl Altern Med 1:5
Mahady GB (2001) Global harmonization of herbal health claims. J Nutr 131:1120S–1123S
Marcus DM, Grollman AP (2002) Botanical medicines the need for new regulations. N Engl J Med 347:2073–2076
Ness J, Sherman FT, Pan CX (1999) Alternative medicine: what the data say about common herbal therapies. Geriatrics 54:33–38
O'Mathuna DP (2001) Pharmacognosy. What nurses need to know about herbal remedies. J Christ Nurs 18:18–21
Pinn G, Pallett L (2002) Herbal medicine in pregnancy. Complement Ther Nurs Midwifery. 2002 8:77–80
Pitetti R, Singh S, Hornayak D, Garcia SE, Herr S (2001) Complementary and alternative medicine use in children. Pediatr Emerg Care 17:165–169
Snodgrass WR (2001) Herbal products: risk and beneffits of use in children. Curr Ther Res Clin Exp 62:724–737
Tomassoni AJ, Simone K (2001) Herbal medicines for children: an illusion of safety? Curr Opin Pediatr13:162–169
Winslow LC, Kroll DJ (1998) Herbs as medicines. Arch Intern Med 158: 2192–2199

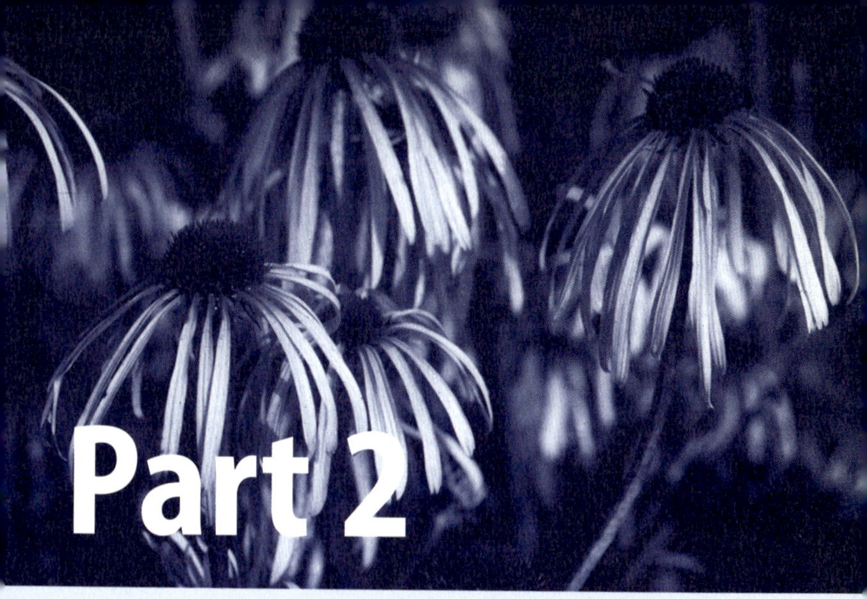

Part 2

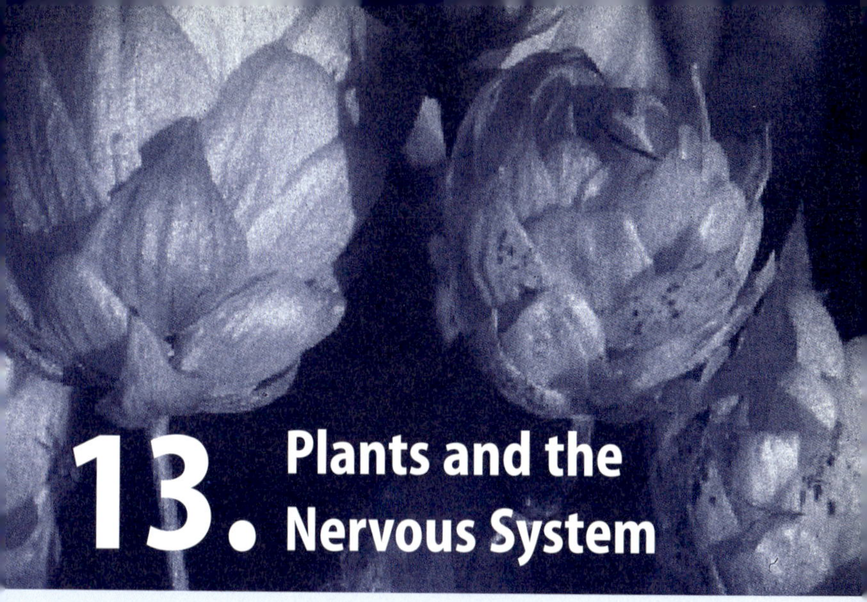

13. Plants and the Nervous System

Introduction

The nervous system controls conscious and unconscious motor and sensory as well as emotional and intellectual functions. It is divided in the *central nervous system* (CNS) and the *peripheral nervous system* (PNS) (Figure 13.1). The CNS consists of the brain and spinal cord. Afferent neurons which connect the peripheral tissues to the spinal cord constitute the part of the PNS that allows perception of external sensation and body function. Efferent neurons which connect the spinal cord to the peripheral tissues constitute the part of the PNS that regulates the activity of peripheral tissues. The efferent section is sub-divided into the *somatic* and *autonomic nervous systems*. The somatic part is involved in voluntary activity such as contraction of the skeletal muscle.

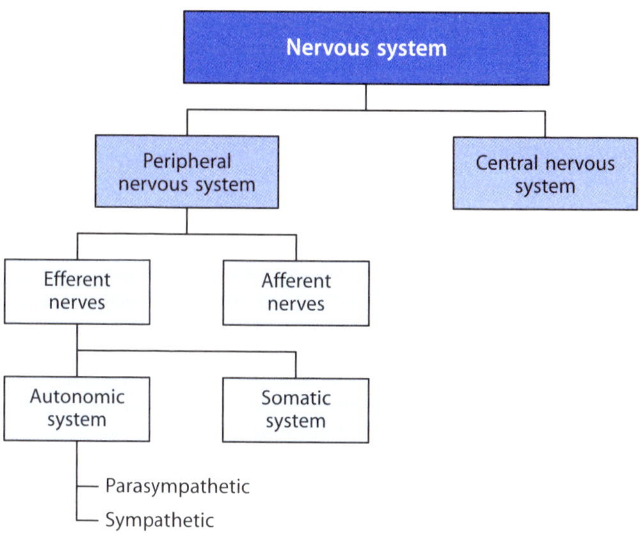

Figure 13.1 ▲ **Organization of the nervous system**

The autonomic system is an involuntary system that functions to control the everyday needs and requirements of the body without the conscious participation of the mind. The autonomic system has two parts, the cranio-sacral (*parasympathetic*) and thoraco-lumbar (*sympathetic*) divisions. The sympathetic and parasympathetic systems generally antagonize each other. The sympathetic system prepares the body for action whereas the parasympathetic system is concerned with the body at rest.

The neuron is the basic unit of both the CNS and PNS. The connection between two neurons occurs through the synapse. Generally, neuronal signals are transmitted via the release of chemical messengers (neurotransmitters) by the presynaptic neuron, and its subsequent binding to a macromolecular receptor on the postsynaptic neuron. Neurotransmitters of the central nervous system include glutamate, γ-aminobutyric acid (GABA), glycine, acetylcholine, 5-hydroxytryptamine (5-HT) and noradrenaline.

Anxiety and Insomnia

Clinical Picture

- **Anxiety** is common and includes psychological symptoms such as insomnia, apprehension, tension or uneasiness, often accompanied by physical symptoms (headache, perspiration, palpitations, upset stomach and tightness in the chest). Anxiety may be a result of a traumatic life event (bereavement, divorce, scholastic or professional failures, financial losses) or it may be devoid of any apparent cause. However, the sensation of anxiety may become exaggerated compared to the casual stimulus or the unknown stimulus and the symptoms may start to interfere with the normal life of the patient. Then the anxiety is pathological and needs an appropriate therapy based principally on the type and degree of anxiety.
- The two neurotransmitters most commonly implicated in the etiology of anxiety are GABA and 5-HT. In particular, GABA is the major inhibitory neurotransmitter in the central nervous system. It acts on $GABA_A$ and $GABA_B$ reeceptors. Benzodiazepines exert their anxiolytic effects by potentiating the action of GABA on $GABA_A$ receptor. Norepinephrine also has a role, particularly in panic disorders.
- **Insomnia** is a sleep non-specific disorder that may be reported by 40–50% of people at any given time. It is due to psychiatric illness (30–35%), psychophysiological problems (1–20%), alcohol or drugs (15–20%), periodic limb movement disorder (10–15%), sleep apnea (5–10%), medical illness (5–10%). Insomnia may also be due to a physical cause (pain, cough) or to environmental factors like noise. The central control of sleep involves serotonergic, noradrenergic and acetylcholine-containing neurons. The electrical activity of sleep when recorded on an EEG shows five stages: stages 1–4 is a period of non-rapid eye movement (NREM) sleep,

while stage 5 is the period of rapid eye movement (REM) sleep. Deprivation of REM sleep often causes irritability and lethargy.

- The treatment of insomnia depends upon the underlying cause. In many cases reducing caffeine intake, changing alimentary and sleep habits, or pain relief might be more appropriate than a sedative medicine. Early morning wakening is one of the biological features of depression: in this case an antidepressant might by more appropriate. In the absence of a cause, insomnia is often treated with one of the benzodiazepines.

Herbal Anxiolytics/Hypnotics

Anxiolytics/hypnotics of botanical origin are listed in Table 13.1. While these herbal remedies are "mild" in their action they do not involve risk of tolerance, habituation or addiction and the risk of overdose is low.

Table 13.1

Herbal medicines used to treat anxiety and/or insomnia

Common name	Latin name	Part(s) of plant used	Key constituents	Daily dose
Bugleweed**	*Lycopus virginicus*	Aerial parts	Caffeic acid derivatives, flavonoids, volatile oil	1–2 g
California poppy	*Eschscholtzia californica*	Aerial parts	Isoquinoline alkaloids	2 g
German chamomile	*Matricaria recutita*	Flower heads	Coumarins, flavonoids, volatile oil, mucilages	5 g
Hops**	*Humulus lupulus*	Glandular hairs	Bitter acids, volatile oil, resins, phenolic acid, flavonoids	1–2 g
Kava**	*Piper methysticum*	Rhizome	Kava lactones, flavonoids	1.5–3 g
Lavender**	*Lavandula angustifolia*	Flowers	Volatile oil, tannins, coumarins, caffeic acid derivatives	20–80 mg of the oil
Lemon balm**	*Melissa officinalis*	Leaves	Volatile oil, glycosides, caffeic acid derivatives, flavonoids	1.5–4.5 g
Passion flower**	*Passiflora incarnata*	Aerial parts	Flavonoids, cyanogenic glycosides, volatile oil	4–8 g
St. John's wort*	*Hypericum perforatum*	Aerial parts	Anthracene derivatives, flavonoids, phloroglucinol derivatives	2–4 g
Valerian**	*Valeriana officinalis*	Roots	Volatile oil, valepotrietes	2–3 g

* supported by the German Commission E

** supported by the German Commission E for nervousness and insomnia

Kava

Botany/Key constituents ▶ Kava (sometimes referred to as kava kava) consists of the dried rhizomes and roots of *Piper methysticum* Forst (Fam. *Piperaceae*), a perennial sub-shrub which grows in the islands of Western Polynesia (Fiji, Samoa, New Guinea, Tonga, Papua, Vanuatu) and Tahiti. Its subterranean parts have been used by the natives of Australia in the preparation of a beverage obtained by soaking in water rhizome or roots fragments after grinding them with a pestle or chewing them. Kava contains starch and a resin from which several lactones (kava pyrones or kava lactones; e.g. yangoin and kawain) can be isolated. Flavonoids (lavokavins) also exist in kava root. The resinous content of kava can change from 3 to 20% depending on cultivars and part of the plant used (rhizome, lateral root).

Mode of action ▶ Kava extract and its components show anticonvulsant, local anaesthetic and skeletal muscle relaxant properties. These activities might be explained by inhibition of voltage-dependent Na^+ channels in the brain, which lead to a reduced neuronal excitability. The kava pyrone kavain is believed to be the main active ingredient responsible of this activity. There is controversy as to whether or not GABA receptors are involved in the action of one or more kava components. However, recent studies indicate that kava pyrones mediate anxiolytic effects by way of $GABA_A$ receptor binding (Figure 13.2).

Clinical efficacy ▶ Today many researchers consider kava as an alternative to benzodiazepines and tricyclic antidepressants for the treatment of various types of anxiety (phobias, panic disorders, obsessive-compulsive disorders) and sleep disorders. Kava is supported by German Commission E for the treatment of insomnia and nervousness. The evidence reported in the literature suggest that kava is relatively safe and more efficacious than placebo in the symptomatic treatment of anxiety. A recent systematic review/meta-analysis retrieved seven double-blind randomized clinical trials and all seven studies showed superiority of kava extract over placebo.

Adverse effects/Contraindications ▶ Adverse effects from ingestion of kava are not generally expected when used within the recommended dosage. Two postmarketing surveillance studies, each involving more than 3000 patients, found adverse events in 2.3% and 1.5% of patients during treatment with kava extract. Adverse events reported frequently were gastrointestinal complaints, allergic skin reactions, headache, and photosensitivity. Taken for long periods of time at a high dose level kava can cause reversible yellow discoloration of the skin. In some cases an ichthyosiform skin rash, known as kava dermopathy can occur. The onset typically begins on the face and moves in a descending fashion towards the feet, with subsequent desquamation and cracking in a scaly pattern. In many European countries (e. g. Germany, France, Italy) kava has been suspended from sale because of clinical cases of severe liver disease thought to have

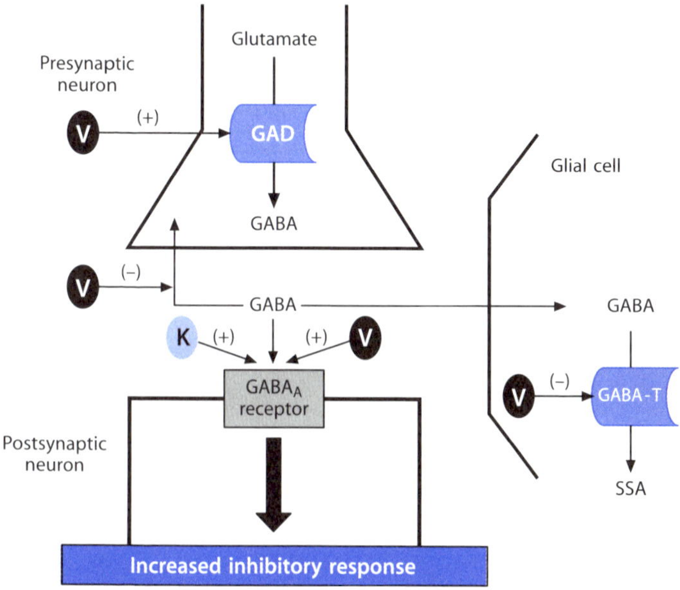

Figure 13.2 ▲ **Possible site of action of valerian and kava**
Constituents of valerian (V) have been shown to: (i) activate the enzyme glutamate decarboxylase (GAD) which is involved in GABA synthesis in presynaptic nerves, (ii) inhibit GABA re-uptake in glial cells or neurons, (iii) inhibit the enzyme GABA transaminase (which is involved in GABA catabolism), (iv) bind to GABA$_A$ receptors. These effects lead to a potentiation of the action of GABA, the primary inhibitory neurotransmitter in the central nervous system. Kava pyrones (K), active ingredients of kava, can activate GABA$_A$ receptors resulting in an inhibitory effect on neuronal activity

been caused by this herbal medicine. Case reports have also highlighted the possibility of interaction with the benzodiazepine alprazolam (resulting in a lethargic and disoriented state) and the anti-Parkinson drug levodopa (resulting in diminution of the efficacy of levodopa).

Preparations/Dosage

The following doses are recommended: 1.5–3 g per day of dried root in decoction or 3–6 ml per day of liquid extract (1:2). About 25 pharmaceuticals based on standardized extracts (i.e. 35–120 mg kava pyrones) are currently marketed especially in Germany. WS1490 is a well-known kava extract containing 70% kava pyrones. The daily dose of kava pyrones used in clinical studies is in the range 60–240 mg (divided in three daily doses). As a sleep aid 180–210 mg of kava lactones, in the form of extract, can be taken one hour before bedtime.

Valerian

Botany/Key constituents ▶ Valerian is the common name given to the crude drug consisting of the dried rhizome, roots and stolons (subterranean organs) of species of *Valeriana* (Fam. *Valerianaceae*). In Northern Europe the official drug in the British and European Pharmacopoeias is derived from *V. officinalis* L. but other species are used as crude drugs in other part of the world, the most notable being Indian Valerian, *V. wallichii* DC, and Chinese and Japanese Valerian, *V. angustifolia* Tausch or *V. fauriei* Briq. A related species which has an important place in traditional medicine in the Indian subcontinent and the Middle East is nard (*Nardostachys jatamansii*) DC. The best known valerian, *V. officinalis* is a perennial herb very common in damp woods, ditches and along the streams all over Europe. The roots and rhizome are carefully dried at a temperature below 40°C. It contains a volatile oil (containing valerenic acid and other compounds), valepotriates (iridoid compounds such as valerenic acid, valtrate and dihydrovaltrate), lignans and alkaloids (Box 13.1).

Box 13.1

Chemical constituents of valerian

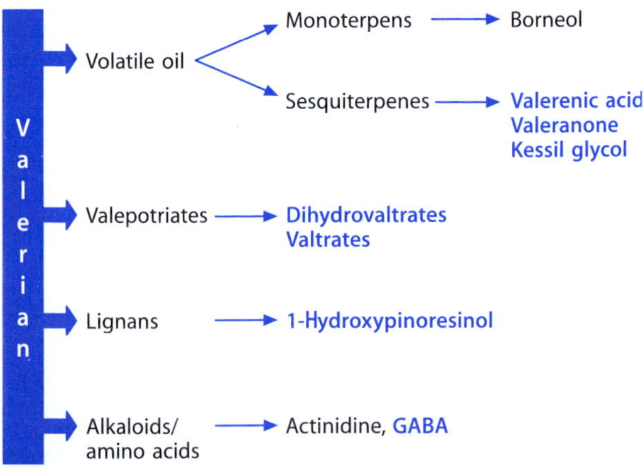

Compounds which have shown to posses hypnotic-sedative activity in experimental studies are highlighted in blue. Chemical constituents of valerian include:

(i) Volatile oil. The volatile fraction represents 2–20 ml/kg dried plant material. Chemical components include: monoterpenes, chiefly consisting of borneol and sesquiterpenes which are distinctive and which have received most attention regarding their biological activity. Three major types of sesquiterpene skeleton are found and these are exemplified by valerenic acid, valeranone and kessyl glycol. Valerenic acid has so far been found in no other organism apart from *Valeriana officinalis* whilst valeranone is found to be the major component of the oil of *Valeriana wallichiana* and the related plant nard (*Nardostachys jatamansii*). Compounds with the kessyl ring system are the major constituents in the volatile oil of Japanese valerian *Valeriana fauriei* but are also found in *Valeriana officinalis.*

(ii) Valepotriates (iridoid compounds) include dihydrovaltrate and valtrates and isovalerenic acid. The valepotriates, whose level generally ranges from 0.8–1.7% are unstable and occur only in the fresh drug or in material dried at temperatures under 40°C. They decompose under the influence of moisture, heat (40°C) or acidity (pH 3). A valerian tincture, stored at 20°C for two weeks after preparation, contains about 1/3 of valepotriates initially found. The process of degradation of dihydrovaltrate and valtrate, both by physical means in tinctures and by microbial transformation in the gut, results in products such as homobaldrinal. Baldrinals, including homobaldrinal are considered the active forms of valepotriates. Valepotriates possess cytotoxic effects *in vitro* and consequent potential carcinogenicity and these findings have made the presence and use of valepotriates in valerian undesirable factors. However, *in vivo* studies have failed to show carcinogenic effects, even at high doses. Isovaleric acid (a carboxylic acid) is commonly esterified to dihydrovaltrates and valtrates and the ester link is easily hydrolyzed resulting in the characteristic odor of the dried crude drug which is, however, not detected in fresh plant samples.

(iii) Lignans are present in small amounts. 1-hydroxypinoresinol has little effect on benzodiazepine receptor, but it inhibits 5-HT binding to its receptor.

(iv) Alkaloids/amino acids. Alkaloids (i.e. actinidine) are present in small amounts and are not presently considered to make a significant contribution to its overall effect. The valerian extract contains high levels of GABA and glutamine (which could be metabolized to GABA). The amount of GABA present in valerian is sufficient to induce release of GABA *in vitro* and may also inhibit GABA re-uptake. However, since GABA does not readily cross the blood-brain barrier, the relevance of these findings to central sedating effects is questionable.

Mode of action ▶ The specific active principles of valerian have not been conclusively determined. Valerian represents the classic example of a herbal drug where the overall effect is due to several types of constituents. However, the considerable variation in its composition and content as well as the instability of some of its constituents pose serious problems for standardization. Research on the mechanism of action has yielded contradictory findings. Extracts of valerian have affinity for $GABA_A$ receptor, stimulate synthesis and release of GABA and inhibit its re-uptake and catabolism (Figure 13.2). Other postulated mechanisms of action include affinity for the 5-HT_A receptor by 5-hydroxypinoresinal and binding to adenosine receptors.

Clinical efficacy ▸ The evidence available from a systematic review which retrieved nine randomized, placebo-controlled, double-blind trials (n = 390 subjects) indicates that the efficacy of valerian for improving sleep is promising but not fully conclusive. The results of some trials suggest that valerian may have both acute and cumulative effects on sleep, but not all studies have produced positive findings. The same conclusion was reached by the United States Pharmacopoeia (USP) in 1998, which decided that there is insufficient evidence in the scientific literature to warrant use of valerian as short-term treatment for insomnia. Nevertheless valerian is supported by German Commission E for the treatment of insomnia and nervousness.

Adverse events/Contraindications ▸ Adverse events associated with the short term use of valerian are scarce and similar to those experienced with placebo in randomized clinical trials. The short-term safety of valerian has been confirmed in a post-marketing surveillance study which monitored 3447 patients taking valerian preparations. At high doses, valerian has been associated with cardiac function disturbance and depression of the central nervous system, making potentiation of other central nervous depressants a possibility. Addiction to valerian preparations has not been reported. The ESCOP monograph (1997) states that valerian should be used with caution in children under three years of age, in pregnant or lactating women (iridoids are cytotoxic and mutagenic agents). Like other herbal anxiolytics/hypnotics, valerian could potentiate the effect of other central depressants, including ethanol.

Preparations/Dosage

Valerian may be administered in the form of tea (infusion or decoction) prepared from 2–3 g crude drug (two-three times daily or at bedtime), powder (0.1–1 g crude drug two-three times daily) or tincture (20% concentration by volume in a 70% ethanol solution: 1–3 ml three times daily). Valerian is frequently associated with hawthorn, passion flower, and other sedative drugs. Valerian is believed to be more stable in dry extracts incorporated into solid oral dosage forms. The dry extract must contain 0.25–0.35% total sesquiterpenic acids (expressed as valerenic acid) and administered (dose: 400–900 mg) 30–60 min before bedtime.

Passion flower

Botany/Key constituents ▸ Passion flower consists of the dried flowering and fruiting top of a perennial climbing vine, *Passiflora incarnata* L. (Fam. *Passifloraceae*)

(Plate 13.1). The drug also includes fragments of lignified stem with slender and smooth tendrils. The plant grows wild in the bushes of the south of the United States and Mexico. Passion flower contains flavonoids (e.g. vitexin), cyanogenic glycosides, alkaloids (e.g. harman, harmaline) and maltol.

Mode of action ▸ The constituents responsible for the pharmacological activities and the mode of action of passion flower are not known. Maltol is a depressant but its concentration in the plant is insignificant. The concentration of alkaloids (i.e. harman) is very low and they are CNS stimulants and some of them also hallucinogens. A flavone isolated from *P. coerulea*, 5,7-dihydroxyflavone, possesses anxiolytic effect but some experiments carried out on passion flower extract demonstrate that there are two active components and neither of them corresponds to any flavonoid or alkaloid structure described to date in passion flower.

Clinical efficacy ▸ Passion flower preparations were recognized as having medicinal effects as early as 1840 and by 1898 this botanical remedy was used as a "sedative". Passion flower is cited by the German Commission E for the treatment of nervous restlessness and sleep disturbances. No clinical studies of passion flower alone have been found although one randomized, controlled trial that used a commercial preparation containing passion flower in addition to valerian showed benefit in the treatment of adjustment disorder with anxious mood.

Adverse events/Contraindications ▸ The drug is reputed to be harmless; however hypersensitivity, vasculitis and altered consciousness have been reported with products containing passion flower. No safety details exist regarding the use of this drug in pregnancy and lactation. Like other herbal anxiolytics/hypnotics, passion flower could potentiate the effect of other central depressants, including ethanol.

Preparations/Dosage

Passion flower is used in the form of tea (infusion) prepared from 4–8 g crude drug in 150 ml (three times daily). The drug is also used as a dried powder (0.25–1.0 g three times daily), liquid extract (1:1 in 25% alcohol; 0.5–1 ml three times daily) or tincture (1:8 in 45% alcohol; 0.5–2 ml three times daily). The drug is very seldom given alone, but rather frequently combined with valerian and other anxiolytic/hypnotic herbal medicines.

Hops

Botany/Key constituents ▸ Hops are the dried pistillate inflorescence (= strobiles) of *Humulus lupulus* L. (Fam. *Cannabaceae*), a climbing perennial herb, 6 m high, that grows wild in the hedges and wood skirts of Europe and North America

(Plate 13.2). The plant is widely cultivated. The drug contains flavonoids, chalcones, volatile oil including humulene, myrcene, beta-caryophyllene, an oleoresin including alfa-bitter acids (humulone, cohumulone, adhumulone), bitter acids (lupulone, colupulone, adlupulone) and their oxidative degradation products (2-methyl-3-buten-2-ol), tannins, estrogenic substances.

Mode of action ▶ The mode of action of hops is not known. The sedative action of hops is attributed to 2-methyl-3-buten-2-ol, but there is insufficient information to confirm this; moreover, the isovaleric acid residues present in hop may contribute to the sedative action.

Clinical efficacy ▶ Although hops are used by the brewing industry to produce beer, this plant is stated to possess a mild sedative property and is indicated in the management of insomnia and agitation/restlessness. Hops are cited by the German Commission E for the treatment of restlessness and sleep disturbances. However, there are no clinical studies of its use as a single agent to treat specific symptoms or illnesses, such as insomnia. Hops, in combination with valerian have been documented to improve sleep disturbances, reduce anxiety and nervousness.

Adverse events/Contraindications ▶ Adverse events might include allergy and disruption of menstrual cycles. It is stated that hops should not be taken by individuals suffering from depressive illness, as the sedative effect may accentuate symptoms, nor during pregnancy, in view of its antispasmodic activity. Although there are currently no documented case examples, care should be taken when using hops with sedative-hypnotic agents and alcohol, as potentiation of their effect may be seen.

Preparations/Dosage

Hops may be administered several times daily as a tea prepared from 1–2 g of the dried strobiles. Hops is also used as a dried strobiles 0.5–1.0 g liquid extract 0.5–1 ml (1:1, 45% of ethanol) or a tincture 1–2 ml (1:5, 60% ethanol) three times daily and before bed.

Chamomile

Botany/Key constituents ▶ Chamomile consists of the dried flower heads of *Matricaria recutita* L. (= *Matricaria chamomilla* L.) (**German chamomile**) or *Chamaemelum nobile* (L.) All. (= *Anthemis nobilis* L.) (**Roman chamomile**) (Fam. *Asteraceae/Compositae*). Key constituents include coumarins, flavonoids (e.g. apigenin) and an essential oil whose main components are alfa-bisabolol and chamazulene (1–15%).

Mode of action ▶ The sedative properties of chamomile may be attributed to certain flavonoids because it has been referred that apigenin has an affinity for central benzodiazepine receptors and exerts a distinct anxiolytic action. A possible presence of tryptophan, the precursor of 5-HT, and GABA in the flowers could, at least in part, justify the hypnotic effect of chamomile.

Clinical efficacy ▶ Chamomile has a strong tradition in Latin countries as a mild sedative drug. It is often used to treat anxiety and insomnia. However, no randomized clinical trials have been performed to confirm the anxiolytic/sedative properties of chamomile.

Adverse events/Contraindications ▶ Chamomile is a safe herb. The presence of lactones in the drug preparations may cause allergic reactions (urticaria, edema, obstruction of the respiratory tract) and in rare cases anaphylactic reactions. Therefore, individuals with allergic conditions should use chamomile products with caution. In view of the documented allergic reactions and cross-sensitivities, chamomile should be avoided by individuals with a known hypersensitivity to any member of the *Asteraceae/Compositae* family (e.g. feverfew, calendula).

Preparations/Dosage

The most popular dosage form of chamomile is an infusion prepared from 5 g dried flowers in 150 ml boiling water (a cup three times daily). Other forms of administration are: liquid extract (1:1, 45% ethanol), 1–4 ml three times daily; tincture (1:5, 45% ethanol), 3–10 ml three times daily; dried flowers heads (2–4 g) three times daily.

▶ *See Chapter 23 for the dermatological use of chamomile*

Lavender

Botany/Key constituents ▶ Lavender consist of the flower of *Lavandula angustifolia* Miller (Fam. *Lamiaceae*), gathered shortly before fully unfolding. Flowering shoots are harvested when the middle section of the spike is flowering. *L. angustifolia* is indigenous to the Mediterranean region but is common in most of Southern Europe and is cultivated extensively. Key constituents include a volatile oil (1–3%, main constituents are linalyl acetate and linalool), hydroxycoumarins, tannins (13%) and caffeic acid derivatives.

Mode of action ▶ The sedative action of lavender is well documented in animal experiments. The essential oil showed anticonvulsant effects, inhibitory effects on spontaneous motor activity, and prolonged the duration of sleep induced by barbiturics. Linalool and linalyl acetate are believed to be, at least in part, responsible of such actions. The mode of action is not known.

Clinical efficacy ► The anxiolityc/hypnotic effects of lavender are better documented by empirical medicine and experimental studies than the effects of hops and passion flower. However there is a lack of randomized clinical studies. In its monograph on lavender flowers, the German Commission E described the indication for internal use as "states of unrest, difficulty in falling asleep, and functional upper abdominal complaints."

Adverse events/Contraindications ► No health hazards or side effects are known in conjunction with the proper administration of designated therapeutic dosages. The volatile oil possesses a weak potential for sensitization. Contraindicated during pregnancy and lactation.

Preparations/Dosage

The whole drug is used for infusions or as an extract. Lavender oil can also be used. The German Commission E recommends 1–2 teaspoons of dried herb per cup of tea or 1–4 drops of lavender oil (about 20–80 mg) taken with a sugar cube.

Depression

Clinical Picture

- Depression is an emotional disorder accompanied by feelings of helplessness and lack of self-worth. Intense sadness, asthenia, reduced ability to concentrate and make decisions, alteration of appetite and recurrent thoughts of death or suicide are major symptoms. Depression is less frequent in males (9–15%) than females (20%); the mean age of onset is 45–50 years (after involutional changes of the gonads, menopause, male climacteric) although onset can be at any age. Depression usually reveals itself with episodes lasting 5–10 months tending to periodicity. Environmental stress and life events (e.g. loss of job, etc.) are associated with an increased risk of developing depression.
- The etiology of depressive disorder is not clear. The original hypothesis of depression suggested that depression was due to a functional deficit of a transmitter amine (e.g. noradrenaline, dopamine, 5-HT), partly because well-known antidepressant drug such as tricyclic antidepressant and monoamine oxidase (MAO) inhibitors facilitated neurotransmission in

central neurons. Other systems that may be involved in depression include the GABA system and some of the neuropeptide systems like vasopressin and endogenous opioids.

Herbal Antidepressants

Herbal medicines that are reported to be antidepressants are listed in Table 13.2. St John's wort is the only plant supported by German Commission E and it has been shown to alleviate the symptoms of mild to moderate depression in many controlled clinical studies. However, St John's wort is not effective in treating major depression. In many countries, such as the USA and UK, St John's wort and other putative herbal antidepressants are marketed as a "dietary supplement" and hence are available for self-medication. The possible use of herbal remedies by patients suffering from depression (especially major depression) is worrying. Depression is a serious and common disorder which can lead to severe suffering, social dysfunction, and, in severe form, suicide. Hence, herbal antidepressants must be used only after an appropriate diagnosis of the severity of depression has been made.

Table 13.2

Herbal medicines traditionally used to treat depression. With the exception of St John's wort, no scientific claim justifies their use

Common name	Latin name	Part(s) of plant used	Key constituents	Daily dose
Corydalis	*Corydalis cava*	Tubers	Isoquinoline alkaloids	1 g
Lemon balm	*Melissa officinalis*	Leaves	Volatile oil, glycosides, caffeic acid derivatives	1.5–4.5 g
Mugwort	*Artemisia vulgaris*	Roots	Volatile oil, sesquiterpene lactones, flavonoids	1.5–6 g
Passion flower	*Passiflora incarnata*	Aerial parts	Flavonoids, cyanogenic glycosides, volatile oil	4–8 g
Scarlet pimpernel	*Anagallis arvensis*	Flowering plant	Triterpene saponins, cucurbitacins, flavonoids	6–8 g
St. John's wort*	*Hypericum perforatum*	Aerial parts	Anthracene derivatives, flavonoids, phloroglucinol derivatives	2–4 g
Sweet marjoram	*Origanum majorana*	Aerial parts	Volatile oil, flavonoids, triterpenes	a

* supported by the German Commission E

a. reliable data not available

St John's wort

Botany/Key constituents ► St John's wort consists of the leaves and flowering tops of *Hypericum perforatum* L. (Fam. *Clusiaceae*), a five-petaled, yellow-flowered perennial weed that grows in the neglected fields and along the country roads of Europe and North America (Plate 13.3). The common name of the plant St John's wort apparently relates to the fact that it flowers around St John's day (24 June). The drug contains anthraquinone derivatives (hypericin, pseudohypericin); flavonoids, phloroglucinol derivatives (hyperforin, adhyperforin).

Mode of action ► Inhibition of MAO by hypericin was believed to be the primary mode of action of the antidepressant effect of St John's wort. More recent data, however, suggest that hyperforin is the main active ingredient. Hyperforin inhibits the synaptosomal uptake of serotonin (5-HT), noradrenaline, dopamine, glutamate and GABA in the central nervous system (Figure 13.3). The increase of neurotransmitter levels lead, after chronic treatment, to up-regulation of 5-HT_1 and 5-HT_2 receptors and down regulation of β_1-adrenergic receptors. Changes in receptor expression are believed to be responsible for the antidepressant effect of St John's wort.

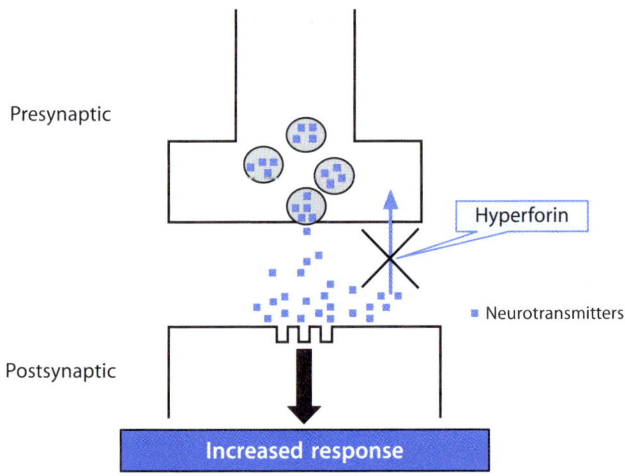

Figure 13.3 ▲ **Mechanism of the antidepressant action of St John's wort**
Hyperforin inhibits the neuronal re-uptake of a number of brain neurotransmitters (serotonin, noradrenaline, dopamine, glutamate and GABA) into presynaptic nerve terminal. By blocking the major route of neurotransmitter removal, hyperforin leads to increased concentrations of neurotransmitters in the synaptic cleft

Clinical efficacy ▶ St John's wort is approved by German Commission E for the treatment of depressive moods and anxiety. The effectiveness of St John's wort in the treatment of mild to moderate depression has been demonstrated in nine systematic reviews (total number of 27 trials including 2291 patients with depressive disorders). Most trials were of 4–6 weeks duration. Data suggest that St John's wort is superior to placebo and as effective as synthetic antidepressants in the treatment of mild to moderate depression. However, St John's wort is not suited for the treatment of major depression. As with other antidepressants, an antidepressive effect is not expected before 10–14 days treatment.

Adverse events ▶ St John's wort has an encouraging safety profile and it is better tolerated than synthetic antidepressants (Table 13.3): adverse reactions are minor, they include gastrointestinal symptoms, dizziness/vertigo, tiredness/fa-

Table 13.3

Comparison between St John's wort (SJW) and several synthetic antidepressants: percentage of patients reporting specific adverse reactions from randomized controlled trials

Adverse effect	SJW	dothiepin	fluoxetine	moclobemide	mirtazepine
Gastrointestinal symptoms	8.5	1.6	8.2	0	6.0
Tiredness/fatigue	4.6	1.2	0	0	0
Dizziness/vertigo	4.5	4.9	12.2	7.8	8.0
Dry mouth	4.0	15.9	19.7	16.6	34.0
Restlessness	2.6	0.7	0	0	16.0
Headache	1.7	1.9	18.6	13.1	10.0
Insomnia	0.9	2.2	13.8	9.8	8.0
Skin reactions	0.9	0.2	0	0	0
Photophobia	0.6	0	0	0	0
Tremor	0.6	4.7	13.2	5.4	6.0
Nausea	0	0	24.1	8.6	6.0
Diarrhea	0	1.5	9.2	3.3	0
Constipation	0	1.6	9.3	6.4	16.0
Drowsiness	0	10.5	19.2	5.4	20.0
Sedation	0	0.7	0	0	13.0
Agitation	0	0	0	3.6	6.0
Nervousness	0	0	15.0	0	0
Anxiety	0	1.9	10.5	2.5	0
Visual disturbance	0	2.9	6.3	3.9	7.0
Sweating	0	2.6	9.1	6.5	5.0
Anorexia	0	0	7.2	0.3	0
Body-weight increase	0	1.4	0.1	0	11.0

Dothiepin, fluoxetine and moclobemide are typically the most frequently dispensed tricyclic antidepressant, selective serotonin re-uptake inhibitor and MAO inhibitor, respectively; mirtazepine represents the newer class of antidepressant drugs: serotonin and noradrenaline re-uptake inhibitors

tigue, dry mouth, restlessness and headache. Photosensitization is an extremely rare clinical event with recommended dosages of St John's wort, while it can occur at high doses. Fair-skinned people are recommended to avoid a prolonged exposure to sunlight. Recent reports have indicate the possibility of important herb-drug interactions with conventional drugs (Table 13.4) which are metabolized by hepatic enzymes or eliminated through induction of P-glycoprotein (Figure 13.4). Moreover, the symptoms of a central serotonergic syndrome (mental status changes, tremor, autonomic instability, gastrointestinal upsets, headache, myalgia and restlessness) described when St John's wort is given in parallel with other 5-HT re-uptake inhibitors (e.g. the antidepressant paroxetine, sertaline or nefazodone) might be due to an additive effect on central 5-HT re-uptake.

Table 13.4

Clinical reports (case reports or clinical studies) of interaction between St John's wort and prescribed drugs

Co-medication	Co-medication use	Results of interaction	Possible mechanism
Cyclosporin	Immunosuppressant	Lowering of blood cyclosporin; rejection episodes	Hepatic enzyme induction; induction of P-glycoprotein
Ethyniloestradiol/ Desogestrel	Oral contraceptive	Breakthrough bleeding	Hepatic enzyme induction
Theophylline	Antiasthmatic	Lowering of plasma theophylline	Hepatic enzyme induction
Phenprocoumon	Anticoagulant	Lowering of plasma phenprocoumon; decreased anticoagulant effect	Hepatic enzyme induction
Warfarin	Anticoagulant	Lowering of plasma warfarin; decreased anticoagulant effect	Hepatic enzyme induction
Amitriptyline	Antidepressant	Lowering of plasma amitriptyline	Hepatic enzyme induction
Indinavir	Antiviral (AIDS)	Lowering of plasma indinavir	Hepatic enzyme induction; induction of P-glycoprotein
Digoxin	Cardiostimulant	Lowering of plasma digoxin	Induction of P-glycoprotein
Nefazodone	Antidepressant	Serotonin syndrome	Synergistic serotonin uptake inhibition
Sertraline	Antidepressant	Serotonin syndrome	Synergistic serotonin uptake inhibition
Paroxetine	Antidepressant	Serotonin syndrome	Synergistic serotonin uptake inhibition

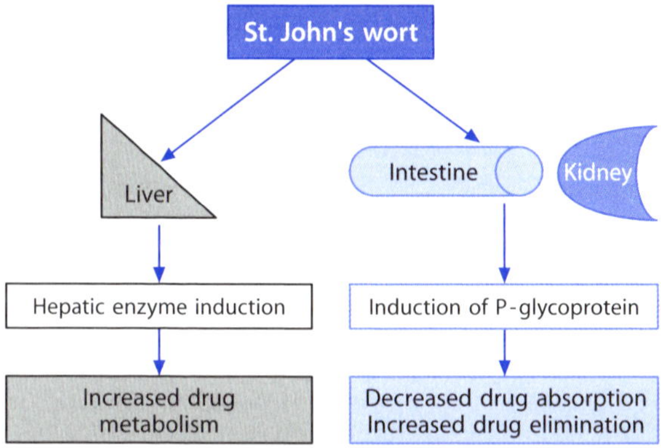

Figure 13.4 ▲ **Mechanism of herb/drug interaction**
St John's wort activates hepatic enzymes of the cytochrome P450 system (leading to increased metabolism of drugs) and can induce P-glycoprotein (leading to increased elimination of drugs and/or decreased intestinal absorption). Concomitant use of St John's wort with cytochrome P450- or P-glycoprotein-eliminated medicines might bring about an accelerated clearance of these compounds that might result in reduced efficacy

Preparations/Dosage

According to the German Commission E monograph the daily dose of St John's wort is 2–4 g crude drug. Preparations include tincture (1:10 in 45% alcohol) 2–4 ml three times daily and a tea, prepared from 2–4 g finely chopped herb per 150 ml boiling water (steeped ten minutes and strained), one cup (240 ml) three times daily. Alcoholic extracts (ethanol or methanol) can contain 0.1–0.3% hypericin, 2–4% flavonoids and up to 6% hyperforin. Such extracts (e.g. LI160) are commonly standardized to 0.3% hypericin. The dose of such tablets or capsules is usually 300 mg three times daily. Even though most preparations are standardized to hypericin content, it is presently believed that the principal active component is hyperforin.

Further Reading

Assemi M (2001) Herbs affecting the central nervous system: gingko, kava, St John's wort, and valerian. Clin Obstet Gynecol 44:824–835

Barnes J, Anderson LA (2001) St John's wort (*Hypericum perforatum* L.): a review of its chemistry, pharmacology and clinical properties. J Pharm Pharmacol 53:583–600

Beaubrun G, Gray GE (2000) A review of herbal medicines for psychiatric disorders. Psychiatr Serv 51:1130–1134

Bilia AR, Gallon S, Vincieri FF (2002) Kava-kava and anxiety: growing knowledge about the efficacy and safety. Life Sci 70:2581–2597

Cavanagh HM, Wilkinson JM (2002) Biological activities of lavender essential oil. Phytother Res 16:301–208

Di Carlo G, Borrelli F, Ernst E, Izzo AA (2001) St John's wort: Prozac from the plant kingdom. Trends Pharmacol Sci 22:292–297

Ernst E. (2002) The risk-benefit profile of commonly used herbal therapies: Ginkgo, St. John's Wort, Ginseng, Echinacea, Saw Palmetto, and Kava. Ann Intern Med 136:42–53

Ernst E, Stevinson C (1999) New data on old herbal remedies. Perfusion 5:192–194

Henderson L, Yue QY, Bergquist C, Gerden B, Arlett P. (2002) St John's wort (Hypericum perforatum): drug interactions and clinical outcomes. Br J Clin Pharmacol 54:349–356

Houghton PJ (1999) The scientific basis for the reputed activity of valerian. J Pharm Pharmacol 51:505–512

McIntyre M (2000) A review of the benefits, adverse events, drug interactions, and safety of St John's wort (Hypericum perforatum): the implication with regard to the regulation of herbal medicines. J Alt Compl Med 6:115–124

Nathan PJ (1999) The experimental and clinical pharmacology of St John's wort (*Hypericum perforatum* L.) Mol Psychiatry 4:333–338

O'Hara M, Kiefer D, Farrel K, Kemper K (1998) A review of 12 commonly used medicinal herbs. Arch Fam Med 7:523–535

Pepping J (1999) Kava: Piper methysticum. Am J Health Syst Pharm 56:957–958

Piscopo G (1997) Kava Kava: gift of the islands. Alt Med Rev 2:535–564

Pittler MH, Ernst E. (2000) Efficacy of kava extract for treating anxiety: systematic review and meta-analysis. J Clin Psychopharmacol 20:84–89

Plushner SL (2000) Valerian: Valeriana officinalis. Am J Health Syst Pharm 57:328–335

Schulz V (2001) Incidence and clinical relevance of the interactions and side effects of Hypericum preparations. Phytomedicine 8:152–160

Stevinson C, Ernst E (2000) Valerian for insomnia: a systematic review of randomized clinical trials. Sleep Medicine 1:91–99

Waddell DL, Hummel ME, Sumners AD (2001) Three herbs you should get to know. Am J Nurs 101:48–53

Wong A, Smith M, Boon HS (1998) Herbal remedies in psychiatric practice. Arch Gen Psychiatry 55:1033–1044

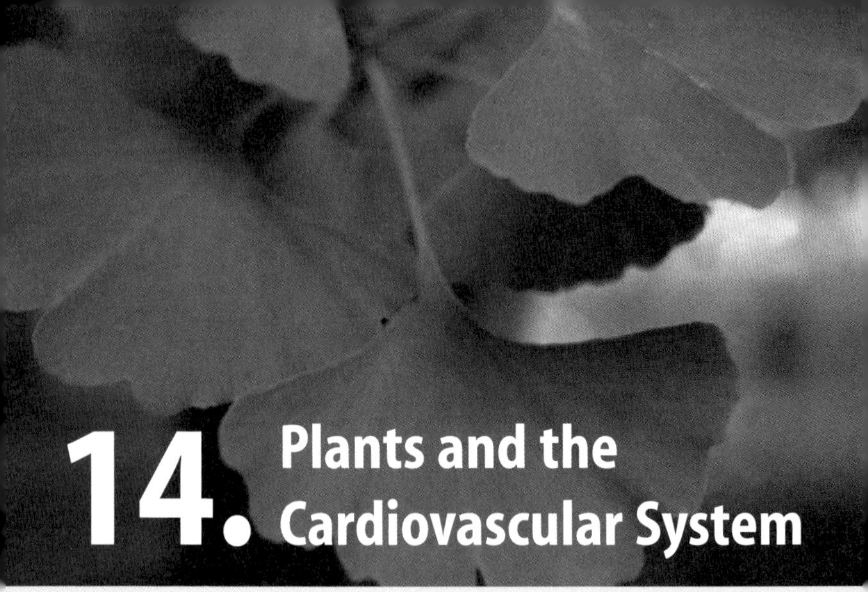

14. Plants and the Cardiovascular System

Introduction

The cardiovascular system consists of the heart and the blood vessels. The heart weighs about 300 g in the adult male. It has two small chambers called the atria, which lie above two larger chambers, the ventricles. The heart is composed of three layers: epicardium (exterior), myocardium (middle) and endocardium (inner layer). Heart valves within the heart ensure that blood flows only in one direction, out to the systemic circulation. The vascular system consists of arteries and veins. The artery's layer that lines the lumen and is in contact with the blood is the endothelium. The endothelium releases vasoactive substances (primarily nitric oxide) that help regulate blood flow and blood clotting.

Blood pressure in a vessel is generated by the output of the heart and the resistance to flow, which depends on vessel caliber, elasticity, geometry and blood viscosity. Blood pressure is expressed as systolic pressure/diastolic pressure and the normal value is 120/80 mmHg.

The relation of the cardiovascular system to cellular homeostasis is that it delivers oxygen, nutrients, and hormones, to the cells of the body, while removing waste products from them. Cardiovascular function must be adaptable to sustain blood flow to the tissues during rest as well exercise. The major cardiovascular diseases, for which botanicals have been used are angina, congestive heart failure, hypertension, cerebral insufficiency, venous insufficiency and arterial occlusive diseases.

Congestive Heart Failure

Clinical Picture

- Congestive heart failure (CHF) is the most common reason for hospitalisation of people over 65 years of age. CHF consists in a gradual reduction in heart function; as a consequence heart does not supply sufficient oxygenated blood to the organs of the body. In CHF there is a progressive systolic and diastolic ventricular dysfunction with a spectrum of symptoms depending upon the severity of heart failure (pallor, cyanosis, tachycardia, shortness of breath, edema peripheral/pulmonary, cardiomegaly, arrhythmias, hypertension).

- The New York Heart Association (NYHA) classifies loss of cardiac output as follows: *class I*: patients with no limitation of activities; they suffer no symptoms from ordinary activities; *class II*: patients with slight, mild limitation of activity; they are comfortable with rest or with mild exertion; *class III*: patients with marked limitation of activity; they are comfortable only at rest; *class IV*: patients who should be at complete rest, confined to bed or chair; any physical activity brings on discomfort and symptoms occur at rest.
- The therapeutic goal for CHF is to increase cardiac output. Therefore CHF is treated with drugs that increase the strenght of the cardiac muscle (i.e. inotropic drugs such as cardiac glycosides, β-adrenergic agonists, vasodilators) and diuretic agents that decrease extracellular fluid volume.

Phytotherapy of Congestive Heart Failure

A number of herbal medicines contain potent cardioactive glycosides, which have positive inotropic actions on the heart and thus are potentially useful for the treatment of CHF (Table 14.1). Cardiac glycosides increase calcium concentration in the cardiac muscle, thereby increasing contraction of the atrial and ventricular myocardium (positive inotropic action) (Figure 14.1). Cardiac glycosides have a low therapeutic index, and hence, the use must be carefully controlled. The best

Table 14.1

Herbal medicines potentially useful to treat congestive heart failure

Common name	Latin name	Part(s) of plant used	Key constituents	Daily dose
Adonis[1]	*Adonis vernalis*	Aerial parts	Cardenolides, flavonoids	1–3 g
Arjun tree	*Terminalia arjuna*	Bark	Tannins, steroids, triterpenes, flavonoids	a
Foxglove	*Digitalis spp.*	Leaves	Cardioactive steroid glycosides	0.1 g
Ginseng	*Panax ginseng*	Roots	Triterpene saponins	1–2 g
Hawthorn[2]	*Crataegus laevigata*	Flowers, leaves, fruits	Flavonoids, triterpenes, proanthocyanidins	5 g
Kombe	*Strophantus hispidus*	Seeds	Cardenolides	0.1 g
Lily of the valley[3]	*Convallaria majalis*	Aerial parts	Cardenolides	0.15 g
Oleander	*Nerium oleander*	Leaves	Cardenolides, pregnanes	0.15 g
Squill[3]	*Urginea maritima*	Bulbs	Bufadienolides	0.1–0.5 g

1 supported by German Commission E for arrhytmia and nervous heart complaints
2 supported by German Commission E for decreasing of cardiac output (Stage II NYHA)
3 supported by German Commission E for arrhythmias, cardiac insufficiency, nervous heart complaints
a. 500 mg bark extract

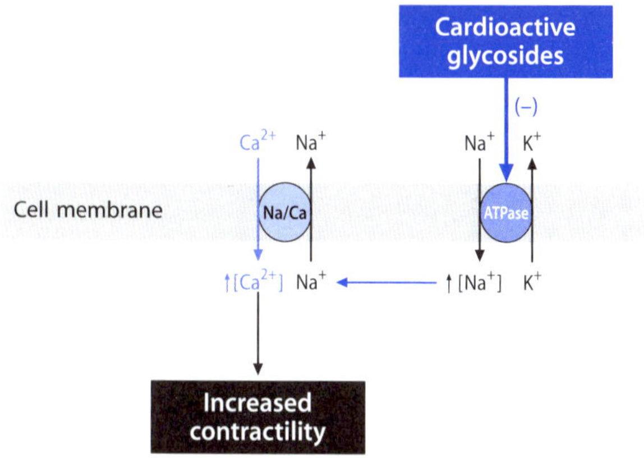

Figure 14.1 ▲ **Mechanism of action of cardioactive glycosides**
Cardioactive glycosides combine reversibly with the sodium-potassium ATPase (ATPase) of the cardiac cell membrane resulting in an inhibition of pump activity. This causes an increase in intracellular sodium concentration. The elevated intracellular sodium concentration favors the transport of calcium into the cell and decreases calcium exodus from the cell, via the sodium-calcium exchange (Na/Ca) mechansim. The final result is an increase in intracellular calcium which causes an increase in the systolic force of contraction

known herb containing cardiac glycosides is foxglove, which consists of the dried leaves of *Digitalis purpurea* or *D. lanata*. Foxglove has been used for about two centuries for the treatment of CHF. Foxglove is an extremely potent herbal medicine and is not easily available in standardized preparations.

Accidental poisonings and even suicide attempts with ingestion of plants containing cardiac glycosides are abundant in the medical literature. Of these, the largest percentage are attributed to oleander (*Nerium oleander*). The clinical manifestations of oleander intoxication is virtually identical to digoxin overdose. Morbidity and mortality are mainly related to cardiotoxic adverse effects that usually include life-threatening ventricular tachyarrhythmias, bradycardia, and heart block. In addition to digitalis, hawthorn stands out as an important cardiostimulant herbal medicine, with efficacy in CHF.

Hawthorn

Botany/Key constituents ▶ Hawthorn consists of the leaves with flowers and/or fruits (berries) of *Crataegus laevigata* (Poiret) DC, *monogyna* Jacq. or *C. oxyacantha* Auct. (Fam. *Rosaceae*). *Crataegus* spp are thorny shrubs or small tree up to 10 m tall common in the temperature areas of the northern hemisphere (Plate

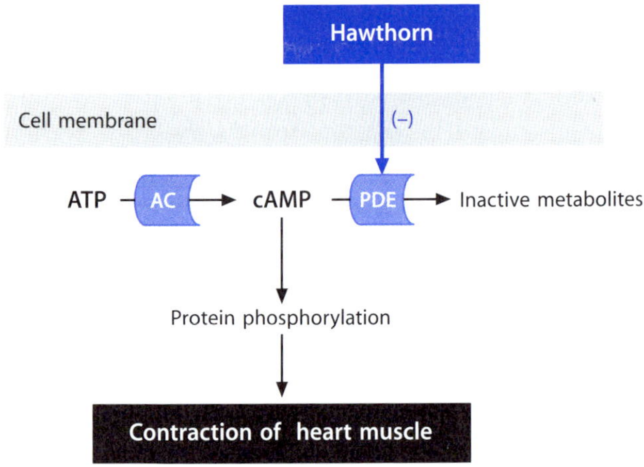

Figure 14.2 ▲ **Possible mode of action of hawthorn**
Cyclic AMP (cAMP) is formed from ATP by the action of the enzyme adenylate cyclase (AC) and it is degraded by the enzyme cyclic AMP phosphodiesterase (PDE). Hawthorn inhibits cyclic AMP phosphodiesterase and thus increases the intracellular concentration of cAMP within the myocardium. The increase in cAMP lead to protein phosphorylation (via protein kinases) and increased in the force of contraction (positive inotropic effect)

14.1). The leaves are broader than long and have 3–5 lobes. The dark red, false fruits are oval and contain a small kernel which is the true fruit. The drug contains proanthocianidins (1–3%), flavonoids (0.1% in the berries and 1% in the aerial parts), aromatic amines, saponins, and cyanogenetic glycosides.

Mode of action ▸ The activity of hawthorn is attributed to flavonoids anthocyanidins and proanthocyanidins (also known as biflavans or procyanidins). Experimental studies have shown that hawthorn possesses many pharmacological effects which are beneficial for the cardiovascular system. It inhibits arrhythmia, dilates coronary blood vessels, reduces serum cholesterol and triglyceride levels, reduces symptoms of angina and CHF and has a hypotensive action due to peripheral dilation of blood vessels. Cardiac improvement is mainly due to inhibition of cyclic AMP phosphodiesterase which leads to a positive inotropic effect (Figure 14.2). An effect on β-adrenergic receptors has been also observed.

Clinical efficacy ▸ Hawthorn has been extensively studied. At least 15 clinical studies involving a total of about 1000 patients have been reported in the literature. Most patients were in Stage II heart failure. Almost all the studies showed therapeutic efficacy of hawthorn, particularly in the subjective symptoms of congestive heart failure such as rapid fatigability, exertional dyspnea, lethargy, exertional cough, decreased exercise tolerance. German Commission E states that hawthorn leaves and flowers are indicated "for declining cardiac performance consistent with stage II failure according to NYHAA".

Adverse events/Contraindications ▸ Hawthorn is devoid of serious adverse effects: gastrointestinal complaints, palpitations, vertigo, headache and flushing may occur. In comparison with the inotropic drug digoxin, hawthorn has a reduced arrhythmogenic risk because of its ability to prolong the effective refractory period. The concomitant use of hawthorn and cardiac glycosides can markedly enhance the activity of glycosides. Although hawthorn is available in the United States and other countries without medical prescription, it should not be used unless under the supervision of a physician.

Preparations/Dosage

Flavonoid (calculated as hyperoside) and oligomeric procyanidins (calculated as epicatechin) are the chemical constituents for testing the pharmaceutical quality of hawthorn. The German Commission E recommends a daily dose of 160–900 mg hawtorn extract with 4–30 mg content in flavonoids and 3–160 mg in oligomeric procyanidins. Most clinical studies used alcoholic extracts in the dose ranging from 180 and 900 mg daily.

Angina

Clinical Picture

- Angina (or angina pectoris), is a radiating chest pain associated with a temporary decrease in the delivery of coronary blood to the heart muscle. Angina may result from a variety of causes: (i) increased physical demands on the heart which cannot be met by the coronary oxygenation; (ii) hypertension (which increases exensively the oxygen demands of the heart); (iii) fever (which elevates cardiac activity); (iv) hyperthyroidism (which increases cardiac activity); (v) aortic stenosis (a narrowing of the aortic valve) and (vi) atherosclerosis. When coronary arteries become completely occluded then blood flow to the heart ceases, and the myocardial tissue dies (myocardial infarction). Occlusion may be due to a thrombus or embolus in one of the coronary arteries. Obviously the effects depend on the size and location of the infarcted area.
- Angina is treated with nitrates, vasodilator compounds able to give rapid relief from acute attacks. Beta-adrenergic receptor antagonists, which increase coronary flow and are useful in effort-induced angina. Calcium channel antagonists are useful in the prophylaxis and/or treatment of vasospastic and effort-induced angina. Individuals with an infarct may

require a coronary vessel bypass surgery. Herbal medicines employed today for the treatment of angina are expected to be not more effective than nitrates, beta-blockers or calcium channel blockers. Overall, there is a lack of randomized clinical trials confirming the clinical efficacy of herbal medicines to treat angina.

Phytotherapy of Angina

The key herb for the treatment of angina is hawthorn (*Crataegus* spp). Hawthorn dilates coronary blood vessels, reduces myocardial oxygen demand and thus reduces symptoms of angina. In traditional Chinese medicine the dried roots of *Panax ginseng* (**ginseng**) are often used in the treatment of patients with angina and coronary artery disease. The ginseng contains ginsenosides, saponins and other active components. Ginseng is considered a calcium, ion channel antagonist in vascular tissue. It dilates coronary arteries, inhibits atherogenesis by interfering with the proliferation of smooth muscle cells, and enhances fibrinolytic activity in the blood. The vasodilatatory effect of ginseng could be due to the release of nitric oxide, a potent vasorelaxant compound. However clinical trials will be necessary to take into consideration the use of ginseng in angina pectoris.

- ► *See chapter 15 for the hypoglycaemic activity of ginseng*
- ► *See chapter 19 for the adaptogenic properties of ginseng*

Similar to *P. ginseng, Salvia miltiorrhiza* (**danshen**) dilates coronary arteries and therefore may be useful in the treatment of angina. *Danshen* has also a protective action on ischemic myocardium,. It protects myocyte mitochondrial membranes from ischemia-reperfusion injury and lipid peroxidation because of its free radical scavenging effects. In vitro danshen inhibits platelet aggregation and serotonin release; decoction of the roots seems as efficacious as the isolated active principles known as tanshinones (diterpene compounds). A clinical observation shows that the concomitant use of danshen and warfarin increases the anticoagulant effects of warfarin. However further studies will be necessary to evaluate the efficacy and safery of this drug.

Hypertension

Clinical Picture

- Hypertension is a condition of increasing blood pressure associated with an increased risk of heart failure and stroke. It occurs when the muscle and elastic components of arterial wells are replaced by fibrous tissue. Hypertension occurs when blood pressure goes beyond the normal value (between 120/80 mm Hg and 150/90 mm Hg systolic/diastolic for a 20 year old to a 70 year old man). In about 10% of all cases, hypertension results from other imbalances and so is called secondary hypertension.

- Causes include excessive renin release as occurs with kidney damage, hypersecretion of aldosterone and cortisol, or hypersecretion of antidiuretic hormone. In about 90% of hypertensive individuals no secondary causes can be determined, since it is almost certainly multifactorial: this form is referred to as primary or essential hypertension.
- Drugs used for treating hypertension include diuretics (which decrease blood volume), sympatholytics (which block the effect of the vasoconstrictor noradrenaline), direct-acting vasodilators (which decrease peripheral resistance), calcium channel blockers (which inhibit calcium ion influx into the vascular smooth muscle cells, thus decreasing peripheral resistance), and angiotensin converting enzyme (ACE) inhibitors (which induce vasodilation by blocking the enzyme that cleaves angiotensin I to form the potent vasoconstricor, angiotensin II).

Phytotherapy of Hypertension

Most of the herbal treatments for hypertension probably act as a peripheral vasodilators. In general there is a lack of clinical data to justify the use of herbal medicine. Important herbs for their traditional use are here described. These herbs are listed in Table 14.2.

Table 14.2
Antihypertensive herbal medicines

Common name	Latin name	Part(s) of plant used	Key constituents	Daily dose
Evodia	*Evodia rutaecarpa*	Fruits	Alkaloids (rutaecarpine), tannins	3–9 g
Garlic*	*Allium sativum*	Bulb	Alliins	4 g
Ligusticum	*Ligusticum wallichii*	Roots	Alkaloids (tetramethylpyrazine, perlolyrine, leucylphenylalanine), essential oil	5 g
Onion*	*Allium cepa*	Bulb	Alliins, flavonoids	20 g
Scotch broom*	*Cytisus scoparius*	Aerial parts	Quinolizidine alkaloids, biogenic amines, flavonoids	1–2 g
Snakeroot*	*Rauwolfia serpentina*	Roots	Alkaloids (reserpine, ajmaline)	a
Stephania	*Stephania tetrandra*	Roots	Alkaloids (tetrandrine)	b
White hellebore	*Veratrum album*	Rhizome, roots	Steroid alkaloids	0.02–0.1 g

* supported by German Commission E
a. 600 mg drug/6 mg total alkaloids
b. reliable data not available

Garlic. The hypotensive effect of garlic (bulb, composed of bulbules of *Allium sativa*, Fam. *Liliaceae*) has been demonstrated in experimental studies, although the exact mode of action is not known. Other cardiovascular effects of garlic are shown in Box 14.1. A meta-analysis on the effect of garlic on blood pressure identified seven randomized controlled trials (all using the same dried garlic powder, 600–900 mg/daily; duration of treatment: at least 4 weeks) including a total of 415 subjects. Of the seven trials, three showed a significant reduction in systolic blood pressure and four in diastolic blood pressure. The results suggest that garlic powder preparation may be of some clinical use in subjects with mild hypertension. However, there is still insufficient evidence to recommend it as a routine clinical therapy for the treatment of hypertensive subjects.

Box 14.1
Cardiovascular properties of garlic

Antioxidant effects
It is widely accepted that lipid peroxidation plays an important role in atherosclerosis initiation and formation. Some garlic constituents are known to have oxygen radical scavenging and antioxidant properties in vitro. However, despite clear experimental evidence, the clinical impact of garlic on lipoprotein oxidation and its potential role in inhibiting atherosclerosis remains an open question

Effects on platelet aggregation
Garlic has been shown to inhibit platelet aggregation caused by several agonists. A number of mechanisms have been proposed by which garlic is thought to exert this action. These include inhibition of thromboxane synthesis, intraplatelet mobilization of calcium uptake, inhibition of calcium uptake into platelets and inhibition of the exposure of fibrinogen receptors on platelet membranes. Dried powder preparations seem to be the strongest platelet inhibitiors while garlic oils and aged garlic extracts are much weaker or even devoid of any activity. The organosulphur compounds (mainly ajoene) seem responsible of this activity

Effect on serum lipoproteins and lipid metabolism
Garlic reduces serum cholesterol, serum triglyceride, and low density lipoprotein (LDL) and increases high density lipoprotein (HDL). It has been suggested that an increase in HDL may enhance the removal of cholesterol from arterial tissue. The hypolipidemic effect of garlic is thought to involve (i) inhibition of cholesterol biosynthesis, (ii) increased degradation of triglycerides, (iii) reduction of LDL.

▶ *See chapter 15 for the antilipidaemic properties of garlic*

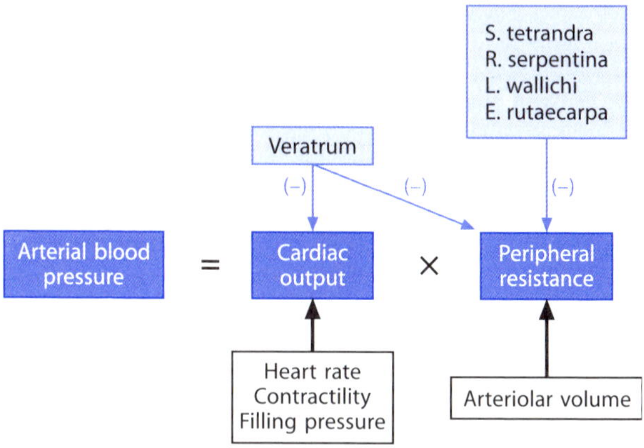

Figure 14.3 ▲ **Mechanisms for controlling blood pressure and site of action of antihypertensive herbal medicines**
Arterial blood pressure is directly proportional to the product of the cardiac output and the peripheral vascular resistance. Antihypertensive drugs lower blood pressure by reducing cardiac output and/or decreasing peripheral resistance.
Rauwoulfia serpentina (snakeroot), *Ligusticum wallichi*, *Evodia rataecarpa* and *Stephania tetrandra* contain active vasorelaxant compounds (see text for details) and hence reduce peripheral vascular resistance. *Veratrum* alkaloids activate vagus nerve causing bradycardia and also cause vasorelaxation

Snakeroot (or **rauwolfia**) (the root of *Rawolfia serpentina*, (L.) Benth, ex Kurz; Fam. *Apocynaceae*), the natural soruce of the alkaloid reserpine, has been a Hindu Ayurvedic remedy since ancient times. Both standardized whole root preparations of R. *serpentina* and its reserpine alkaloid are officially monographed in the United Stated Pharmacopeia. Reserpine was one of the first drugs used on a large scale to treat hypertension. Reserpine causes a depletion of noradrenaline levels in the adrenergic neurons. Thus, sympathetic function is impaired. Snakeroot is supported by German Commission E for the treatment of hypertension. Due to unacceptable side effects (difficulty in sleeping, nightime hallucinations, depression, suicidal tendencies), the use of reserpine as well as preparations of *R. serpentina* has dramatically diminished.

White hellebore consists of the rhizome and roots of *Veratrum* plants, perennial herbs growing in many parts of the world. Varieties include *V. viride* from Canada and the eastern United States, *V. californicum* from the western United States, *V. album* from Alaska and Europe, and *V. japonicum* from Asia. All *Veratrum* plants (Fam. *Liliaceae*) contain alkaloids which act on the posterior wall of the left ventricle and the coronary sinus baroreceptors, causing reflex hypotension and bradycardia via the vagus nerve (Bezold-Jarisch reflex). *Veratrum* alkaloids are toxic and are known to cause vomiting, bradycardia, hypotension and rarely seizures. Although once a treatment for hypertension, the use of white hellebore has lost favour owing to a low therapeutic index and unacceptable toxicity.

Stephania tetrandra (**stephania**, **Han Fang Ji**) is an herb sometimes used in traditional Chinese medicine to treat hypertension. Tetrandrine, from *S. tetrandra* roots, has been shown to be a calcium ion channel antagonist. Tetrandrine is not a safe compound; it has been shown that it causes liver necrosis in dog; moreover, tetrandine has been implicated in an outbreak of rapidly progessive renal failure, termed Chinese herb nephropathy.

The root of **Ligusticum wallichi** (**ligusticum**, **Chuan Xiong**) is used in traditional Chinese medicine. Tetramethylpyrazine, the active constituent of *L. wallichii*, vasodilates blood vessels through antagonism of calcium channels and α-adrenergic receptors. The vasodilatatory effect does not involve the release of vasoactive substances (i.e. prostacyclin, nitric oxide) from the endothelium Currently, there is insufficient information to evaluate the safety and efficacy of this herbal medicine.

Evodia rutaecarpa (**evodia**, **wu-chu-yu**) is a Chinese herbal drug that has been used as a treatment for hypertension. The fruits contain an active vasorelaxant component called rutaecarpine. Efficacy and safety data are not available.

Chronic Venous Insufficiency

Clinical Picture

- Chronic venous insufficiency is among the most common conditions afflicting humans (10–15% of men and 20–25% of women are afflicted). It is more than a mere "cosmetic problem" because patients often require hospital admission and surgical treatment. At least two thirds of leg ulcers have evidence of venous disease in the affected limb. One of the most common manifestations of venous insufficiency are varicose veins
- Varicose veins are largely the result of the destruction of the network of proteoglycans in the elastic tissue of the vein wall by lysosomal enzymes. This situation causes an abnormal dilatation of the vein and a passage of electrolytes, proteins and water through the venous well and then oedema formation.
- Varicose veins are treated with sclerotherapy (injection of sodium tetradecyl sulfate into the vein which usually occludes the vein) or surgery. Herbal medicines used in the treatment of varicous veins may provide only relief of the unpleasant symptoms by increasing capillary resistance and venous tone but not reverse changes in organic structures. These include horse chestnut, butcher's broom, hydrocotile, bilberry and witch hazel (see also Table 14.3). By increasing venous tone, these herbal medicines are also useful to treat hemorrhoids.

Table 14.3
Herbal medicines used to treat chronic venous insufficiency

Common name	Latin name	Part(s) of plant used	Key constituents	Daily dose
Bilberry	*Vaccinium myrtillus*	Fruits	Tannins, anthocyanins, flavonoids	20–50 g
Buckwheat	*Fagopyrum esculentum*	Aerial parts	Flavonoids, anthracene derivatives	1.5–2 g
Butcher's broom*	*Ruscus aculeatus*	Roots, rhizome	Steroid saponins (ruscogenin), benzofuranes	a
French maritime pine	*Pinus pinaster*	Bark	Procyanidins, phenolic acids	b
Gotu kola	*Centella asiatica*	Leaves, stem	Triterpenes, flavonoids, volatile oil	1.8 g
Grape seeds	*Vitis vinifera*	Seeds, leaves	Procyanidins	c
Horse chestnut*	*Aesculus hippocastanum*	Seeds	Flavonoids, triterpene saponins (aescin)	d
Sweet clover*	*Melilotus officinalis*	Aerial parts	Coumarins, flavonoids, triterpene saponins	e
Witch hazel*	*Hamamelis virginiana*	Leaves, bark	Tannins, procyanidins	f

* supported by German Commission E

a. 300–600 mg extract

b. 90–360 mg extract

c. 150–600 mg seeds extract or 360–420 mg leaves extract

d. 35–150 mg of aescin per day

e. 3 to 30 mg of coumarin

f. Decoctions of 5–10 g of crud drug/250 ml water for rinses

Phytotherapy of Chronic Venous Insufficency

Horse chestnut

Botany/key constituents ► Horse chestnut consists of the seeds of *Aesculus hippocastanum* L. (Fam. *Hippocastanaeae*), an ornamental tree cultivated in different countries (see plate 14.2). It is a deciduous tree with grey bark which grows to 25 m. The fruit has a leathery, prickly capsule and contains 1–2 brown seeds with large whitish scar. The drug contains coumarins (e.g. aesculetin), flavonoids, saponins (a mixture of saponins collectively referred as aescin) and tannins.

Mode of action ► Several mechanisms have been proposed to explain the effect of aescin. These include (i) the ability to inhibit lysosomal enzyme activity and the transcapillary filtration of water and proteins by reducing the number and/or diameter of capillary pores; (ii) the ability to increase the tone of the veins, thus improving return blood flow to the heart; (iii) reduction of the activity of pro-

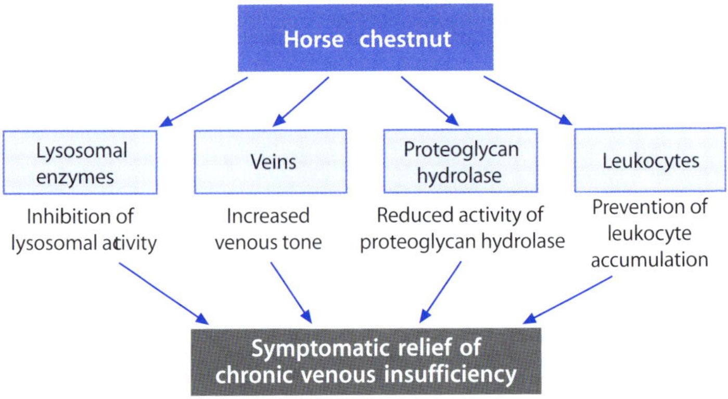

Figure 14.4 ▲ **Actions of horse chestnut which can contribute to relief the symptoms of chronic venous insufficiency** (see text for details)

teoglycan hydrolase (i.e. yaluronidase and elastase enzymes) and (vi) prevention of leukocyte accumulation in chronic venous insufficiency-affected limbs (Figure 14.4). Aescin is less potent than horse chestnut. In fact, there are evidence that the combination of aescin with flavonoids (present in horse chestnut extracts) is superior to aescin alone.

Clinical efficacy ▸ Horse chestnut is supported by German Commission E for the treatment of symptoms of chronic venous insufficiency, for example pain and sensation of heaviness in the legs, nocturnal cramps in the calves, pruritus and swelling of the legs. A recent systematic review retrieved 13 double-blind randomized controlled trials of horse chestnut seed extract in 1083 patients with chronic venous insufficiency. The treatment period ranged from 20 days to 8 weeks. The superiority of horse-chestnut is suggested by all placebo-controlled studies. The use of horse-chestnut is associated with a decrease of the lower-leg volume and a reduction in leg circumference at the calf and ankle. Symptoms such as leg pain, pruritus, and feeling of fatigue and tenseness are reduced. Four comparative trials against the reference drug indicate that horse chestnut and O-(β-hydroxyethyl)-rutosides are equally effective. One trial suggests a therapeutic equivalence of horse chestnut and compression therapy.

Adverse events/Contraindications ▸ Horse chestnut treatment is safe. Pruritus, nausea, gastrointestinal tract symptoms, headache and dizziness are the main adverse events which occur in clinical trials. In a recent observational study involving more than 5000 patients, adverse events occurred in 0.6% of patients.

Gastrointestinal tract symptoms and calf spasm were reported more frequently. A case of liver damage has been reported

Preparations/Dosage

Horse chestnut seed extract containing from 16% to 21% triterpene glycosides, calculated as aescin, is normally used. Initially daily oral dosage is 90–150 mg of aescin but following improvement this may be reduced to 35–70 mg daily. Aescin is a registered drug in German and is the active ingredient in a number of preparations used either topically or orally for the treatment of peripheral vascular disease, in particular that related to altered capillary permeability and resistance.

French maritime pine (Pycnogenol®)

Botany/Key constituents ▸ French maritime pine is the bark of *Pinus pinaster* Aiton, subsp. Atlantica des Villar (also named *Pinus maritima* Lamk., Fam. *Pinaceae*), a specie of pine tree that is cultivated in the forest of the Landes of Gascogne (South-western France). Chemical identification studies have shown that French maritime pine is primarily composed of procyanidins (e.g. catechin, taxifolin and oligomers with 7 or more flavonoid subunits) and phenolic acids (i.e. derivatives of benzoic and cinnamic acids).

Mode of action ▸ French maritime pine possesses a number of pharmacological effects which could contribute to its efficacy in the treatment of chronic venous insufficiency. French maritime pine protects against oxidative stress by increasing the synthesis of anti-oxidative enzymes and by acting as a potent scavenger of free radicals. Anti-inflammatory activity, protection against UV-radiation, anti-allergic and immunostimulant effects, reduction of capillary permeability and beneficial effects on microcirculation have been also described.

Clinical efficacy ▸ Six placebo-controlled, double-blind studies involving a total of 189 patients have demonstrated that the administration of French maritime pine significantly improves pain, occurrence of cramps, heaviness in the legs and significantly reduces swelling in the lower leg and ankle after 30–60 days treatment. These results are encouraging, although more studies are required to fully elucidate and confirm the potential value of French maritime pine.

Adverse effects/Contraindications ▸ According to documented clinical experience with 2000 patients, the rate of unwanted effects is 1.5%. These consist mainly of gastrointestinal disturbances, dizziness, nausea and headache. The majority of unwanted effects are considered to be minor. French maritime pine has also been tested for dermal toxicity: no irritation of the skin or the eyes has been noted.

Preparations/Dosage

In many countries, including the United States, a standardized water-soluble hydroalcoholic extract of the bark of the French maritime pine is sold under the trade mark Pycnogenol®; this extract has been evaluated in clinical studies. Pycnogenol® is given in oral doses ranging from 90 to 360 mg/daily (divided into three daily doses).

Butcher's broom

Botany/key constituents ▸ Butcher's broom is the rhizome and roots of *Ruscus aculeatus* L. (Fam. *Liliaceae*), a lignified plant which grows wild in woods and underwoods in all of Europe. The drug contains steroidal saponins (6%, mainly ruscogenin and neoruscogenin), flavonoids, benzofuranoid derivatives, essential oil.

Mode of action ▸ Ruscogenin and neoruscogenin, two steroidal saponins, are thought to be the pharmacological active components of butcher's broom. The drug and its components (ruscogenins) cause constriction of venules without appreciably affecting arterioles. The vascular effects of saponins, which are efficiently absorbed when given orally, is thought to be linked in part to activation of α_1-adrenergic receptors and calcium channels on the smooth muscle cells. *Ruscus* extract also shows anti-elastase activity, in contrast to horse chestnut. The extract has little effect on hyaluronidase.

Clinical studies ▸ Butcher's broom is supported by German Commission E for the treatment of hemorrhoids and venous conditions. Butcher's broom is used as supportive therapy for discomfort of chronic venous insufficiency, such as pain and heaviness, as well as cramps in the legs, itching, and swelling. Butcher's broom also is used as therapy for haemorrhoid complaints such as itching and burning. Preliminary trials have shown patients with chronic venous insufficiency given oral drug extract maintained venous tone and improved venous emptying in comparison to placebo-treated patients.

Adverse events ▸ If used properly, no adverse effects are expected. The drug very seldom may cause nausea and gastritis.

Preparations/Dosage

Capsules or tablets containing about 300 mg each of dried extract are available (one or two capsules daily). Sometimes a capsule may contain *Ruscus* extract (75 mg) associated to rosemary oil (2 mg). A 4–6 g of cream containing 64 to 96 mg of Ruscus extract is used in in leg venous insufficiency. Oral forms of ruscogenins (or the extract) are associated with other venous tonics (sweet clover, hesperidin, *Black currant* extract)

Gotu kola (hydrocotyle)

Botany/Key constituents ▸ Gotu kola consists of the leaves and stems of *Centella asiatica* L. Urban (Fam. *Apiaceae*), an herbaceous plant of the tropical areas today cultivated in the Oriental countries (see plate 14.3). The drug contains terpenoids (i.e. asiaticoside, centelloside, madecassoside), flavonoids, aminoacids, volatile oil and other constituents. The active constituents are believed to be the pantacyclic triterpene derivatives. Studies have been conducted in particular to investigate the madecassosides and asiacosides.

Mode of action ▸ Gotu kola has been reported to improve the blood circulation in the lower limbs through a stimulation of collagen and mucopolysaccharides synthesis in the vein wall. As a consequence there is an increase in vein elasticity and a reduction in the capacity of the vein to distend. Hydrocotile is also useful in case of cutaneous ulcers of venous origin, surgical wounds, fistulas, gynaecological wounds. Gotu kola is stated to act like cortisone with respect to wound healing.

Clinical efficacy ▸ Gotu kola has been subjected to quite extensive clinical investigations. Three double-blind randomized clinical trials have shown it to have a positive effect in the treatment of venous insufficiency. Gotu kola also appears to be effective in accelerating wound healing. At present time, clinical studies aimed at investigating the sedative, analgesic, antidepressant, antimicrobial, antiviral and immunomodulatory effects that have been demonstrated experimentally, are still lacking.

Adverse events/Contraindications ▸ Adverse reactions following the use of Gotu kola include allergic contact dermatitis after topical application, gastric complaints and nausea after oral administration.

Preparations/Dosage

The drug is available in capsule containing each 60 mg of dry extract which contains not less 5% of total triterpenes for the treatment of chronic venous insufficiency (one capsule two times daily and for four-five weeks). Ointments may also be used for the treatment of wounds, cellulitis and hemorrhoids.

Bilberry

Botany/Key constituents ▸ Bilberry fruit is well known as a food from *Vaccinium myrtillus* L. (Fam. *Ericaceae*). The plant is deciduous, dwarf shrub with sharp-edged, green branches 15 to 50 cm high. It is particularly abundant in the woods that grow on siliceous soils in the mountains of the northern hemisphere.

Bilberry fruits are deep violet with crescent-shaped seeds. Key constituents include anthocyanins, tannins and flavonoids

Mode of action ▸ Anthocyanins improve functional disturbances of the fine blood vessels, especially capillaries and also stimulate capillary repair. They are more protective than flavonoids. Anthocyanins have antiplatelet activity; they inhibit collagen- or ADP-induced platelet aggregation and stimulate the activity of prostacyclin (an antiplatelet agent) of the vascular walls.

Clinical studies ▸ There is a paucity of reports dealing with the clinical efficacy of bilberry fruits in peripheral vascular disorders and venous disorders. Uncontrolled studies demonstrated the efficacy of bilberry in chronic venous insufficiency. Preliminary double-blind, placebo-controlled trials also seem to confirm the clinical efficacy of bilberry fruits

Adverse events/Contraindications ▸ No significant adverse effects are expected. A surveillance study conducted on over 2000 patients with venous and retinal disorders showed mild side effects in about 4% of patients. Ingestion of the whole fresh fruit may irritate the intestinal lining in sensitive individuals. Digestive complaints due to the high tannin content could occur.

Preparations/Dosage

Preparations include dried or fresh fruit as an infusion, liquid extract (3–6 ml of 1:1 liquid extract per day) and tables for internal use. Tablets providing 50–120 mg of anthocyanins per day (equivalent to about 20–50 g of fresh fruit) have been typically used in clinical trials. Infusion or extracts for topical use are also available.

Hemorrhoids

Clinical Picture

- Hemorrhoids are dilated, enlarged, and often inflamed venous plexuses of the rectum and anal canal. External hemorrhoids are dilatations of the inferior rectal plexuses: they originate in the anal canal and do not present symptoms. Except an occasional burning sensation when a constipated motion is passed. Internal hemorrhoids are dilatations of the superior/middle rectal plexuses and occur in the part of the bowel and anal canal: they may cause pain, bleeding and itching.
- Hemorrhoids are aggravated by constipation and straining at stool. Hemorrhoids are also common in pregnancy due to the rise in intra-abdominal pres-

Table 14.4
Main herbal medicines supported by German Commission E to treat hemorrhoids

Common name	Latin name	Part(s) of plant used	Key constituents	Daily dose
Aspen (poplar)	*Populus alba* (*P. nigra, P. tremula*)	Bark and leaves	Glycosides and esters yielding salicylic acid	10 g
Butcher's broom	*Ruscus aculeatus*	Roots, rhizome	Steroid saponins (ruscogenin), benzofuranes	a
Horse chestnut	*Aesculus hippocastanum*	Seeds	Flavonoids, triterpene saponins (aescin)	b
Sweet clover	*Melilotus officinalis*	Flowering tops	Coumarins, flavonoids, triterpene saponins	c
Peruvian balsam	*Myroxylon balsamum*	Balsam from trunks	Cinnamein (an exter mixture), resins, volatile oil	d
Witch hazel	*Hamamelis virginiana*	Leaves, bark	Tannins, procyanidins	e

a. 600 mg extract
b. 40 to 150 mg of aescin per day
c. 3 to 30 mg of coumarin
d. Galenic preparations containing 5 to 20 % Peruvian balsam
e. Suppositories (0.1-1 g drug) can be used 1 to 3 times a day

sure, that causes venous engorgement by compressing the gut. Some herbal medicines supported by German Commission E for the treatment of hemorrhoids are listed in Table 14.4. In general, treatment of hemorrhoids include:

- increase diatary fibre and treatment of constipation
- Mucilage-containing herbs (e.g. psyllium) to keep the stool soft
- Oral treatment using herbs to improve venous tone such as horse-chestnut and butcher's broom. These herbs are also available as a cream for topical application
- Topical treatment with astringent herbs such as witchhazel

Phytotherapy of Hemorrhoids

Witch hazel

Botany/key constituents ▶ Witch hazel consists of the leaves (or bark) of *Hamamelis virginiana* (Fam. *Hamamelidaceae*), an up to 7 m high shrub or tree occurring in eastern North America. Key constituents are a mixture of tannins (3–10%) including gallotannins, hamamelitannins and procyanidins.

Mode of action ▸ Witch hazel is known to possess astringent (vasoconstrictive) and hemostatic properties, which have been attributed to the tannin constituents. The anti-inflammatory activity could be due, in part, to a vasoconstrictor activity. Moreover hamamelitannins and procyanidins possesses anti-inflammatory activity through inhibition of 5-lipoxygenase and PAF biosynthesis, respectively.

Clinical efficacy ▸ Witch hazel is supported by German Commission E for the treatment of hemorrhoids and venous conditions (chronic venous insufficiency). The clinical efficacy of witch hazel is promising, although it need more rigorous clinical trials. A reduction of symptoms (greater reduction in itching and soreness, less frequent bleeding) in patients with hemorrhoids or varicose veins has been observed.

Adverse events/Contraindications ▸ Contact dermatitis caused by the topical use of witch hazel has been reported in rare cases. In a study of 1032 consecutively tested patients, four were found to react to an ointment containing a 25% extract of witch hazel. Two of these patients reacted positively to the wool fat in the ointment base. Oral preparations can cause gastric upsets.

Preparations/Dosage

Dried bark and leaves as a decoction and extract for topical use are available. The recommended dosage is 2 g of leaf or bark by infusion three times daily; 2–4 mL three times daily of *Hamamelis* liquid extract (1:1 in 45% alcohol) and *Hamamelis* Water (BPC 1973) for local application. For the treatment of hemorrhoids 0.1–1 g in suppositories is used 1–3 times daily. The drug is also used in cosmetic formulation as hamamelis water or distilled hamamelis extract and used as an astringent.

▸ *See chapter 23 for the dermatological use of witch hazel*

Arterial Occlusive Disease

Clinical Picture

- Arterial occlusive disease are a result of abnormalities of the vessels, blood flow or blood itself. Such abnormalities may produce a reduction in the blood flow and consequently ischemia. Depending on its severity, location and duration, it may cause central (e.g. dizziness, depression, tinnitus, weakened memory and even dementia) and peripheral symptoms (e.g. intermittent claudication)

Box 14.2
Main pharmacological properties of ginkgo

Antioxidant properties
Ginkgo has been shown to induce the destruction of various free radicals and to inhibit lipid peroxidation. The flavone component may mediate ginkgo's ability to protect from reactive oxygen species. This may be useful in treating the effects of blood lipoprotein oxidation that result in the deposition and aggregation of atherosclerotic plaques.

Anti platelet activating factor (anti-PAF) activity
Ginkgolides are competitive antagonists of PAF. This finding is important due to the role played by PAF in the pathophysiology of inflammation and hypercoagulable states

Anti-ischemic properties
Ginkgolides prevent the metabolic damage caused by experimental cerebral ischeamia. They reduce the infarct size in experimental myocardial occlusion. Bilobalide has demonstrated a potent neuroprotective effect against ischemic damage, which is stronger than ginkgolide B. Ginkgo possesses neuroprotective properties under conditions such as hypoxia/ischemia and nerve damage.

Effect on metabolism
Ginkgo produces changes in glucose utilization in various areas of the rat brain, including the frontoparietal somatosensory cortex. This may help explain the clinical effectiveness of ginkgo in treating problems associated with deficient somatosensory processing (e.g. impairment of vigilance) and vestibular mechanisms (e.g. vertiginous syndromes).

Phytotherapy of Arterial Occlusive Diseases

Ginkgo

Botany/Key constituents ▸ Ginkgo consists of the leaves of the Chinese tree *Ginkgo biloba* L. (Fam. *Ginkgoaceae*). The *Ginkgo biloba* tree, cultivated in various parts of the world including France, USA, Japan, Korea and China, is the oldest tree on the earth: more than 200 million years old. Individual ginkgo trees sometimes lives more than 1.000 years. The leaves are fanshaped with bifurcated ribs and glabrous (see plate 14.4). They are fresh green to golden yellow in autumn. Ginkgo contains terpenoids (bilobalide, ginkgolides), flavonoids and other compounds like amino acids.

Box 14.3

Clinical evidence of ginkgo from randomized clinical trials. Analysis of systematic reviews or meta-analysis

Dementia

Dementia is defined as "acquired global impairment of intellect, memory, and personality, but without an impairment of consciousness. Pharmacological treatments for dementia are still being developed. Conventional drugs used (e.g. cholinesterase inhibitors) have given modest clinical benefits and serious adverse effects. The results of a recent systematic review[1] which included nine double-blind, randomised, placebo-controlled trials suggest that ginkgo is more effective for dementia than placebo. The findings are encouraging and warrant large scale confirmatory and comparative trials.

Alzheimer's Disease

Alzheimer's disease is the most common cause of dementia, accounting for 50–60% of all cases. Pharmacological tratment for Alzheimer's disease includes drugs which increase the endogenous levels of acetylcholine (acetylcholine precursors, releasers or inhibitors of its degradation). Serious adverse effects have been noted, including severe liver toxicity. Of more than 50 articles identified, the overwhelming majority were excluded primarily because of lack of clear diagnoses of Alzheimer's dementia. Only 4 studies involving a total of 424 subjects were analysed[2]. Based on a quantitative analysis of these studies there is a small but significant effect of 3- to 6-month treatment with 120 to 240 mg of ginkgo extract on objective measures of cognitive function in Alzheimer's disease.

Tinnitus

Tinnitus is the perception of sound in the absence of an external source. Causes include musculoskeletal and vascular sounds porducing tinnitus, and disorders of the peripheral and central auditory system, which usually produce tinnitus. Anti-tinnitus drugs include oral local anesthetics (tocainide), which can have serious adverse effects on the heart, benzodiazepines, which should be used sparingly because they can be habituating and tricyclic antidepressants, which have antimuscarinic and cardiac adverse effects. The results of a recent systematic review[3] which included five double-blind, randomized, placebo-controlled trials (n = 541 subjects) suggest that ginkgo is more effective than placebo. Although not fully conclusive, the findings are promising and warrant large scale confirmatory studies.

Intermittent claudication

Intermittent claudication is a condition caused by sclerosis of the arteries of the leg; it is characterised by a cramping pain in the calf muscles brought on by walking a short distance. Treatment is usually conservative and consists largely of regular physical exercise (regular walking is effective, but compliance is often poor) and pharmacological interventions (pentoxyfylline has a modest clinical effect). A recent meta-analysis[4] identified eight randomized, placebo-controlled, double blind trials involving a total of 415 patients . The results suggest that ginkgo extract (120–160 mg/daily for 24 weeks) is superior to placebo in the symptomatic treatment of intermittent claudication. However, the size of the overall treatment effect is modest.

Ginkgo and memory in healthy subjects

Ginkgo is promoted as a "smart" drug and hence used by healthy individuals. A recent systematic[6] review identified nine controlled trials of the cognitive effects of ginkgo in young subjects (n = 224 subjects; 20–40 years old) without cognitive deficits. All the trials were double-blinded and eight used a randomized design. The duration of the treatment was in general short (the longest had a treatment period of 30 days). In the nine studies reviewed, there is no evidence for a consistent positive effect of ginkgo upon any particular aspect of cognitive performance in healthy people. The use of ginkgo as a "smart" drug cannot be recommended on the basis of the evidence available to date, and there is a particular need for longer-term trials.

Macular degeneration

Loss of vision occurs frequently with advancing age. Age-related macular degeneration, the most common cause of visual loss in the elderly, is thought to result in part from oxidative damage to the retina. One published trial has been identified[5]. Although a beneficial effect was observed, as only 20 people were enrolled in the trial, and assessment of outcome was not masked, its results must be considered equivocal.

References

1. Ernst E, Pittler E (1999) Ginkgo biloba for dementia. Clin Drug Invest 17:301–303
2. Oken BS, Storzbach DM, Kaye JA (1998) The efficacy of Ginkgo biloba on cognitive function in Alzheimer disease. Arch Neurol 55:1409–1415
3. Ernst E, Stevinson C (1999) Ginkgo biloba for tinnitus: a review. Clin Otoryngol 24:164–167
4. Pittler M, Ernst E (2000) Ginkgo biloba extract for the treatment of intermittent claudication: a meta-analysis of randomized trials. Am J Med 108:276–280
5. Evans JR (2000) Ginkgo biloba extract for age-related macular degeneration. Cochrane Database Syst Rev 2:CD001775
6. Canter PH, Ernst E (2002) Ginkgo biloba: a smart drug? A systematic review of controlled trials of the cognitive effects of ginkgo biloba extracts in healthy people. Psychopharmacol Bull 36:108–123

Mode of action ▶ The well-documented activities of ginkgo (Box 14.2) in its enhancement of cerebral and peripheral blood flow and its anti-oxidant and free radical scavenging properties, together with its know antagonism of the activity of the pro-inflammatory agent, platelet-activating factor (PAF) are compatible with its widely reported therapeutic benefits in the treatment of both cerebral and peripheral vascular disease. Further, the recent observation of a reduced incidence of Alzheimer's disease in elderly arthritic patients self-administering high doses of anti-inflammatory drugs is also compatible with the importance of Ginkgo's anti-inflammatory role in ameliorating the disease process in Alzheimer's disease.

Clinical efficacy ▶ The German Commission E states that ginkgo is indicated for memory impairment (both vascular and degenerative dementia), concentration difficulties, depression, vertigo or tinnitus of vascular or involutional origin, headache, and intermittent claudication. Many systematic review/meta-analysis have been performed (Box 14.3). Most of these reviews concluded that ginkgo extracts were significantly more effective than placebo in reduce symptoms of intermittent claudication, dementia and cerebral insufficiency. One review found that ginkgo extracts might be effective in the treatment of tinnitus and another found insufficient evidence for efficacy in patients with macular degeneration.

Adverse events/Contraindications ▶ Ginkgo has generally been safe. Adverse effects most often reported in clinical studies were stomach complaints, nausea, headache, dyspepsia and allergic skin reactions. Because ginkgo acts as an anti-PAF, caution should be used when it administered with anticoagulants or anti-platelet drugs. In fact documented herb/drug interactions include spontanous bleeding when taken with aspirin and intracerebral hemorrhage when taken with warfarin.

Preparations/Dosage

Ginkgo is available in many countries in several pharmaceutical forms (tablets, liquids and parenteral preparations) and in a variety of dosages. In most studies the dosage of ginkgo was 40 mg three times daily of an extract standardized to contain 24% flavone glycosides and 6% terpenoids. This can be incorporated into liquids or tablets at 40 mg per ml or 40 mg per tablet. The German Commission E lists two special extracts made from *Gingko biloba* leaves (acetone-and-water extracts with an average herb-to extract ratio of 50:1) generally designed as Egb 761 or LI 1370

▶ *See Chapter 18 for the antiasthmatic properties of gingko*

Further Reading

Briankhaus B, Lindner M, Schuppan D, Hahn EG (2000) Chemical, pharmacological and clinical profile of the East Asian medical plant *Centella asiatica*. Phytomedicine 7: 427–448

Canter PH, Ernst E (2002) *Ginkgo biloba*: a smart drug? A systematic review of controlled trials of the cognitive effects of *ginkgo biloba* extracts in healthy people. Psychopharmacol Bull 36:108–123

Chang Q, Zuo Z, Harrison F, Chow MS (2002) Hawthorn. J Clin Pharmacol 42:605–612

Curtis-Prior P, Vere D, Fray P (1999) Therapeutic value of *Ginkgo biloba* in reducing symptoms of decline in mental function. J Pharm Pharmacol 15: 535–541

Diamond BJ, Shiflett SC, Feiwel N, Matheis RJ, Noskin O, Richards JA, Schoenberger NE (2000) *Ginkgo biloba* extract: mechanisms and clinical indications. Arch Phys Med Rehabil 81: 668–678

Ernst E, Stevinson C (1999) *Ginkgo biloba* for tinnitus: a review. Clin. Otolaryngol. 24: 164–167.

Ernst E, Pittler MH (1999) *Ginkgo biloba* for dementia. A systematic review of double-blind, placebo-controlled trials. Clin Drug Invest 17: 301–308

Evans JR (2000) *Ginkgo biloba* extract for age-related macular degeneration. Cochrane Database Syst Rev 2: CD001775

Kris-Etherton PM, Hecker KD, Bonanome A, Coval SM, Binkoski AE, Hilpert KF, Griel AE, Etherton TD (2002) Bioactive compounds in foods: their role in the prevention of cardiovascular disease and cancer. Am J Med 113 Suppl 9B:71S–88S

Mashour NH, Lin GI, Frishman WH (1998) Herbal medicine for the treatment of cardiovascular disease. Arch Intern Med 158: 2225–2234

Morelli V, Zoorob RJ (2000) Alternative therapies: Part II. Congestive heart failure and hypercholesterolemia. Am Fam Physician 62:1325–1330

Miller AL (1998) Botanical influences on cardiovascular disease. Altern Med Rev 3: 422–431

Pittler MH, Ernst E (1998) *Horse-Chestnut* seed extract for chronic venous insufficiency. Arch Dermatol 134: 1356–1360

Pittler MH, Ernst E (2000) *Ginkgo biloba* extract for the treatment of intermittent claudication: a meta-analysis of randomized trials. Med 108:276–281

Rohdewald P (2002) A review of the French maritime pine bark extract (Pycnogenol), a herbal medication with a diverse clinical pharmacology. Int J Clin Pharmacol Ther 40:158–168

Silagy CA, Neil HA (1994) A meta-analysis of the effect of garlic on blood pressure. J Hypertens 12: 463–464

Valli G, Giardina EG (2002) Benefits, adverse effects and drug interactions of herbal therapies with cardiovascular effects. J Am Coll Cardiol 39:1083–1095

Wang HX, Ng TB (1999) Natural products with hypoglycemic, hypotensive, hypocholesterolemic, antiatherosclerotic and antithrombotic activities. Life Sci 65: 2663–2677

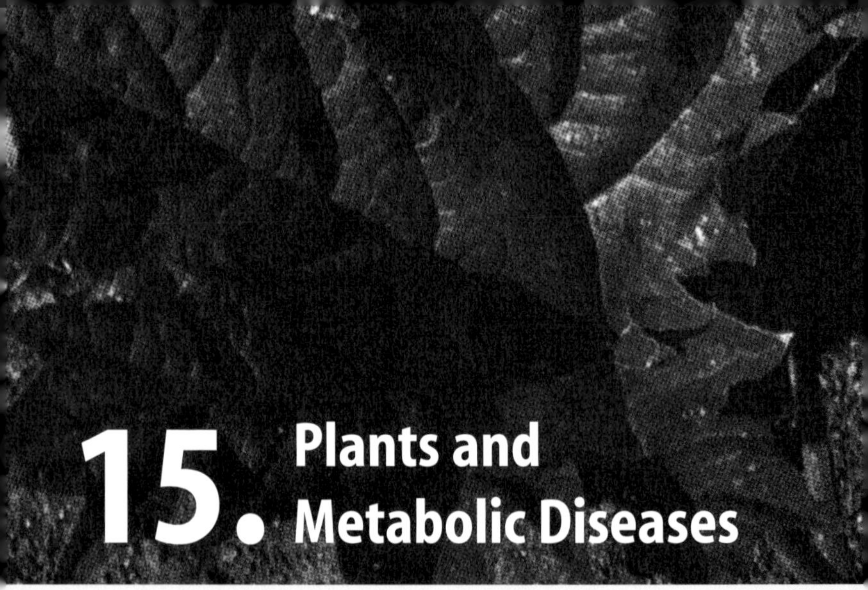

15. Plants and Metabolic Diseases

Introduction

Hyperlipidemia, obesity and diabetes are complex metabolic disorders affecting millions of people in the world. In the United States about 98 million people have elevated cholesterol levels, 58 million have weight problems and 16 million have diabetes. The cause of these diseases is not always known; it is assumed that they have a genetic component because they often run in families. Other factors involved are: age, diet, physical activity, ethnic background, environmental and psychological factors, and perhaps hormonal disorders. These diseases greatly increase the risk of premature death; in addition, they are the major risk factors for developing heart disease, stroke, high blood pressure, gallbladder disease and some forms of cancer. Most people with diabetes, weight problems or hyperlipidemia can lead normal lives and dramatically reduce the risk of serious complications by carefully balancing their diet and by increasing physical activity. In some cases, the use of drugs may help to normalize metabolic functions.

Lipid Metabolism

Clinical Picture

- Ingested fats are the main source of stored fuel in the body. These fats, and those that are synthesized endogenously, form a variety of functionally important compounds such as cell membrane components, bile, steroid hormones, and intercellular signaling molecules (e.g. lipid mediators such as prostaglandins, leukotrienes and PAF).
- Because lipids are insoluble in aqueous solutions, they must be transported in the plasma from tissue to tissue bound to proteins, hence the name, lipoprotein. The processes of dietary fat intake, hepatic synthesis of fat molecules, and delivery to target tissues are known collectively as lipoprotein metabolism (Box 15.1).
- Hyperlipidemias are common disorders in many countries. The most commonly encountered conditions are elevations of LDL, VLDL, or both lipoproteins produced by a combination of familial tendencies and dietary

Box 15.1

Lipoprotein metabolism and site of action of herbal medicines

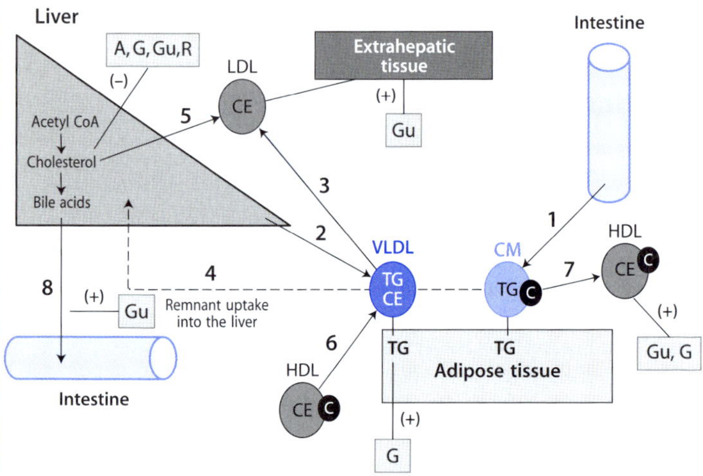

Movement of triglycerides (TG)

1. Ingested fatty acids are converted to triglycerides (TG), combined with apoproteins and covered by a phospholipid monolayer to form chylomicrons (CM).
2. Similarly, TG synthesized in the liver are combined with apoproteins to form very low density lipoprotein (VLDL). CM and VLDL have the highest TG content and therefore the lowest density.
3. While circulating through peripheral vascular beds, lipoprotein lipase in adipose tissues removes TG from VLDL and CM. Thus, the TG content is progressively lost and the density increases with the formation of intermediate density lipoprotein (IDL, not shown in figure) and low density lipoprotein (LDL).
4. CM and VLDL remnants are taken up by a hepatic uptake mechanism. Apoproteins serve as a cofactor for lipase activity in adipose tissues and for recognition for remnant uptake into the liver.

Movement of cholesterol

5. The liver synthesizes LDL particle for delivery of cholesterol to peripheral tissue. Extrahepatic tissues receive cholesterol ester (CE) through a recep-

tor mediated mechanism. Defects of the LDL receptor lead to familiar hypercholesterolemia.

6. The liver also synthesizes components of the HDL particle that contain apolipoproteins which facilitate cholesterol esterification and transfer of cholesterol esters to TG-rich particles. HDL cannot deliver cholesterol to peripheral tissues.
7. HDL also recovers non-esterified cholesterol (C) from CM and VLDL remnants for reuse by new TG-rich particles. This represents a mechanism for removing cholesterol from the peripheral circulation and reusing it in triglyceride-rich lipoprotein particles, which are less atherogenic than LDL.
8. Lastly, cholesterol is also the precursor of bile acids synthesized in the liver and delivered in the intestine. This represents the only way of elimination of cholesterol from the body.

Site of action of herbal medicines

Gugulipid (Gu) (i) increases the uptake of LDL into the liver, (ii) inhibits cholesterol synthesis into the liver, (iii) increases biliary excretion of cholesterol and (iv) increases the blood levels of HDL.

Garlic (G) (i) inhibits cholesterol biosynthesis, (ii) increases the degradation of TG via increased lipase activity in adipose tissues and (iii) increases HDL.

Artichoke (A) inhibits cholesterol synthesis into the liver.

Fenugreek (F) increases biliary excretion of cholesterol and also inhibits cholesterol re-absorption from the intestine (see also Figure 15.3)

Red yeast rice (R) inhibits cholesterol synthesis.

excess. They can be designated either primary or secondary depending on their causes:

- **Primary hyperlipidemias** can be divided into two groups: (1) those resulting from a single inherited gene defect, or more commonly (2) those caused by a combination of genetic and environmental factors. Specific deficiences include:
- defective LDL receptors (familial hypercholesterolemia)
- deficiency in lipoprotein lipase (Type I hyperlipidemia)
- deficient remnant particle clearance (Type III hyperlipidemia)
- **Secondary hyperlipidemias** are the results of more generalized metabolic problems, such as diabetes mellitus, excessive alcohol intake, hypothyroidism, or biliary cirrhosis. Therapeutic strategies for treating hyperlipidemia caused by one of these disorders include dietary inter-

vention plus a regimen of drugs used to treat the primary cause of the hyperlipidemia.

- Drug treatment of hyperlipidemia includes a variety of agents that (1) decrease production of a lipoprotein by the tissue, (2) increase catabolism of a lipoprotein in the plasma, or (3) reduce synthesis of cholesterol or increase its removal from the body.

Antihyperlipidemic Drugs

A large number of herbal medicines are promoted for hypercholesterolemia, including some of the top selling supplements. Table 15.1 lists some of these plants. Clinical evidence is promising for artichoke, gugulipid, garlic, fenugreek and red yeast rice which have demonstrated reduction in total serum cholesterol levels ranging from 10–33% in randomized trials. These herbal medicines are discussed here.

Artichoke

Botany/Key constituents ► The aerial part (globe) of *Cynara scolymus* L. (Fam. *Asteraceae*) is a natural source of food while the leaf is used in traditional medicine as diuretic, choleretic and hypolipidemic. It contains 1% caffeic acid deri-

Table 15.1
Antilipidaemic herbal medicines

Common name	Latin name	Part(s) of plant used	Key constituents	Daily dose
Artichoke	*Cynara scolymus*	Leaves	Caffeic acid derivatives, flavonoids sesquiterpene lactones	4–9 g
Fenugreek	*Trigonella foenum graecum*	Seeds	Steroid saponins, flavonoids, fibers	6 g
Garlic*	*Allium sativum*	Bulb	Alliins	4 g
Ginseng	*Panax ginseng*	Roots	Triterpene saponins	1–2 g
Gugulipid	*Commiphora mukul*	Resin from the bark	Volatile oil, triterpenes, mucilages,	a
Psyllium	*Plantago psyllium*	Seeds	Mucilages, fatty oil, iridoids (aucubin), proteic substances	12–40 g
Soy*	*Glycine max*	Soya lecithin from soy beans	Phospholipids, fatty oil, phytosterols	b

* supported by German Commission E
a. 75 mg guggulsterones
b. 3.5 g of phospholipids

vatives [e.g. 1,5-dicaffeoylquinic acid (cynarin), 5-caffeoylquinic acid (chlorogenic acid)], 1% flavonoids (luteolin, apigenin), volatile oils and sesquiterpene lactones (cynaropicrin). The root and fully developed fruit and flowers are devoid of cynaropicrin.

Mode of action ▸ The mechanism of action of artichoke has been investigated in a number of experimental studies; the final result is that more than a single mechanism contribute to the hypolipidemic activity (Box 15.1). Artichoke (i) inhibits the oxidation of LDL, (ii) inhibits the incorporation of acetate, thus reducing cholesterol biosynthesis and (iii) inhibits the enzyme hydroxymethylglutaryl CoA (HMGCoA) reductase, a key enzyme in the cholesterol biosynthesis (Figure 15.1). Cynarin has been suggested as the principle active component of artichoke. More recent findings indicate a role for the flavonoid luteolin in the inhibiting effects of artichoke on cholesterol synthesis.

Clinical efficacy ▸ Several studies published in the last thirty years report marked decrease in blood cholesterol and triglycerides in humans after the administration of artichoke extracts. However, a recent systematic review indicated the existence of only one randomized placebo-controlled clinical trial which assessed 44 subjects; it gave positive results in subjects with total cholesterol levels of 210 mg/d or above. This positive result has been confirmed in another double blind, randomized, placebo-controlled, multi-center clinical trial. Overall, the clinical effectiveness for lowering serum cholesterol is promising, but requires more controlled clinical trials.

Adverse events/Contraindications ▸ The safety data for the extract indicate only mild and infrequent adverse effects. Two rigorous trials report the absence of serious adverse effects and no changes in safety parameters in patients treated with 1.9 g per day of artichoke leaf extract compared to placebo. Artichoke could cause allergic contact dermatitis (the sesquiterpene lactone cynaropicrin is a potentially allergenic molecule), with cross-sensitivity to other *Compositae/Asteraceae plants* (e.g. feverfew, chamomile, calendula). A rare case of allergy after ingestion of artichoke has been described in patients affected by allergic rhinitis and asthma. Artichoke is contraindicated in patients with a blockade of the bile duct. Colic may occur if the patient suffers from gallstones.

Preparations/Dosage

The dose needed to achieve a clinical relevant reduction in cholesterol levels is 4–9 g dried leaves per day. This dose can be formulated into liquid extract (3–8 ml of 1:2 liquid extract). The usual dose in clinical studies is 640 mg artichoke extract three times daily.

▸ *See Chapter 22 for the cholagogue/choleretic properties of artichoke*

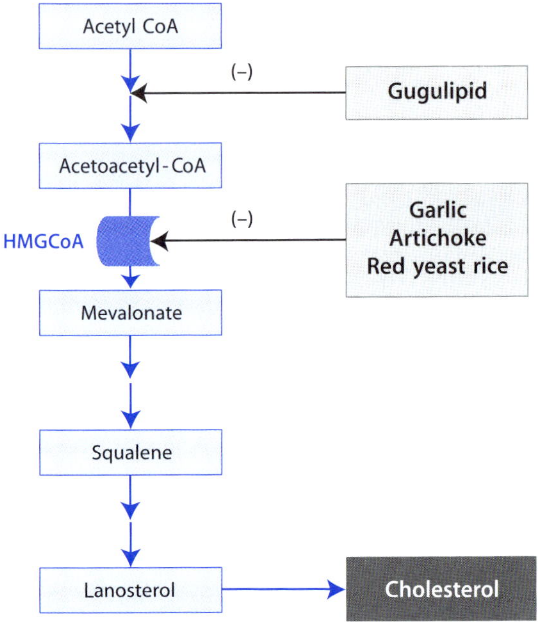

Figure 15.1 ▲ **Effect of herbal medicines on cholesterol biosynthesis in the liver**
Gugulipid reduces the incorporation of acetate. Garlic, artichoke and red yeast rice inhibit the enzyme hydroxymethylglutaryl (HMG)CoA, the rate-limiting enzyme in cholesterol biosynthesis. Ajoene, luteolin and monocolin K are the active ingredients, respectively

Gugulipid

Botany/Key constituents ▸ Gugulipid is a standardized neutral fraction extract of gum guggul (Box 15.2), a yellowish oleoresin obtained by the guggul (or guggulu) plant, (*Commiphora mukul* Hook., Fam. *Burseraceae*), a small, thorny tree native to Arabia, Pakistan and Northwest India. When tapped during the winter, the tree yields about 700–900 g resin per tree. Guggul plays an important role in Ayurvedic medicine in the treatment of rheumatoid arthritis, obesity and disorders of lipid metabolism.

Mode of action ▸ The exact mechanism of hypolipidemic and hypocholesteremic action of gugulipid is unknown, but several attempts have been made to unravel it. Thus, gugulipid (i) lowers serum levels of triglycerides and cholesterol by increasing the uptake of the lipoprotein VLDL and LDL into the liver; (ii) inhibits

Box 15.2

Chemical components in gugulipid

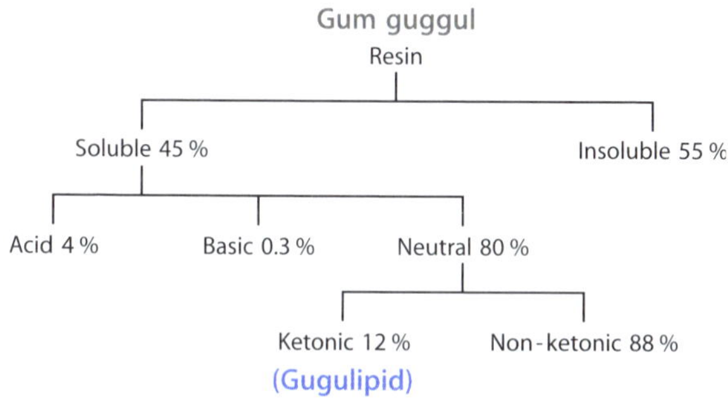

The resin is fractioned, first by mixing it with ethyl acetate, a non-polar solvent, to yield a soluble fraction and an insoluble fraction. The insoluble fraction contains the carbohydrate residues, which are toxic. The soluble portion is further subfractionated into acid, basic and neutral fractions. The acid fraction contains the anti-inflammatory components (i.e. ferulic acid, phenols, and other nonphenolic aromatic acids). The neutral fraction is further divided into ketonic and nonketonic subfractions, with the active components residing in the ketonic fraction. The ketonic subfraction contains lignans, diterpenes and alcohols. The active ketonic fraction consists of C21 and C27 sterols, mainly Z- and E-guggulsterones. Gugulipid is a standardized neutral fraction extract of gum guggul that contains a minimum of 50 mg guggulsterones per gram of extract.

the hepatic biosynthesis of cholesterol by reducing the incorporation of acetate; (iii) increases biliary excretion of cholesterol and (iv) increases the blood level of HDL, resulting in a cardioprotective effect (Box 15.1; Figure 15.1). Gugulipid can also act by stimulating the thyroid function. Active components of the hypolipidemic action are believed to be a series of sterols, named guggulsterones.

Clinical efficacy ▶ The clinical efficacy of gugulipid in reducing the serum cholesterol level is promising. A recent systematic review retrieved five randomized clinical trials, involving patients with hypercholesterolemia, hyperlipidemia, obesity and coronary artery disease. Four were placebo-controlled while one compared guggul to two reference compounds. A reduction in total serum cholesterol and triglyceride levels has generally been observed.

Adverse events/Contraindications ▶ Gugulipid is a fairly non-toxic product. In doses used for clinical efficacy, there may be mild skin rashes, headache, itching and gastrointestinal upset/diarrhea; it does not adversely affect liver or kidney function, hematological tests or blood sugar levels in diabetic patients. Gugulipid must be used with caution in the case of liver disease or gut disorders (diarrhea). Gugulipid also decreases the plasma level of the calcium antagonist diltiazem and the β_2-adrenergic antagonist propranolol.

Preparations/Dosage

Preparations include tablets (500 mg) containing 25 mg guggulsterones. The usual clinical effective dosage of gugulipid is 1500 mg daily (in three doses), which correspond to 75 mg guggulsterones.

Garlic

Botany/Key constituents ▸ Garlic (*Allium sativum* L. Fam. *Liliaceae*) has a rich history. It is mentioned in the Bible and was used by Hippocrates, Galen, Pliny the Elder, and Dioscorides. It originated from Central Asia, but nowadays it is known only in cultivated form. The subterranean garlic bulb consists of 4–20 cloves, each enclosed within a dry, white leaf skin. Garlic constituents are commonly divided into two groups: sulfur-containing compounds including alliin, alliicin, and non-sulfur containing compounds (enzymes such as alliinase). Alliicin is produced enzymatically from alliin and spontaneously degraded into a variety of other active sulfur-containing compounds (Figure 15.2).

Mode of action ▸ When garlic is crushed, alliin comes into contact with alliinase, which converts alliin to alliicin. This is considered (together with ajoene) to be the main active constituent of garlic's pharmacological properties. Garlic (i) inhibits cholesterol biosynthesis (Figure 15.1), (ii) increases the degradation of triglycerides via increased lipase activity in adipose tissues, and (iii) reduces LDL and (iv) increases HDL (Box 15.1).

Clinical efficacy ▸ The German Commission E states that garlic preparations are indicated "as an adjunct to dietary measures in patients with elevated blood lipids and for the prevention of age-related vascular changes". A recent meta-analysis, which included 13 randomized clinical studies suggested that compared with placebo, garlic reduces total cholesterol levels in people whose levels are elevated. Compared with conventional methods of lipid lowering, the reduction for garlic (4–6% reduction in cholesterol level) is unimpressive and the clinical significance uncertain. In comparison, dietary interventions have been shown to decrease total cholesterol by 5.3% after 6 months and statin drugs have reported reductions in total cholesterol level between 17% and 32%. The duration of the treatment ranged between 8 and 24 weeks.

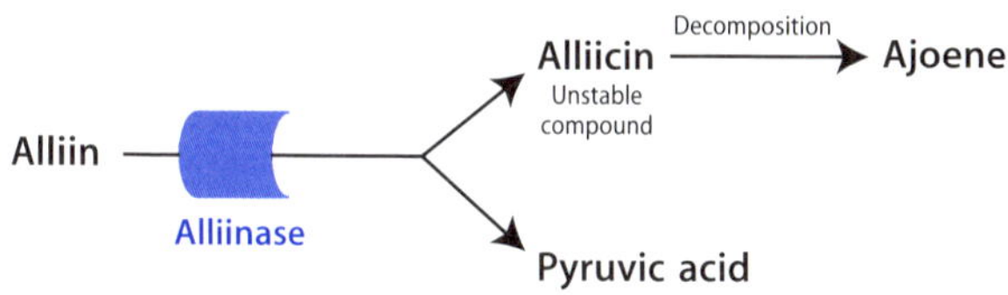

Figure 15.2 ▲ **Formation of alliicin and ajoene**
Intact cells of garlic bulbs contain alliin and the enzyme alliinase. When garlic is crushed, alliin comes into contact with alliinase, which converts alliin into alliicin. Alliicin spontanously degrades into ajoene. Both alliicin and ajoene are believed to be active ingredients. The enzyme alliinase can be inactivated by gastric pH and heat (50°C).

Adverse events/Contraindications ▶ Few adverse events were reported in clinical trials. German Commission E indicates that the side effects of garlic preparations are "infrequent gastrointestinal complaints, allergic reactions, and a garlic odor of the breath and skin". Hypotensive circulatory reactions can occur in less than 1% of patients. Theoretically, garlic may interact with anticoagulant therapy, resulting in a greater than desired anticoagulant effect.

Preparations/Dosage

The German Commission E recommends a daily dose corresponding to 4 g fresh garlic clove. Preparations include standardized powder (600–900 mg/daily), spray-dried powder (700 mg daily), essential oil (0.25 mg/kg body mass) and steam-distilled oil (10 mg/daily). These dried garlic preparations lack alliicin but contain alliin and the enzyme alliinase. Since alliinase is inactivated in the stomach, dried garlic preparations should be enteric coated so that they pass through the stomach into the small intestine where alliin can be enzymatically converted to alliicin. On the contrary, fresh garlic releases alliicin in the mouth during the chewing process.

▶ *See Chapter 14 for the antihypertensive properties of garlic*
▶ *See Appendix B for the use of garlic in cancer prevention*

Fenugreek

Botany/Key constituents ▶ Fenugreek is the seed of *Trigonella foenum-graecum* L. (Fam. *Fabaceae*), an annual herb native to South-eastern and Western Asia (Plate 15.1). Today the plant is cultivated on the Mediterranean rim. The seeds have been used as a condiment and food supplement since ancient times. It contains a high amount of fiber (48%), proteins (30%), lipids (7%), flavonoids and saponins. These saponins are present in the form of glycosides, such as diosgenin and fenugreekine.

Mode of action ▸ Several mechanisms for the hypocholesterolemic effect have been postulated. Fenugreek increases the excretion of bile acids with depletion of cholesterol stores in the liver. Moreover saponins may form complexes with cholesterol in the intestine, reducing its absorption; also the fiber content may reduce the rate of diffusion towards the mucosal surface and thus reduce cholesterol absorption (Figure 15.3).

Clinical efficacy ▸ There is good evidence in the literature of the clinical efficacy of fenugreek. A recent systematic review reports six randomized clinical trials. All six studies reported a reduction in serum cholesterol levels.

Adverse events/Contraindications ▸ There are not many adverse events associated with the use of fenugreek. Mild gastrointestinal symptoms such as increased flatulence, nausea, fullness and diarrhea are adverse events reported in clinical trials. Reduction of serum potassium levels and allergic reactions have also been reported. The drug is contraindicated during pregnancy. There is a potential for fenugreek to exaggerate the effect of concomitantly administered hypoglycemic drugs.

Preparations/Dosage

The daily internal dose of the crude drug is 6 g. Whole and powdered drug is available in the form of teas and compound preparations. Aqueous extract (2.8 g/daily) and defatted powder have been used in clinical studies.

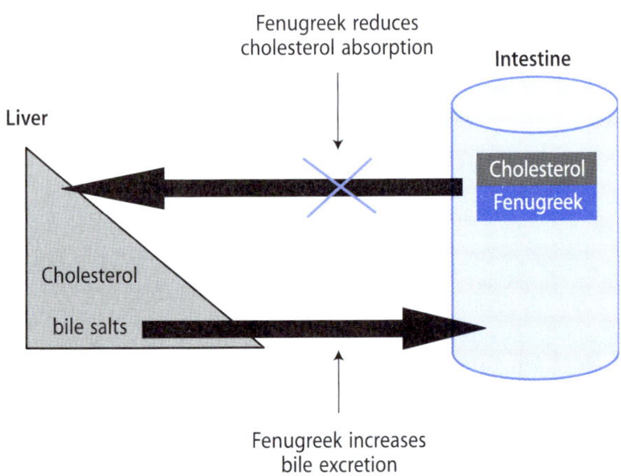

Figure 15.3 ▲ **Antihyperlipidemic action of fenugreek**
(see text for details)

Red yeast rice

Preparation/Composition ▶ Red yeast rice is produced by solid state fermentation of washed and cooked rice (*Oryza sativa* L., Fam. *Poaceae*) using the fungus *Monascus purpureus*. It has been used in Asia as a food preservative and colorant and for its medicinal properties since the Tang Dynasty (800 AD). Red yeast rice contains up to ten monacolins, sterols, isoflavones and fatty acids.

Mode of action ▶ Experimental studies have shown that monacolin K inhibits HMGCoA reductase (Figure 15.1) and thus cholesterol synthesis (Box 15.1). However, there is much debate and controversy surrounding the involvement of monacolin K in the mechanism of action of red yeast rice as the quantity of monacolin K present in red yeast rice is inadequate to fully explain the hypocholesterolemic action. Thus, other substances (including other monacolins) may be involved.

Clinical efficacy ▶ There is good evidence in the literature of the clinical efficacy of red yeast rice. On the other hand, monacolin K is an approved prescription drug in the USA under the name lovastatin (Mevacor). Three randomized clinical studies have been retrieved in a recent systematic review. All three studies reported significant reduction of total cholesterol level and LDL cholesterol in patients receiving red yeast rice. In two studies increases in HDL levels were observed.

Adverse events/Contraindications ▶ Adverse events experienced in clinical trials include stomachache, heartburn, dizziness and flatulence. Elevated increase of liver enzymes can also occur. A case of anaphylaxis in men who used red yeast rice in preparing sausages has been described. Adverse event of monacolin K (lovastatin) include muscle pain, tenderness, and weakness.

Preparations/Dosage

Red yeast rice is standardized to contain 0.4% monacolin K. Randomized clinical trials have been performed using red yeast rice extract (1.2–2.4 g/daily), sold under the brand name Cholestin.

Obesity

Clinical Picture

- Obesity is a major public health concern in the USA and UK, where the number of obese individuals has almost trebled over the last twenty years. Two-thirds of adults aged 45 years and over are now overweight or obese.

Using the WHO classification of obesity, more than one in five of the general adult population can be classified as obese. Overweight and obesity in children is a considerable public health problem in many Western countries. 5–6% of white boys and 9–10% of white girls are overweight in England. Obesity has become one of the most important avoidable risk factors for morbidity. The problem of tackling overweight and obesity is complex, although even modest weight loss confers significant medical benefit.

- Obesity results from an imbalance between energy intake and energy expenditure. Environmental factors, such as the general availability of high-caloric food or the limited need for physical exercise, and genetic factors that predispose to weight gain contribute to the development of obesity. Drugs used to treat obesity may have one or more of the following mechanism: (i) reduction of energy intake: appetite suppression; (ii) reduction of energy intake: inhibtion of absorption; (iii) increase of energy expenditure; (iv) modulation of fat storage.

Botanical Products for Weight Reduction

Many herbal medicines have traditionally been used to treat obesity; some of them are listed in Table 15.2. However, there is little evidence that herbal medicines are effective for body-weight reduction.

Ephedra consists of the dried aerial parts of *Ephedra sinica* Stapf. (Fam. *Ephedraceae*), a shrub, 60–90 cm high coming from China (Plate 15.2), where it has been used for thousands of years under the name "**ma-huang**" for the treatment of the common cold. Ephedra contains ephedrine and pseudoephedrine, which have stimulant effects on the central nervous system, resembling those of amphetamine, but which are less potent. Ephedrine is more potent than pseudoephedrine. Ephedra does not suppress appetite, but it promotes weight loss by increasing the metabolic rate of adipose tissue. This effect is greatest in individuals with a low basal metabolic rate and/or decreased diet-induced thermogenesis (Figure 15.4). Side effects of ephedra are the same as ephedrine (although to a lesser extent), which raises some doubt about whether this herbal preparation is clinically acceptable. They include increased blood pressure and heart rate, insomnia and anxiety. Drugs containing methylxanthines (coffee, tea, cola nut, guarana, matè) or salicylates (willow) can enhance the thermogenic effects of ephedra. Ephedra has not been extensively studied in clinical trials; a recent randomized clinical study has shown that the herbal mixture of ephedra and guarana effectively promoted short-term weight and fat loss. Dry mouth, insomnia and headache were the adverse symptoms reported most frequently by the mixture.

► *See Chapter 18 for the antiasthmatic properties of ephedra*

Table 15.2
Herbal medicines used to reduce body weight

Common name	Latin name	Part(s) of plant used	Key constituents	Daily dose
Garcinia	*Garcinia cambogia*	Pericarp of the fruit	Hydroxycitric acid	3 g
Guarana	*Paullinia cupana*	Seeds	Purine alkaloids (caffeine), tannins	1–3 g
Guar gum	*Cyamopsis tetragonolobus*	Endosperm of the seeds	Galactomannan, proteins	15 g
Kelp	*Fucus vesiculosus*	Thallus	Inorganic iodine salts, organic-bound iodine, polysaccharides	15–30 g
Ma-huang	*Ephedra sinica*	Aerial parts	Ephedrine, pseudoephedrine	a
Maté	*Ilex paraguariensis*	Leaves	Purine alkaloids (caffeine), caffeic acid derivatives, flavonoids	3 g
Psyllium	*Plantago psyllium*	Seeds	Mucilages, fatty oil, iridoids (aucubin), proteic substances	12–40 g
Rhubarb	*Rheum palmatum*	Rhizome, root	Anthraquinones derivatives, tannins, flavonoids	1–2 g

a. The average single dose is 15 to 30 mg total alkaloid, calculated as ephedrine, for a total dose of 120 mg per day

Guarana is prepared from the seeds of *Paullinia cupana* Kunth ex H.B.K. (Fam. *Sapindiaceae*). The plant is indigenous to the Amazon basin. Guarana contains 4–8% caffeine and 8% catechin-type tannins. Because of its caffeine content, it is widely used in Brazil to make a stimulating drink. As with many central stimulants, guarana is believed to reduce appetite, thus reducing food intake. As stated above, a clinical study has shown the effectiveness of guarana in combination with ephedra. In another double-blind, placebo-controlled, parallel trial with guarana, in combination with maté (leaves of *Ilex paraguariensis*, another caffeine-containing drug) and damiana (leaves of *Turnera diffusa* var *aphrodisiaca*), a significant weight loss over 45 days in overweight patients was induced. As a monotherapy, no clinical studies have been performed on guarana.

Guar gum is obtained from the endosperm of the seed of *Cyamopsis tetragonolobus* L. Taubert (Fam. *Fabaceae*), a 60 cm high plant cultivated in India and nowadays also grown in the USA. The main constituent of guar gum is a galactomannan (molecular weight ca 220.000). Experimental studies have shown that guar gum reduces the glucose and cholesterol blood serum levels. Because of its fiber content, it also reduces food absorption from the intestine. Whether guar gum is an option for the treatment of obesity has been assessed in a meta-analysis. Analysis of 20 double-blind, placebo-controlled randomized clinical trials including 392 patients suggested that, contradictory to other reports in medical literature, guar gum is not effective for reducing body-weight. Considering the adverse events associated with its use (i.e. abdominal pain, flatulence, diarrhea

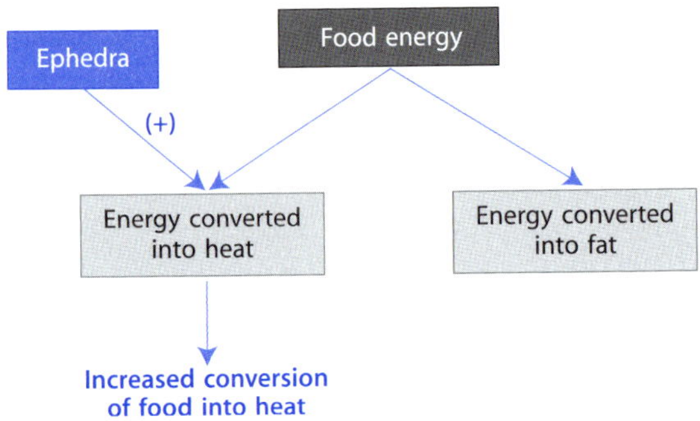

Figure 15.4 ▲ **Effect of ephedra on thermogenesis**
Thermogenesis is the direct conversion of ingested food into heat. A lean individual may produce a 40% increase in heat production, whereas an obese individual may only produce a 10% increase in heat production. In these people, the food energy is stored instead of converted to heat. Ephedrine increases thermogenesis, resulting in weight loss

and cramp), the risks of taking guar gum outweigh the benefits for this indication.

Kelp (also named bladderwrack or fucus) is the thallus (whole plant) of the seaweed *Fucus vesiculosus* L. (Fam. *Fucaceae*). The most important active component in kelp is iodine (up to 0.76% dry weight). This element plays an important role in the treatment of obesity. Nowadays, it is no longer used because of the untoward effects on thyroid activity when treatment ceases. The highest suggested dose of kelp will not lead to any of these problems, although it is unable to significantly increase basal metabolism (Figure 15.5.). There is a lack of clinical trials on the effect of kelp in treating obesity. Because of its iodine content, hypo- or hyperthyroidism can occur.

Rhubarb is the peeled and dried rhizome and root of *Rheum palmatum* L. (Fam. *Polygonaceae*), a perennial herb native to the mountainous regions of China (Plate 15.3). Key constituents include anthraquinones and tannins. Rhubarb is a component of the obesity-reducing Chinese herbal preparation Jiang-Zhi Jian-Fei Yao. There is a lack of pharmacological studies dealing with the effect of rhubarb on body-weight. Three randomized clinical trials (unblinded) involving a total of 472 obese patients (272 patients were children) without endocrinological or metabolic disorders have shown that the efficacy of rhubarb in treating simple obesity was similar to that of fenfluramine, but fewer adverse effects were observed. These findings are of potential interest, but the complete lack of double-blind trials is an obvious flaw.

► *See Chapter 21 for the laxative properties of rhubarb*

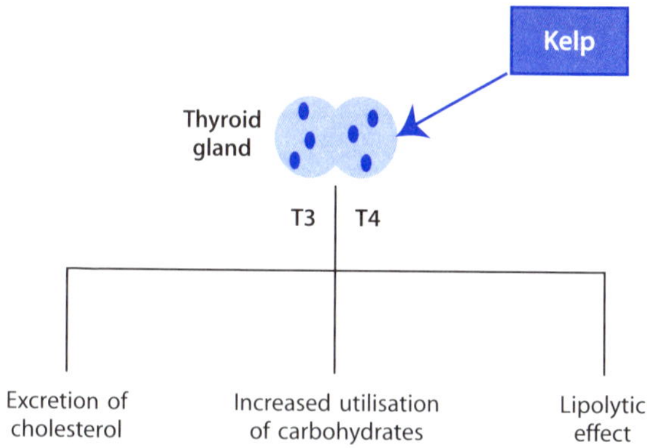

Figure 15.5 ▲ **Possible site of action of kelp**

Fucus contains high amounts of iodine, which is implicated in the synthesis of the thyroid hormones T_3 and T_4. Thyroid hormones are known to have a number of metabolic effects including:

(i) Stimulation of cholesterol metabolism to bile acids

(ii) Enhancement of lipolytic responses of fat cells to other hormones

(iii) Accelerated utilization of carbohydrates, presumably secondary to increased caloric demand

Garcinia (malabar tamarind) is the dried and cured pericarp of the fruit of *Garcinia cambogia*, which grows primarily in Southeast Asia. Garcinia contains up to 30% hydroxycitric acid (HCA). HCA may promote weight reduction through suppressed *de novo* fatty acid synthesis, increased lipid oxidation and reduced food intake. One potential mechanism accounting for the satiety effect of HCA may involve inhibition of citrate lyase (Figure 15.6). This would limit the availability of acetyl coenzyme A for lipid synthesis during carbohydrate feeding. As a result carbon is diverted to glycogen synthesis. Because HCA does not appear to enter the brain, it does not elicit CNS side-effects that may limit its acceptability. A high quality double-blind randomized clinical trial investigated the effects of garcinia extract for body weight reduction in 135 overweight individuals. They received either 1 g garcinia extract (50% hydroxycitrate) 3 times daily or placebo for 12 weeks. The results suggested no beneficial effect regarding weight loss beyond that observed with placebo. Moreover, another double-blind randomized clinical trial also reported no significant effect in subjects treated with 400 mg garcinia extract and 25 mg caffeine (guarana and green tea). Thus, the benefit of *cambogia* in reducing body-weight seems unlikely.

Psyllium (Plantago seeds) The crude drug consists of the ripe seed of *Plantago psyllium*, annual herb growing in the Mediterranean area. The seed is small (2–3 mm long), dark brown and looks like a flea (hence the name psyllium = flea). The epidermis of the seed coat contains mucilage that swells when the seed is

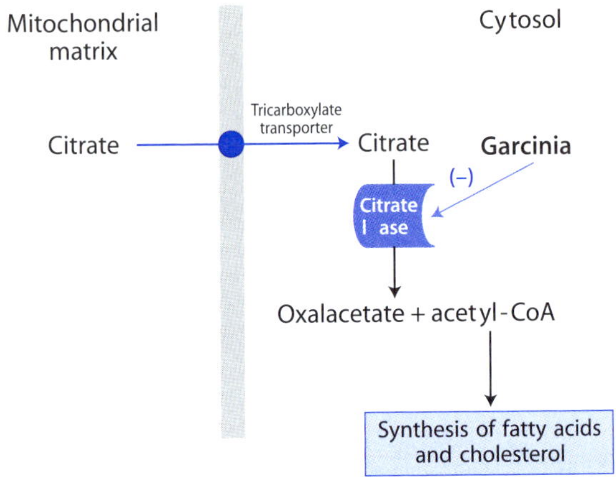

Figure 15.6 ▲ **Effect of garcinia on lipid synthesis**
Hydroxycitrate from garcinia inhibits the enzyme citrate lyase, which transform citrate into oxalacetate and acethyl-CoA. The reduced production of acetyl-CoA in the cytosol leads to a decreased synthesis of fatty acids

soaked in water. Ground seeds should not be employed, because the pigment of the seed coat may be absorbed and accumulated in the kidney tubules. The mucilage increases the fecal elimination of cholesterol and bile acids and decreases the intestinal reabsorption by binding them. It also increases the viscosity in the gut and slows down the resorption of sugar. Psyllium has been tested in a randomized, double-blind trial including 125 Type II diabetic patients. 15 g psyllium daily or placebo was administered for 6 weeks in addition to a low-fat diet. There was no significant reduction in body-weight in either group. Other clinical trials have shown that the consumption of psyllium lead to a modest decrease in total cholesterol. Rare cases of allergic reactions have been reported.

► *See Chapter 21 for the laxative properties of psyllium*

Diabetes Mellitus

Clinical Picture

- Diabetes is not a single disease; instead, it is a heterogeneous group of syndromes all characterized by an elevation of blood glucose, caused by a relative or absolute deficiency of insulin, the hormone secreted by the β cells of the endocrine pancreas. Based on the requirement for insulin, there are two types of diabetes mellitus:

- **Insulin-dependent diabetes mellitus (Type I diabetes).** This type of diabetes is thought to result from an autoimmune destruction of pancreatic β cells, with the consequent inability to secrete insulin. As a result of the destruction of β cells, the pancreas fails to respond to ingestion of glucose. Type I diabetic patients require exogenous insulin to control hyperglycemia and ketoacidosis. Type I diabetes mellitus usually occurs in people under the age of 30, (hence also named "juvenile onset" diabetes mellitus) and constitutes 10–20% of the diabetic patients. The disease occurs most commonly among juveniles, but it can occur among adults.
- **Non-insulin-dependent diabetes mellitus (Type II diabetes).** In these patients insulin is secreted, but is ineffective in normalizing plasma glucose. The cardinal finding is that increments in plasma insulin do no lead to the expected increases in glucose disposal. The decreased responsiveness to both endogenous and exogenous insulin is termed "insulin resistance". In some cases, insulin resistance can be due to a decreased number of insulin receptors. Patients with Type II disease constitute 80–90% of the diabetics and are often obese. The metabolic alterations observed are milder than those described for the insulin-dependent form of the disease. The goal in treating Type II diabetes is to maintain blood glucose concentration within normal limits and to prevent the development of long-term complications of diabetes mellitus. Weight reduction and dietary modification often correct the hyperglycemia. Hypoglycemic agents or insulin therapy may be required to achieve satisfactory serum glucose levels.

Phytotherapy of Diabetes

Herbal medicines are frequently used as treatment for diabetes in most cultures. More than 1200 species of plants have traditionally been used for their alleged hypoglycemic effects. Some of these plants are listed in Table 15.3. However, no convincing data exist demonstrating effectiveness for any of the remedies in question.

Theoretically, plant medicines could act as hypoglycemic agents through a variety of mechanisms. In the case of plants with high fiber content, glucose absorption might get retarded. For herbal medicines, however, this seems an unlikely mechanism of action. The volume consumed is simply not sufficient to cause such an effect. Other remedies might modify gastrointestinal peptides involved in insulin secretion. Further possible mechanisms might involve alterations in the sensitivity to or synthesis of insulin, inhibition of insulin or its enzymatic breakdown, interference with mitochondrial fatty acid oxidation or with gluconeogenesis.

Gymnema consists of the leaves of *Gymnema sylvestre* (Retz.) R. Br. Ex Schultes (Fam. *Asclepiadaceae*), a woody, climbing shrub that grows in the tropical forests of India. This plant has been used for over 2000 years in Ayurvedic medicine to treat "excess blood sugars" or "sweet urine", now recognized as diabetes. By chewing the leaves, the ability to discriminate the "sweet" taste is destroyed, giving its common name, gurmar, or "sugar destroyer". Key constituents include two resins, gymnemic acids, saponins, flavonoids and amino acids. Several mechanisms could contribute to the gymnema antidiabetic effects; experimental studies have shown that gymnema increases the release of insulin from β cells in the pancreas, increases the uptake of glucose into the cells, and reduces glucose absorption from the intestine (Figure 15.7). Moreover, sugar intake could also be reduced by the presence in gymnema extract of gurmarin, a protein which depresses the taste response to sugar. Gymnemic acid, which causes secretion of insulin and saponins (gymnesians), which reduces intestinal absorption, are believed to be in part responsible for the antihyperglycemic effect of gymnema.

Table 15.3
Antidiabetic herbs used in traditional medicine

Common name	Latin name	Part(s) of plant used	Key constituents	Daily dose
Aloe	*Aloe vera*	Dried juice of the leaves	Anthraquinone derivatives, flavonoids	0.1–0.2 g
Artichoke	*Cynara scolymus*	Leaves	Caffeic acid derivatives, flavonoids	4–9 g
Bitter melon	*Momordica charantia*	Seeds	Polypeptide-P	a
European goldenrod	*Solidago virgaurea*	Flowering tops	Triterpene saponins, flavonoids, volatile oil	6–12 g
Fenugreek	*Trigonella foenum-graecum*	Seeds	Steroid saponins, flavonoids, fibers	6 g
Garlic	*Allium sativum*	Bulb	Alliins	4 g
Ginseng	*Panax ginseng*	Roots	Triterpene saponins	1–2 g
Gymnema	*Gymnema sylvestre*	Leaves	Resins, gymnemic acid, saponins, flavonoids	b
Goat's Rue	*Galega officinalis*	Leaves	Guanidine derivatives, quinazoline alkaloids	2 g
Guar Gum	*Cyamopsis tetragonolobus*	Endosperm of the seeds	Galactomannans, proteins	15 g
Jambolan	*Syzygium cumini*	Seeds	Tannins, fatty acids	2–4 g
Onion	*Allium cepa*	Bulb	Alliins	20 g
Opuntia	*Opuntia streptacantha*	Cladodes	Polysaccharides	3 g

a. reliable data not available
b. the typical therapeutic dose of ethanolic extract, standardised to contain 24 % gymnemic acid, is 400-600 mg daily

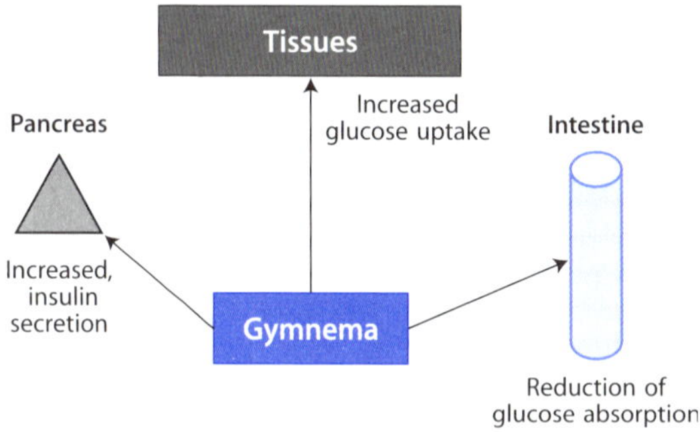

◀ Figure 15.7
Hypoglycemic action of gymnema
(see text for details)

Clinical studies have provided positive results in diabetic patients, but these studies are too preliminary to establish firm conclusions. The typical therapeutic dose of ethanolic extract, standardized to contain 24% gymnemic acid, is 400–600 mg daily. No significant adverse effects have been reported, aside from the expected hypoglycemia.

Opuntia consists of the cladodes of *Opuntia streptacantha* (Fam. *Cactaceae*), a cactus which traditionally has been used in Mexico for treating diabetes. Opuntia contains high molecular weight polysaccarides (up to 50%) and other substances which reduce absoption of glucose and cholesterol from the gastrointestinal tract. The daily dose is 3 g dried drug. There is only one randomized clinical study described in the literature. It showed that broiled stems of *O. streptocantha* lowers the glucose and insulin levels in non-insulin-dependent diabetic patients but not in healthy volunteers. The response was potentially meaningful, but these results are too preliminary.

Bitter melon (karela) consists of the seeds of *Momordica charantia* (Fam. *Cucurbitaceae*). It contains a polypeptide, named polypeptide-P, which elicited hypoglycemia in humans when injected subcutaneously. Other two polypeptides exhibit insulin-like activity. No randomized clinical trials have been performed. Non-randomized, non-blinded studies have generally shown decreased serum glucose levels. Bitter lemon is hepatotoxic in rats; two cases of hypoglycemic coma have been described after an overdose of bitter melon, while another case report indicated that bitter melon may increase the hypoglycemic effect of chlorpropamide.

Ginseng (*Panax ginseng*) contains ginsenosides that promote an insulin release and increases the number of insulin receptors. Ginseng also contains glycans designated panaxans A to E, which have hypoglycemic activity through an increase of insulin secretion from pancreatic islets. There is only one randomized clinical study described in the literature. It shows that ginseng reduced blood glucose levels in patients with Type II diabetes mellitus.

► *See Chapter 14 for the use of ginseng in the treatment of angina*
► *See Chapter 19 for the adaptogenic properties of ginseng*

Aloe vera (syn *Aloe barbadensis*) is a cactus-like plant that grows readily in hot, dry climates and, because of demand, is currently cultivated in large quantities. Cosmetic and some medicinal products are made from aloe vera gel derived from the mucilaginous tissue in the center of the Aloe vera leaf. The peripheral bundle sheath cells of Aloe vera produce an intensely bitter, yellow latex, commonly termed aloe juice, or sap. Aloe vera juice (laxative) and aloe vera gel (cosmetic) are often confused. Experiments in rats have shown that *A. vera* leaf pulp was inactive, *A. vera* gel extract was hyperglycemic, while *A. vera* leaf pulp extract displayed hypoglycemic activity. A recent systematic review suggests that aloe vera juice might be effective in reducing blood glucose in diabetic patients; however, the results are too preliminary.

► *See Chapter 23 for the dermatological use of aloe vera*
► *See Chapter 21 for the stomatic properties of aloe vera*

Further Reading

Ackerman RT, Mulrow CD, Ramirez G, Gardner CD, Morbidoni L, Lawrence VA (2001) Garlic shows promise for improving some cardiovascular risk factors. Arch Intern Med 131:813–824

Banerjee SK, Maulik SK (2002) Effect of garlic on cardiovascular disorders: a review. Nutr J 1:4

Berthold HK, Sudhop T (1998) Garlic preparations for prevention of atherosclerosis. Cur Op Lipidology 9:565–569

Boozer CN, Nasser JA, Heymsfield SB, Wang V, Chen G, Solomon JL (2001) A herbal supplement containing Ma Huang-Guarana for weight loss: a randomized, double-blind trial. Int J Obes Metab Disord 25:316–24

Chagan L, loselovich A, Asherova L, Cheng JW (2002) Use of alternative pharmacotherapy in management of cardiovascular diseases. Am J Manag Care 8:270–285

Chattopadhyay RR (1998) Possible mechanism of antihyperglycemic effect of *Gymnema sylvestre* leaf extract, Part I. Gen Pharmacol 31:495–496

Chattopadhyay RR (1999) Possible mechanism of antihyperglycemic effect of *Azadirachta indica* leaf extract, Part V. J Ethnopharmacol 67:373–376

Englisch W, Beckers C, Unkauf M, Ruepp M, Zinserling V (2000) Efficacy of artichoke dry extract in patients with hyperlipoproteinemia. Arzneimittelforschung 50:260–265

Ernst E (1997) Plants with hypoglycemic activity in humans. Phytomedicine 4:73–78

Gebhardt R (1998) Inibition of cholesterol biosynthesis in primary cultured rat hepatocytes by artichoke (*Cynara scolymus* L.) extracts. J Pharmacol Exp Ther 286:1122–8

Grosvenor PW, Gothard PK, McWilliam NC, Supriono A, Gray DO (1995) Medicinal plants from Riau province, Sumatra, Indonesia, Part I: Uses. J Ethnopharmacol 45:75–95

Grover JK, Yadav S, Vats V. (2002) Medicinal plants of India with anti-diabetic potential. J Ethnopharmacol 81:81–100

Heymsfield SB, Allison DB, Vasselli JR, Pietrobelli A, Greenfield D, Nunez C (1998) *Garcinia cambogia* (hydroxycitric acid) as a potential antiobesity agent: a randomized controlled trial. JAMA 280:1596–600

Jappe U, Bonnekoh B, Hausen BM, Gollnick H (1999) Garlic-related dermatoses: case report and review of the literature. Am J Contact Dermat 10:37–39

Morelli V, Zoorob RJ (2000) Alternative therapies: Part II. Congestive heart failure and hypercholesterolemia. Am Fam Physician 62:1325–1330

Moro CO, Basile G (2000) Obesity and medicinal plants. Fitoterapia 71:S73–S81

Pittler MH, Ernst E (2001) *Guar gum* for body weight reduction: meta-analysis of randomized trials. Am J Med 110:724–730

Shapiro K, Gong WC (2002) Natural products used for diabetes. J Am Pharm Assoc (Wash) 42:217–226

Stevinson C, Pittler Max H, Ernst E (2000) Garlic for treating hypercholesterolemia. Ann Intern Med 133:420–429

Thomson Coon J, Ernst E (2003) Herbal medicinal products for the treatment of hypercholesterolemia: a systematic review. Perfusion 16:40–55

Wang HX, Ng TB (1999) Natural products with hypoglycemic, hypotensive, hypocholesterolemic, antiatherosclerotic and antithrombotic activities. Life Sci 65:2663–2677

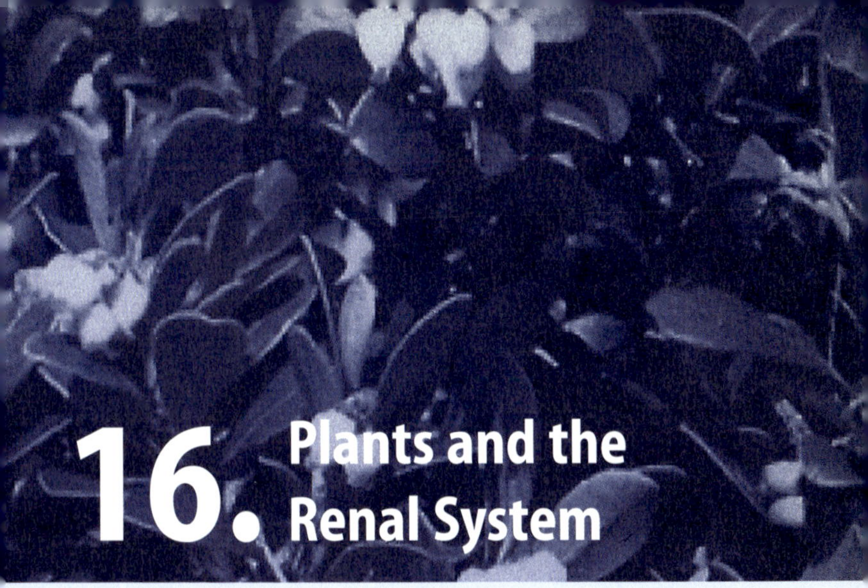

16. Plants and the Renal System

Introduction

The kidneys are the principal funtional unit of the renal system. They remove the breakdown products of protein metabolism, electrolytes, water and many drugs and their metabolites. The kidneys also regulate the volume of extracellular fluid, the concentration of extracellular electrolytes, pH of the body fluids and the blood pressure. Other components of the renal system include the bladder, the ureters and the urethra.

The most common problems with the renal system arise from: (a) renal infection, (ii) renal obstruction, (iii) renal failure or (iv) bladder infection. A prompt diagnosis and appropriate therapy are fundamental to preventing or eliminating glomerulonephritis (inflammation of the glomeruli), pyelonephritis (bacterial infection of renal tubules, interstitium and the renal pelvis), hydronephrosis (accumulation of urine within the renal pelvis), renal failure (slow progressive decline in glomerular filtration rate and hence in kidney function) and bladder infection.

The effect of herbal medicines on these disorders is for the most part limited to facilitating diuresis, preventing or treating urinary tract infections or treatment of urinary stones (Tables 16.1–3).

Infections of the Urinary Tract

Clinical Picture

- Urinary tract infections are among the most common bacterial infections, and the most common manifestations are cystitis (infection of the lower urinary tract) and pyelonephritis (infection of the upper urinary tract). Pyelonephritis is usually preceded by cystitis.
- Urinary tract infections are more prevalent in women than men. Apart from gender, several other factors predispose to urinary tract infections. Typical symptoms of a urinary tract infection include (i) a burning sensation when passing urine, (ii) increased frequency on micturition, (iii) increased nocturnal micturition, (iv) pyrexis.
- The majority of urinary tract infections are caused by organisms that originate from the patient's own intestinal flora. *Escherichia coli* is the

most common urinary tract pathogen, responsible for 80% of all urinary tract infections acquired outside a hospital. Infection of the urinary tract is treated with urinary antiseptics.

Herbal Urinary Antiseptics

Lower urinary tract infections are generally very responsive to phytotherapy. Several plant constituents can exert their antiseptic action as they are eliminated and concentrated in the urinary tract. Moreover, an increase of urinary flow induced by botanical drugs facilitates the clearing or 'washing out' of the urinary tract, which is believed to have beneficial effects. Plants used to treat lower urinary tract infections are listed in Table 16.1. In general, there is a paucity of randomized clinical trials dealing with the efficacy of herbal medicine in treating urinary infections.

Bearberry

Botany/Key constituents ▸ Bearberry or uva ursi consists of the dried leaves of *Arctostaphylos uva-ursi* (L). Spreng (Fam. *Ericaceae*), a small shrub growing in the mountains of the Northern hemisphere (Plate 16.1). The plant grows from stems and leaves and has bright red globular, edible berries. The leaf blade is coriaceous and shows a network of fine pinnate veins. Key constituents include phenolic glycosides (arbutin 6–10%, methylarbutin) gallotannins (pentagalloylglucose 15–20%) and flavonoids.

Mode of action ▸ The medicinal properties of the plant probably arise mainly from its arbutin content. It is well known that arbutin is hydrolyzed in the gut to yield a diphenol which is immediately oxidized to hydroquinone (Figure 16.1) Once absorbed hydroquinone is conjugated as the glucuronide and sulfate excreted in urine. In order for the antiseptic activity to occur the urine must be alkaline (> pH 8) to allow hydrolysis of the conjugates and to maintain the hydroquinone concentration > 60 µg/ml. To mantain the alkaline pH of urine, it is better to use a diet rich in milk and vegetables or to consume 6–8 g of sodium bicarbonate daily.

Clinical efficacy ▸ Bearberry has been widely used to treat urinary tract infections until 1950 and claims of its efficacy derive from non-controlled clinical studies, documented experience and experimental studies. Bearberry is approved by German Commission E for the treatment of infections of the urinary tract. However, no randomized clinical studies have been performed with the single herb preparation. A double-blind, placebo-controlled, randomized clinical trial showed that bearberry, in combination with dandelion (*Taraxacum officinale*) reduced the recurrence of cystitis in elderly women.

Table 16.1
Herbal mediciness used as urinary antiseptics

Common name	Latin name	Part(s) of plant used	Key constituents	Daily dose
Angelica*	*Angelica archangelica*	Fruits	Furanocoumarins, phytosterols, volatile oil	4.5 g
Asparagus*	*Asparagus officinalis*	Rhizome, roots	Steroid saponins, fructans, amino acids	45–80 g
Bean Pod*	*Phaseolus vulgaris*	Pods, beans	Lectins, saponins, L-pipecolic acid, flavonoids, chromium salts	5–15 g
Bearberry*	*Arctostaphylos uva-ursi*	Leaves	Hydroquinone glycosides, tannins, phenol acids	3 g
Birch*	*Betula spp.*	Leaves	Flavonoids, proanthocyanidins, triterpene alcohol esters	2–3 g
Buchu	*Barosma betulina*	Leaves	Flavonoids, mucilages, essential oil	3–6 g
Canadian goldenrod*	*Solidago canadensis*	Flowering tops	Triterpene saponins, polysaccarides, flavonoids, volatile oil	6–12 g
Cranberry	*Vaccinium macrocarpon*	Fruits	Fructose, acids, anthocyanins, flavonoids	a
Echinacea*	*Echinacea purpurea*	Aerial parts	Flavonoids, polysaccharides, flavonoids	0.9 g
European goldenrod*	*Solidago virgaurea*	Flowering tops	Triterpene saponins, polysaccarides, flavonoids, volatile oil	6–12 g
Horseradish*	*Armoracia rusticana*	Root	Gucosinolates (sinigrin and gluconasturtin)	20 g
Horsetail*	*Equisetum arvense*	Aerial parts	Flavonoids, caffeic acid ester, silicic acid, pyridine alkaloids	6 g
Java Tea*	*Orthosiphon spicatus*	Leaves	Volatile oil, flavonoids, caffeic acid derivatives, triterpene saponins	6–12 g
Lovage*	*Levisticum officinale*	Rhizome, roots	Volatile oil, coumarins	4–8 g
Nasturtium*	*Tropaeolum majus*	Whole plant	Glucosilonates, ascorbic acid, fatty oil, cucurbitacins	30 g
Parsley*	*Petroselinum crispum*	Aerial parts, roots	Myristicin, flavonoids, coumarins, volatile oil	6 g
Sandalwood*	*Santalum album*	Bark, wood	Volatile oil, tannins, resins	10 g
Spiny rest harrow*	*Ononis spinosa*	Roots, flowering branches	Isoflavonoids, volatile oil, triterpenes	6–12 g
Stinging nettle*	*Urtica dioica*	Flowering plant, roots	Flavonoids, silicic acids, volatile oil, amines	8–12 g
Witch grass *	*Agropyron repens*	Rhizome	Carbohydrates, volatile oil, flavonoids, saponins, minerals	6–9 g

* supported by German Commission E

a. 600–800 mg daily of standardized extract

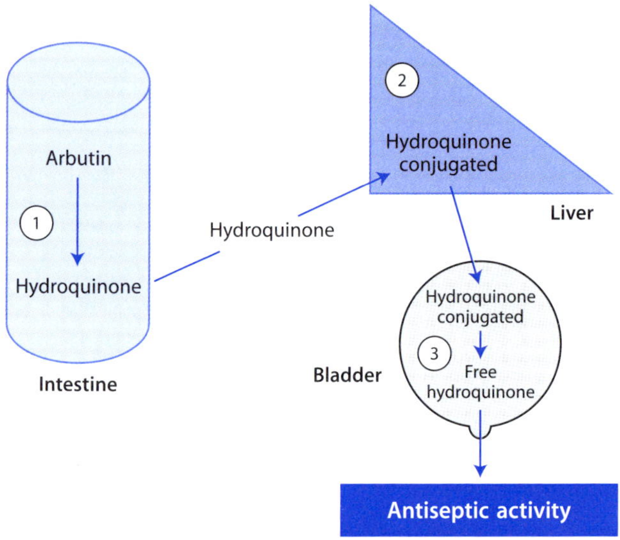

Figure 16.1 ▲ **Pharmacokinetic of arbutin, the active ingredient of bearberry**

1. Arbutin is a glycoside (i.e. formed by a sugar part and a non-sugar part, the aglycone) which is hydrolized in the gut to yield hydroquinone
2. Hydroquinone is absorbed in the plasma and conjugated as the glucuronide and sulphate in the liver
3. Conjugated hydroquinone is hydrolized in the urine (pH > 8) and thus the free hydroquinone can exert the antiseptic activity

Adverse effects/Contraindications ▸ There is very low risk associated with the short-term use of bearberry. Due to its content in tannins, the drug may cause nausea and vomiting in individuals with gastric sensitivity. According to the German Commission E, bearberry is contraindicated in pregnancy and lactation and for children under 12 years of age.

Preparations/Dosage

Normally it is used in the form of infusion (2.5 g dried drug in 150 ml boiling water; allow it to infuse for 15 min before straining and drinking). The treatment (3 g, that is 400–700 mg arbutin) must not be consumed for more than one week or administered more than 5 times per year because hydroquinone is toxic at a dose of 1 g. Bearberry preparations must not be taken at the same time as substances that can acidify the urine, as this will diminish the antibacterial activity.

Cranberry

Botany/Key constituents ▸ This is the American name of the fruit of *Vaccinium macrocarpon* Aiton (Fam. *Ericaceae*), a small shrub which grows abundantly in Eastern North America, from the Carolinas to Canada. It produces red berries (fruit), consumed as such and as juice (pure or as a cocktail sweetened with corn syrup). Cranberry is rich in fructose, acids (malic, quinic, citric, benzoic) and anthocyanins (3-O-galactosides and 3-O-arabinosides of cyanidin and peonidin); it also contains flavonoids and condensed tannins (proanthocyanidins).

Mode of action ▸ The activity was first attributed to the fact that the urine became more acid after eating large amounts of cranberries. It has successively been shown that the urine pH remained unchanged. Most recently it has been postulated that the antibacterial activity is due to the inhibition of bacterial adhesion to mucous membranes of the urinary tract (Figure 16.2). *E. coli* adhesion activity is inhibited by fructose and by a polymer of a procyanidin type.

Clinical efficacy ▸ Cranberries (particularly in the form of cranberry juice) have been used widely for several decades in the prevention and treatment of urinary tract infections. A recent systematic review found four randomized placebo-controlled clinical trials. Data from three out of the four trials indicated that cranberries were effective. No randomized trials were found which assessed the effectiveness of cranberry juice in the treatment of urinary tract infections.

Side effects/Contraindications ▸ Cranberry is considered to be a safe herbal medicine. Results of clinical studies indicate that cranberry juice may not be acceptable over long periods of time. Capsules may be more acceptable. Contraindications are not recorded.

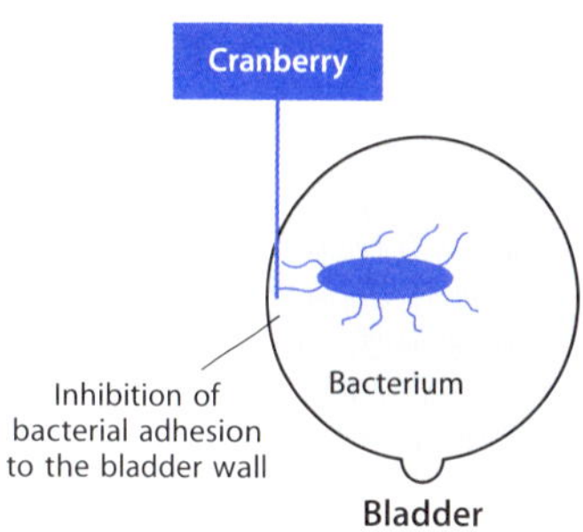

Figure 16.2◂ **Mechanism of the urinary antiseptic action of cranberry**
Cranberry is believed to inhibit the bacterial adesion to mucous membrane of the urinary tract

Preparations/Dosage

The drug is used as standardized extract (300–400 mg twice daily) as dilute juice (150–600 ml daily) or as dried juice capsules (300–400 mg twice daily).

Buchu

Botany/Key constituents ▸ Buchu consists of the dried leaf of *Barosma* (= *Agathosma*) *betulina* (Berg.) Bartl. and Wendl. (short buchu), *B. crenulata* (L.) Hook (oval buchu) and *B. serratifolia* Willd. (long buchu). All of these plants are small shrubs widespread at high altitudes around Cape Town in South Africa. The leaves contain flavonoids (diosmin), mucilage and an essential oil.

Mode of action ▸ *In vitro* studies have demonstrated some activity in the alcoholic extract of buchu against microflora typical of urinary tract infections. However, only the essential oil showed considerable activity against all the test organisms.

Clinical efficacy ▸ Buchu possesses a mild diuretic action and it is traditionally used to enhance diuresis in benign urinary disorders. However, no clinical studies of the urinary antiseptic and diuretic effects traditionally attributed to buchu are available.

Adverse events/Contraindications ▸ Buchu is a safe herbal medicine; however, occasionally it may cause gastrointestinal irritation if taken on an empty stomach. Like some other herbal diuretics buchu may cause hypokalemia, which can be avoided by supplementing the diet with foods rich in potassium. Buchu is stated to be contraindicated during pregnancy because of the presence of the irritant molecule pulegone.

Preparations/Dosage

Buchu is normally taken as an infusion prepared from the dried leaf (3–6 g per day).

Diuretics

Clinical Picture

- Diuretics increase renal excretion of sodium (Na) and water. The effect of most diuretics is to reduce the reabsorption of Na, with increased water loss being a secondary effect. Many synthetic diuretics are available. They show a different mode of action but the clinical indications are basically the same and include acute renal failure (they are administered to increase urine production), hypertension and edematous states.

Herbal Diuretics

Several botanical drugs containing flavonoids, saponins and/or volatile oil are able to increase the volume of urine without retarding the resorption of Na^+ and Cl^-. As a consequence these electrolytes are not excreted along with the water and therefore such diuretics are not useful for the treatment of edema or hypertension.

There is a lack of clinical studies dealing with the diuretic activity of herbal products. Examples in the literature of plants with direct diuretic effects producing consistent activity in controlled conditions are rare. Plant remedies traditionally used as diuretics are listed in Table 16.2. Some of these plants are described below. Herbal diuretics are contraindicated in the case of renal failure or diabetes.

Horsetail consists of the aerial sterile dried parts of *Equisetum arvense* L. (Fam. *Equisetaceae*), a shrub about 2 m high, which grows wild in Europe (Plate 16.2). The plant is fond of moist and swampy soils and also prefers siliceous clay. It presents two types of stems: fertile stems appearing in the spring, have no

Table 16.2
Herbal medicines used as diuretics

Common name	Latin name	Part(s) of plant used	Key constituents	Daily dose
Asparagus	*Asparagus officinalis*	Aerial parts	Flavonoids, steroid saponins, fructans, amino acids	a
Birch	*Betula spp.*	Leaves	Flavonoids, proanthocyanidins, triterpene alcohol ester	2–3 g
Celery	*Apium graveolens*	Seeds	Flavonoids, furocoumarins, fatty oil	1.2–4 g
Corn silk	*Zea mays*	Styles	Fatty oil, amines, tannins, potassium, saponins, sterols	40 g
European goldenrod	*Solidago virgaurea*	Flowering tops	Triterpene saponins, polysaccarides, flavonoids, volatile oil	2–6 g
Horsetail	*Equisetum arvense*	Aerial parts	Flavonoids, caffeic acid ester, silicic acid, pyridine alkaloids	4 g
Java Tea	*Orthosiphon spicatus*	Leaves	Volatile oil, flavonoids, caffeic acid derivatives, triterpene saponins	6–12 g
Stinging nettle	*Urtica dioica*	Flowering plant, roots	Flavonoids, silicic acid, volatile oil, amines	8–12 g
Witch grass	*Agropyron repens*	Rhizome	Carbohydrates, volatile oil, flavonoids, saponins, minerals	6–9 g

a. reliable data not available

chlorophyll and support a sporangium-bearing oblong spike; the sterile stems appearing later are articulated at the nodes. Whorled leaves of very small size are inserted at the nodes. Horsetail contains flavonoids, sterols, ascorbic acid, phenolic acids (e.g. cinnamic and dicaffeoyltartaric), minerals (SiO_2), alkaloids (nicotine), and saponins (e.g. equisetonine). Traditional medicine has long considered horsetail as a diuretic remedy. The drug is also considered a hemostatic and remineralizing agent. Experimental studies show a slight increase in water excretion. In some countries horsetail is indicated for inflammatory and bacterial disorders of the kidney, bladder and kidney stones. This mild diuretic is also used to solve static and post-traumatic edema. It is contraindicated in edema due to impaired cardiac or renal function. The preparation widely used is an infusion prepared by adding 4 g (four teaspoonfuls) dried drug to 150 ml boiling water. It is better to allow it to steep for 5 min before straining and drinking. Horsetail is also used externally in the treatment of wounds that do not heal well and in cosmetology to prevent cellulite and wrinkles. Horsetail is stated to be contraindicated in patients who have edema due to impaired heart and kidney function.

European goldenrod consists of the flowering tops of *Solidago virgaurea* L. (Fam. *Asteraceae*), a perennial herb (1 m high) common all over Europe, with a round purplish red stem with yellow flowers. Other species used in place of *S. virgaurea* are *S. gigantea* Aiton, *S. serotina* Kuntze and *S. canadensis* L. (**Canadian goldenrod**). European goldenrod contains flavonoids, saponins (virgaurea saponins I and II and other bidesmosides of polygalacic acid), phenolic acids (chlorogenic acid, virgaureoside A, leiocarposide), diterpenes, essential oil, tannins. The diuretic activity of goldenrod is attributed to flavonoids while the glycoside leiocarposide, which is hydrolyzed to salicylic acid in the gut, has shown anti-inflammatory and analgesic properties. However, some studies have demonstrated that leiocarposide possessess diuretic activity and that flavonoids and saponins reduce such activity. The saponins are antifungal *in vitro* and the polysaccharides have antitumor activity. However, there are no human studies to substantiate the properties attributed to this drug. In Europe goldenrod is used orally to enhance urinary functions and to increase urine quantity in the case of bladder and kidney inflammation. It is used in the form of decoction, prepared by adding 2 g dried drug to 150 ml water, bringing it to boil and allowing for 2–4 min before straining and drinking. The daily dose ranges from 2–6 g of drug.

Witch grass (Couch grass) is the rhizome, free of adventitious roots, of *Agropyron repens* (L.) P. Beauv. (Fam. *Poaceae*). It grows everywhere. The plant contains up to 10% carbohydrates (fructose, glucose, inositol, mannitol, fructosan), 0.05 % essential oil (agropyrene 95%), flavonoids, saponins and minerals. The presence of sugar molecules may account for a gentle diuretic effect throughout an osmotic mechanism (Figure 16.3). Witch grass is traditionally used to facilitate the renal elimination of water and as an adjunct in weight loss diets. Agropyrene is regarded as the main active principle in couch grass on account of its antibiotic

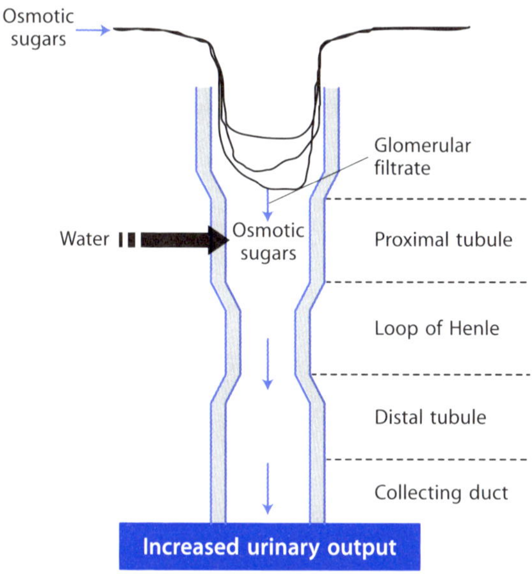

◄ Figure 16.3
Possible mechanism and site of action of witch grass
Osmotic sugars (e.g. fructosan, inulin) present in witch grass are filtered through the glomerulus and undergo little or no reabsorption; the filtered sugars will then carry water with them into the tubular fluid and thus increase the urinary output

effect (infections of the urinary tract). It is used in the form of decoction prepared by adding 50 g dried drug to 100 ml water bringing it to boil for 20–30 min before straining and drinking 150 ml every 3–4 hours/day. Capsules containing dried drug (0.4 g each capsule) are also available. No specific side-effects have been reported.

Corn silk consists of styles (stigma) of *Zea mais* L. (Fam *Graminaceae*), an herbaceous plant extensively cultivated in the world. It contains fixed oils, amines, tannins, not less than 1.5% potassium, saponins and sterols. Corn styles have traditionally been used to enhance the renal functions, to facilitate the renal elimination of water, and as an adjunct in weight loss diets. The drug is used in the form of decoction prepared by adding 40 g dried drug in 1000 ml water, bringing it to boil for 10 min before straining and drinking 200 ml every 3–4 hours/day. Corn silk may cause allergic reactions, including contact dermatitis and urticaria, in susceptible individuals. Specific contraindications are not recorded.

Table 16.3
Main herbal medicines supported by German Commission E to treat urinary stones

Common name	Latin name	Part(s) of plant used	Key constituents	Daily dose
Asparagus	*Asparagus officinalis*	Rhizome, roots	Steroid saponins, fructans, amino acids	45–80 g
Bean Pod	*Phaseolus vulgaris*	Pods	Lectins, saponins, L-pipecolic acid, flavonoids, chromium salts	5–15 g
Birch	*Betula spp.*	Leaves	Flavonoids, proanthocyanidins, triterpene alcohol esters	2–3 g
Canadian goldenrod	*Solidago canadensis*	Flowering tops	Triterpene saponins, polysaccarides, flavonoids, volatile oil	6–12 g
European goldenrod	*Solidago virgaurea*	Flowering tops	Triterpene saponins, polysaccarides, flavonoids, volatile oil	6–12 g
Horsetail	*Equisetum arvense*	Aerial parts	Flavonoids, caffeic acid ester, silicic acid, pyridine alkaloids	6 g
Java tea	*Orthosiphon spicatus*	Leaves	Volatile oil, flavonoids, caffeic acid derivatives, triterpene saponins	6–12 g
Lovage	*Levisticum officinale*	Rhizome, roots	Volatile oil, coumarins	4–8 g
Parsley	*Petroselinum crispum*	Herb, root, fruit	Myristicin, flavonoids, furocoumarins, volatile oil	6 g
Butterbur	*Petasites hybridus*	Roots	Sesquiterpene alcohol esters, volatile oil, alkaloids	4–6 g
Spiny rest harrow	*Ononis spinosa*	Roots, flowering branches	Isoflavonoids, volatile oil, triterpenes	6–12 g
Stinging nettle	*Urtica dioica*	Flowering plant, roots	Flavonoids, silicic acid, volatile oil, amines	8–12 g
Witch grass	*Agropyron repens*	Rhizome	Carbohydrates, volatile oil, flavonoids, saponins, minerals	6–9 g

Urinary Stones

Clinical Picture

- Renal stones develop when poorly soluble substances (calcium oxalate, calcium phosphate, uric acid, cystine) crystallize in the urine and the crystals aggregate to form particles large enough to lodge within the urinary system, in the presence of a low urine volume. Hence diuretics from botanicals may be useful in the prevention of kidney stones.

Phytotherapy of Urinary Stones

Table 16.3 lists some herbal medicines supported by German Commission E to treat urinary stones. Their solvent action on uric acid stones is probably linked to the alkalinizing capacity of the herb and to a possible urinary antiseptic activity. Other Asiatic herbal products have been shown to reduce experimental renal stones formation. In Ayurveda, *Crataeva nurvala* is highly acclaimed for its use in the management of kidney stones.

Further Reading

Hickey J (2000) Managing lower urinary tract infections. What is the best approach? Can Fam Physician 46:1577–1578

Howell AB (2002) Cranberry proanthocyanidins and the maintenance of urinary tract health. Crit Rev Food Sci Nutr 42(3 Suppl):273–278

Jaeger P (1996) Genetic versus environmental factors in renal stone disease. Curr Opin Nephrol Hypertens 5:342–346

Jepson RG, Mihaljevic L, Craig J (2000) Cranberries for treating urinary tract infections. Cochrane Database Syst Rev 2:CD001322

Krieger JN (2002) Urinary tract infections: what's new? J Urol 168:2351–2358

Lowe FC, Fagelman E (2001) Cranberry juice and urinary tract infections: what is the evidence? Urology 57:407–413

Newton M, Combest W, Kosier JH (2001) Select herbal remedies used to treat common urologic conditions. Urol Nurs 21:232–234

Patel N, Daniels IR (2000) Botanical perspectives on health of cystitis and cranberries. J R Soc Health 120:52–53

Reid G (1999) Potential preventive strategies and therapies in urinary tract infection. World J Urol 17:359–363

Reid G. (2002) The role of cranberry and probiotics in intestinal and urogenital tract health. Crit Rev Food Sci Nutr 42(3 Suppl):293–300

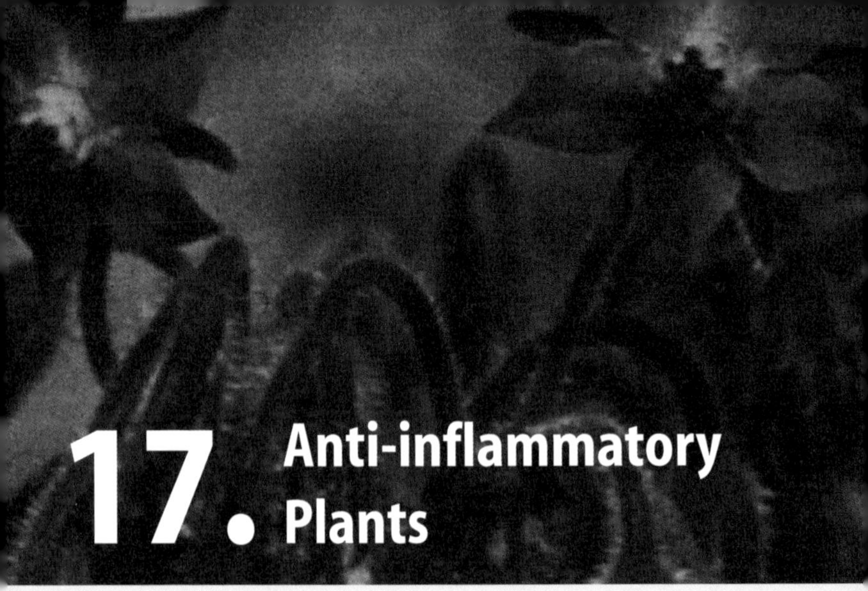

17. Anti-inflammatory Plants

Introduction

Inflammation is a normal, protective response to tissue injury caused by physical trauma, noxious chemicals, or microbiological agents. Inflammation is the body's effort to inactivate or destroy invading organisms, remove irritants, and set the stage for tissue repair. When healing is complete, the inflammatory process usually subsides.

There are certain features of the inflammatory process that are generally agreed to be characteristic. These include fenestration of the microvasculature, leakage of the elements of blood into the interstitial spaces, and migration of leukocytes into the inflamed tissue. On a macroscopic level, this is usually accompanied by the familiar clinical signs of erythema, edema, hyperalgesia, and pain.

Inflammation is triggered by the release of chemical mediators from injured tissues and migrating cells (Figure 17.1). These include amines (histamine, 5-hydroxytryptamine (5-HT), lipids (prostaglandins, leukotrienes, PAF), small peptides (bradykinins) and larger peptides (cytokines). The great variety of chemical mediators can explain why different drugs are effective in treating one form of inflammation but not others.

Inflammatory Diseases

Clinical Picture

- **Rheumatoid arthritis** is a chronic inflammatory disease of joints resulting in joint pain, swelling, and destruction. It is characterized by chronic inflammation in the synovium, which lines the joint. The synovium is inflamed, with an accumulation of leukocytes and mononuclear cells. Proteinases, prostaglandins, leukotrienes, and reactive oxidants have all been implicated as mediators in the inflammatory changes and tissue destruction of the synovial lining. The treatment of rheumatoid arthritis is generally symptomatic and involves the use of anti-inflammatory drugs.
- **Osteoarthritis** is a form of chronic arthritis characterized by cartilagine degradation, mildly inflammatory or non-inflammatory joint fluid, joint-space narrowing and bone sclerosis. Osteoarthritis generally occurs in the

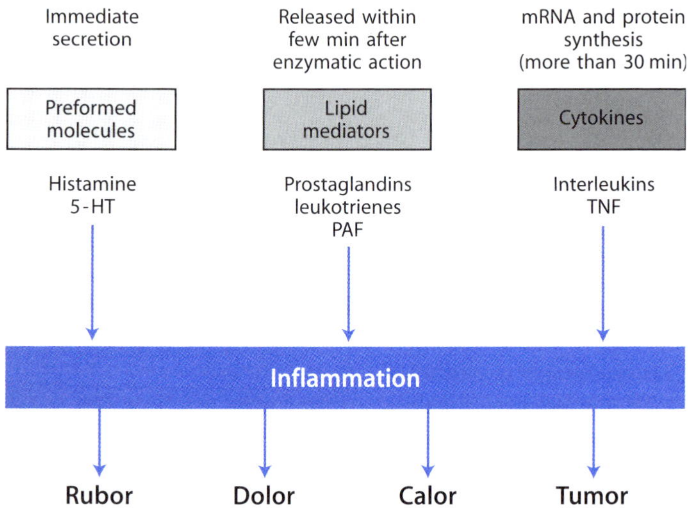

Figure 17.1 ▲ **Mediators of inflammation**
Inflammation is triggered by the release of chemical mediators from injured tissues and migrating cells. Such mediators include amines (histamine, 5-HT), which are preformed and immediately released, lipids (prostaglandins, leukotrienes and PAF), which can be formed upon appropriate stimulus within few minutes, and proteins (cytokines such as interleukins and TNF) which require more than 30 min to be formed. Characteristic signs of the inflammatory response are redness (rubor), pain (dolor), heat (calor) and edema (tumor)

older age group, or in those whose joints have been previously deformed for any reason. The most characteristic feature of osteoarthritis is gradual progressive cartilage loss. Local factors, including lysosomal proteases, neutral metalloproteinases and cytokines (e.g. interleukin-1), are involved in cartilage destruction. Drug treatment of osteoarthritis includes analgesics and non-steroidal anti-inflammatory drugs.

Anti-inflammatory Plants

Plants with anti-inflammatory activity are listed in Table 17.1. Compared to steroidal (e.g. cortisone) and non-steroidal (e.g. aspirin) anti-inflammatory drugs, herbal medicines play only a minor role in the treatment of inflammatory conditions such as rheumatoid arthritis and osteoarthritis. Nevertheless, some of them (e.g. devil's claw, nettle, willow bark) or some herbal formulation (Phytodolor®) have shown promising clinical efficacy associated to mild adverse reactions.

Table 17.1
Antinflammmatory herbal medicines

Common name	Latin name	Part(s) of plant used	Key constituents	Daily dose
Arnica*	*Arnica montana*	Flowers	Sesquiterpene lactones (helenalin), volatile oil, flavonoids	a
Ash	*Fraxinus excelsior*	Bark	Coumarins (isofraxidin), tannins, iridoide monoterpenes	b
Aspen (poplar)	*Populus spp.*	Leaves	Salicylic acid derivatives	10 g
Birch*	*Betula spp.*	Leaves	Flavonoids, proanthocyanidins, monoterpene glucosides	6–9 g
Blackcurrant	*Ribes nigrum*	Oil from the seeds	Fatty oil (gamma-linolenic acid, alpha-linolenic acid)	10 g
Borage	*Borago officinalis*	Oil from the seeds	Fatty oil (gamma-linolenic acid)	c
Cajuput*	*Maleleuca leucadendra*	Oil from leaves and twigs	Cineol, (+)-α-terpineol, (-)-α-terpineol	a
Camphor*	*Cinnamomum camphora*	Oil from the tree	Camphor	a
Chili*	*Capsicum annuum*	Fruits	Capsaicin, flavonoids, steroid saponins	a
Devil's claw*	*Harpagophytum procumbens*	Tubular secondary roots	Iridoids, triterpene, phenols	6–9 g
Eucalyptus*	*Eucalyptus globulus*	Oil from the leaves	Cineole	0.3–0.6 g
European goldenrod	*Solidago virgaurea*	Aerial parts	Triterpene saponins, polysaccarides, flavonoids, volatile oil	6–12 g
European mistletoe*	*Viscum album*	Leaves, branches	Lectins, polypeptides, mucilages, flavonoids	10 g
Evening primrose	*Oenothera biennis*	Oil from the seeds	Fatty oil (gamma-linolenic acid)	c
Feverfew	*Tanacetum parthenium*	Aerial parts	Volatile oil, sesquiterpene lactones (parthenolide), flavonoids	0.25 g
Garlic	*Allium sativum*	bulb	Alliins	4 g
Ginger	*Gingiber officinalis*	roots	Volatile oil, gingerols, shogaols, gingerdiols, starch	
Guaiac*	*Guaiacum officinale*	Resin of the heartwood	Triterpene saponons, resin, isoguajacin, volatile oil	4–5 g
Indian olibaum (boswellia)	*Boswellia serrata*	Resin gum from the tree	Boswellic acids	2–3 g
Larch*	*Larix decidua*	Bark	Volatile oil, resins	a
Rosemary*	*Rosmarinus officinalis*	Oil from the leaves, leaves	Caffeic acid derivatives, diterpenes, flavonoids, volatile oil (cineole, alpha-pinene, camphor)	a

continued on page 178

Table 17.1
Antinflammmatory herbal medicines (continued)

Common name	Latin name	Part(s) of plant used	Key constituents	Daily dose
Scotch Pine*	*Pinus spp.*	Oil from needles	(-)-α-pinene, δ-3-carene, limonene, camphene	a
Spruce *	*Picea spp.*	Oil from needles	Bornyl acetate, limonene, camphene, α-pinene	a
Stinging nettle*	*Urtica dioica*	Flowering plant	Flavonoids, silicic acid, volatile oil, amines	8–12 g
Tipi	*Petiveria alliacea*	Roots, leaves	Volatile oil, tannins	d
Thunder god vine	*Tripterygium wilfordii*	Roots	Saponins, di- and tetra-terpenes, tannins	e
White fir*	*Abies alba*	Timber of the fir	Limonene, α-pinene, camphene, bornyl acetate	a
White mustard*	*Sinapis alba*	Seeds	Glucosinolates, fatty oil, proteins	a
Willow*	*Salix spp.*	Bark	Glycosides and esters yielding salicylic acid, tannins	5–10 g

* supported by Commission E as antirheumatic or for other inflammatory states
a. generally for external use
b. ash is a component of the herbal formula Phytodolor®
c. 0.5–1.5 g gamma-linolenic acid
d. reliable data not available
e. 180–360 mg extract

Devil's claw

Botany/Key constituents ▶ Devil's claw is the tuberized secondary root of *Harpagophytum procumbens* (Burch) DC ex Meisson (Fam. *Pedaliaceae*), an African herb from the Southwest African desert regions. The plant is native to the savannahs of South Africa, Botswana and Namibia, and used in South African traditional medicine for the treatment of a variety of disorders, such as fever, stomach upsets, birthing pain and rheumatic diseases. Main constituents include iridoids (including harpagoside and harpagide), phytosterols, triterpenes (oleanolic acid) and phenols. The iridoids represent 0.5–3% of the weight of the dried drug. It is worth noting that other plant parts (flower, stem and ripe fruit) are devoid of harpagoside.

Mode of action ▶ Experimental studies have shown that devil's claw possesses analgesic and anti-inflammatory activity in rodents. *In vitro* studies have shown that devil's claw, in contrast to aspirin, does not inhibit cycloxygenase, the enzyme responsible for prostaglandins synthesis. Preclinical studies in humans suggest that the anti-inflammatory activity of devil's claw is related to inhibition

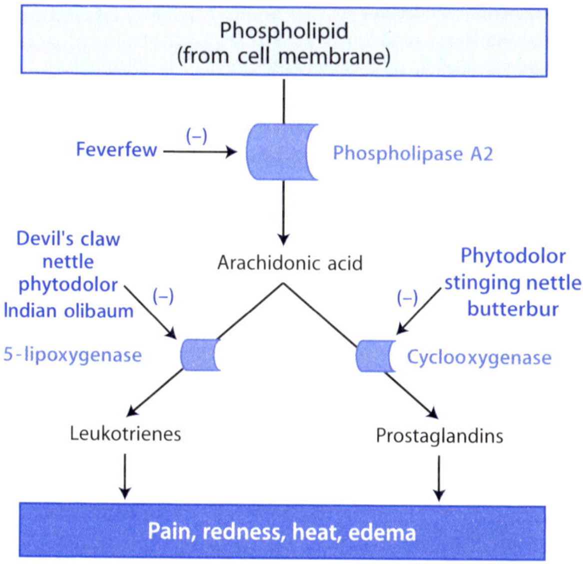

Figure 17.2 ▲ **Effect of some herbal medicines on arachidonic acid metabolism**
Tissue damage and the accompanying plasma membrane distortion activate phospholipase A2 enzyme activity which cleaves free arachidonic acid from its binding sites in membrane phospholipid. This renders it susceptible to enzymatic activity of cycloxygenase (with production of prostaglandins) and lipoxygenase (with production of leukotrienes). Prostaglandins and leukotrienes are pro-inflammatory molecules and thus they can produce inflammation, pain and fever. Inhibition of arachidonic acid metabolism result in an anti-inflammatory effect

of lipoxygenase enzyme (Figure 17.2), the enzyme responsible for leukotriene biosynthesis. Harpagoside is in part responsible for this activity. Other evidence indicates that devil's claw, but not harpagide or harpagoside, reduces TNF release from inflammatory cells.

Clinical efficacy ▶ German Commission E monograph states that devils' claw is indicated for the supportive treatment of degenerative musculoskeletal disorders. A recent systematic review report five randomized, placebo-controlled, double-blind clinical trials for rheumatic diseases (low back pain and osteoarthritis). All trial results indicate more pain-free cases in patients treated with devil's claw (3–4 weeks treatment) compared with placebo. Other evidence indicate that devil's claw is comparable in efficacy and superior in safety to the reference drug diacerhein in the treatment of osteoarthritis, reducing the need for analgesic and non-steroidal anti-inflammatory therapy.

Adverse events/Contraindications ▸ The frequency of adverse events associated with the use of devil's claw is low. The most frequent event reported is diarrhea which occur in about 8% of patients. The German Commission E cites gastric and duodenal ulcers as contraindications. Devil's claw is stated to be contraindicated in diabetics (hypoglycemic action) and in pregnant women; however, no scientific data were located to support these statements.

Preparations/Dosage

The European Scientific Coopertive of Phytotherapy (ESCOP) suggests that the daily dose must not exced 9 g dried root. This can be given as liquid extract (1:1 in 25% alcohol), tincture (1:5 in 25% alcohol) or solid preparations. *Harpagophytum* hydroalchoholic extract (400–1200 mg daily, corresponding to 30–100 mg harpagoside) has been used in most clinical trials. However, it should be noted that in commercial extracts the harpagoside content ranges from 0.8 to 5%. The German Pharmacopoeia prescribes a minimum content of 1% harpagoside based on the dried drug. Galenical forms of devil's claw are used topically (nebulizated) and orally; the latter are more active if used in gastro-resistant formulations.

Stinging nettle (flowering plant)

Botany/Key constituents ▸ The drug consists of the flowering plant of *Urtica* species (e.g. *Urtica dioica* L., Fam. *Urticaceae*), which are perennial plants growing in wasteland areas world-wide. They have a reputation for their savage sting from the hair and bristles present on the leaves and stems. The stinging sensation from contact with the hair is caused by the presence of formic acid and particularly amines (histamine, serotonin and choline). The stinging nettle flowering plant contains flavonoids, silicic acid and a volatile oil.

Mode of action ▸ Stinging nettle displays anti-inflammatory activity through several mechanisms; indeed *Urtica* extract inhibits cyclooxygene and lipoxygenase enzymes (Figure 17.2), responsible of the production of prostaglandins and leukotrienes, respectively. Moreover, nettle inhibits cytokine production. Nettle stew contains high amounts of a phenolic acid, which is an inhibitor of lipoxygenase.

Clinical efficacy ▸ Stinging nettle is a promising anti-inflammatory herbal drug. A 1987 Commission E monograph states that preparations of nettle (leaves and tops) are approved for use in the supportive treatment of rheumatic complaints. A randomized controlled study using a stew concocted from the aerial parts of the plant exhibited clinical efficacy in acute arthritis.

Adverse events/Contraindications ▸ Stinging nettle may have undesirable effects. In a postmarketing survey of 8955 patients, adverse effect occurred in 1% (n = 110).

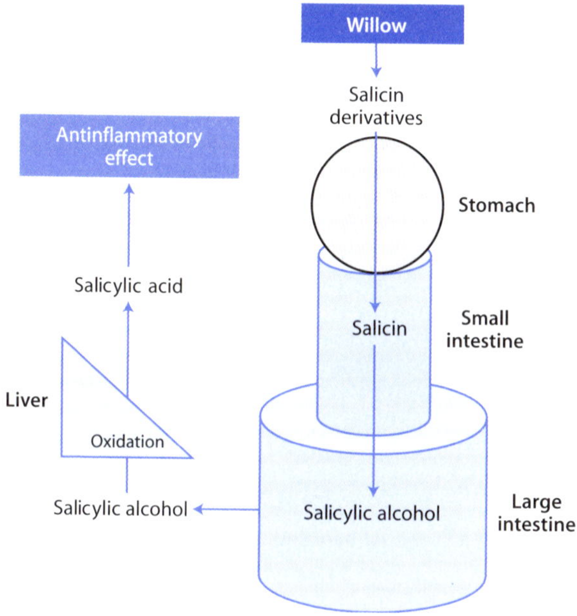

Figure 17.3 ▲ **Pharmacokinetics of salicin and its derivatives**
Salicin derivatives (salicin, salicortin, tremulin, tremulacin) are first converted into salicin in the stomach or small intestine. The salicin may then be absorbed in the small intestine but in humans it is mainly carried to the distal ileum or colon where gut bacteria convert this glycoside into its aglycone, known as salicylic alcohol. The salicylic alcohol is absorbed and oxidized (mainly in the liver) to give salicylic acid, which is the main active form.

They include gastrointestinal complaints (n = 57), allergic reactions (n = 12), pruritus (n = 6) and micturition (n = 11). The drug is contraindicated when there is fluid retention resulting from reduced cardiac or renal function.

Preparations/Dosage

The recommended average daily dose is 8–12 g crude drug. This can be administered by infusion or by liquid extract preparations (1:1 in 25% alcohol). To prepare an infusion, use 1.5 g finely cut herb in cold water, briefly bring it to the boil and steep for 10 min, then strain.

► *See Chapter 20 for the use of stinging nettle root in the treatment of benign prostatic hyperplasia*

Willow

Botany/Key constituents ▸ Willow is the bark of *Salix alba, purpurea* L., *fragilis* L., and other *Salix* species (Fam. *Salicaceae*), common in damp regions all over Europe. The drug is rich in tannins, flavonoids, glycoside and esters yielding salicylic acid (salicin, salicortin, tremulin and tremulacin).

Mode of action ▸ The anti-inflammatory activity of willow is determined not only by salicin but also by other phenolic glycosides (salicortin, tremulin and tremulacin). These compounds act as pro-drugs: they are slowly converted in the liver to salicylic acid (Figure 17.3). For this reason, the onset of drug activity is slower than in conventional salicylic acid derivatives, but has a more prolonged action. Salicylic acid inhibits the formation of inflammatory mediators. However, contrary to aspirin, salicin does not irreversibly inhibit platelet aggregation.

Clinical efficacy ▸ Willow bark is recommended by German Commission E for the treatment of fever, rheumatic disorders and headaches. The efficacy of willow bark in conditions such as low back pain and osteoarthritis is very promising. Results from randomised clinical trials indicate that willow bark may be a useful and safe treatment for low back pain and osteoarthritis (see appendix D).

Adverse events/Contraindications ▸ Willow bark is considered a safe herb. Rare cases of nausea, headache and digestive upset have been reported. It is stated that willow products are contraindicated in individuals with asthma, diabetes, gout, active peptic ulcer disease, hepatic or renal disease and in individuals sensitive to aspirin. Due to the salicin component, caution should be exercised when used in combination with salicylates and other non-steroidal anti-inflammatory drugs.

Preparations/Dosage

Daily doses of willow preparations [5–10 g raw drug; 1–2 ml acqueous extract (1:1, 25% ethanol); 5–8 ml hydroalcoholic tincture (1:5, 25% ethanol)] equivalent to 60–240 mg salicin are recommended. The ESCOP recommends a daily dose of 240 mg salicin per day.

Herbal formula (Phytodolor®) Ash, aspen, European goldenrod

Composition ▸ A standardized herbal preparation of *Populus tremula* leaves and bark (aspen), *Fraxinus excelsior* bark (ash) and *Solidago virgaurea* aerial parts (European goldenrod) (ratio 3:1:1) is sold under the brand name Phytodolor®. This patented formula is a liquid extract standardized to contain salicin 0.75 mg/ml, salicylic alcohol 0.042 mg/ml, isofraxidin 0.015 mg/ml and the flavonoid rutin 0.06 mg/ml.

Mode of action ► Phytodolor's mechanism of action is thought to lie in the inhibition of arachidonic acid metabolism via the cyclooxygenase and lipoxygenase pathways (Figure 17.2). However, Phytodolor may interfere with inflammatory processes in different ways, including by protecting cells from the oxidative stress damage. To this point it should be noted that aspen and ash have activity in experimental models of oxidative stress and oxygen detoxification, while goldenrod was inactive. The active ingredients are a mixture of compounds including salicin, salicyl alcohol, phenolcarbon acids, flavonoids, triterpensaponines and cumarin-derivatives.

Clinical efficacy ► The action of Phytodolor extends from non-inflammatory musculoskeletal pain to inflammatory rheumatic conditions. A systematic review of all double-blind, randomized clinical trials for rheumatic conditions included six trials for the treatment of osteoarthritis. These trials demonstrated significant results for pain reduction and non-steroidal anti-inflammatory drug (NSAID) consumption with administration of Phytodolor. They also suggested that Phytodolor is as effective as NSAID (i.e. diclofenac, indomethacin) but with fewer adverse effects. The notion that Phytodolor is useful for such conditions is furthermore supported by a number of uncontrolled clinical studies.

Adverse events/Contraindications ► Treatment with Phytodolor is not associated with adverse effects. The percentage of patients reporting adverse effects in clinical studies is very low and similar to the placebo. Rare cases of allergic reactions my occur after ingestion of aspen. It is stated that it should not be taken by anyone with known sensitivity to salicylates.

Dosage

The recommended dose is 20 drops three/four times daily mixed in water or in a beverage. The best results are expected 2–4 weeks after starting treatment.

Indian olibaum (boswellia)

Botany/Key constituents ► *Boswellia serrata* Roxb (Fam. *Burseraceae*) is a moderate to large branching tree found in India, Northern Africa and the Middle East. The medicinal part of the tree is the resin gum exuded when incisions are made in the bark of the trunk. Up to 16% of the resin is essential oil, the majority being α-thujene and p-cymene. Pentacyclic terpene acids are also present, with β-boswellic acid being the major constituent.

Mode of action ► Leukotrienes play an important role in inflammation, asthma and inflammatory bowel disease. Extracts from *B. serrata* gum have been shown to inhibit leukotrienes biosynthesis by impairing the 5-lipoxygenase activity (Figure 17.2). Boswellic acids are the chemical compounds responsible of such

Box 17.1

Possible mechanism of the anti-inflammatory action of gamma-linolenic acid (GLA), a component of evening primrose oil, borage oil or blackcurrant oil

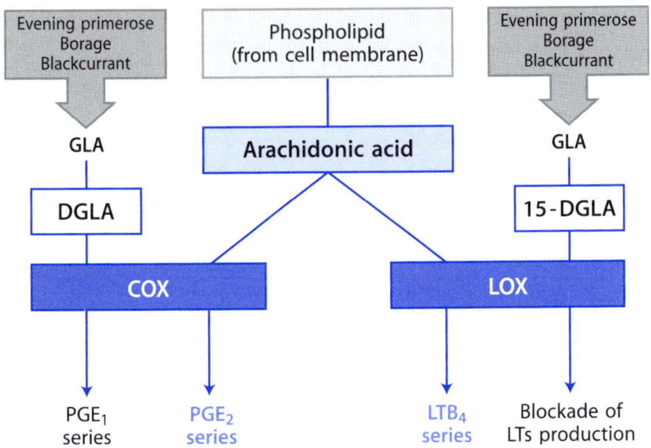

GLA can be metabolically converted into dihomoi-gamma-linolenic acid (DGLA), which is a substrate for cyclooxygenase (COX), the enzyme which generates 2-series prostaglandins (e.g. PGE_2). Great amounts of DGLA can competitively inhibit the action of COX on its natural substrate arachidonic acid, resulting in a reduction of the production of the pro-inflammatory 2-series prostaglandins. Moreover, DGLA through the action of COX can be converted in 1-series prostaglandins (e.g. PGE_1). Like PGE_2, PGE_1 is pro-inflammatory when given acutely. However, it has been suggested that PGE_1 has a negative feedback role in chronic inflammation, initially aiding in the development of the cardinal signs of inflammation (redness, edema, pain and heat) but later suppressing inflammation, and that this anti-inflammatory effect might be useful in a disease characterized by chronic inflammation such as rheumatoid arthritis. In the same way, GLA can be converted into a 15-hydroxyl derivative (15-DGLA) that blocks the transformation of arachidonic acid to leukotrienes.

activity. Indian olibaum has also been observed to inhibit human leukocyte elastase, which may be involved in the pathogenesis of emphysema.

Clinical efficacy ▶ Extracts of *B. serrata* resin gum have traditionally been used in the Ayurvedic system of medicine as an anti-arthritic. However, a preliminary placebo-controlled randomized clinical trial showed that 3.6 g extract daily was not effective in reducing pain or increasing function in 37 patients with rheumatoid arthritis. Preliminary positive results have been reported for the treatment of asthma treatment (see Table 18.1) and ulcerative colitis. Qualified clinical studies are needed to establish the clinical efficacy of Indian olibaum.

Adverse events/Contraindications ▸ No health hazards or side effects are known in conjunction with the proper administration of designated therapeutic dosages. Animal studies in rodents and primates have shown that doses up to 1 g/kg did not produce pathological changes in hematological, biochemical, or histological parameters.

Preparations/Dosage

According to Ayurvedic medicine, the daily dose is 1.5–3 g resin gum (or 56–122 ml bark decoction).

Essential Fatty Acid-containing Plants

Essential fatty acids (EFAs) are considered "essential" because our bodies cannot manufacture them; we must acquire them from external source (i.e. diet or in pharmaceutical preparations). Dietary manipulation of EFAs or supplementation with therapeutic doses of EFAs may be effective in treating inflammatory disorders. The ingestion of EFA [e.g. gamma-linolenic acid (GLA)] may suppress inflammation at least through two distint mechanisms (see also Box 17.1):

- competitive inhibition of the activity of cyclooxygenase and lipoxygenase enzymes, resulting in a decreased production of the pro-inflammatory substances prostaglandins and leukotrienes,
- production of prostaglandin E_1, which, although possessing an acute pro-inflammatory effect, can have inhibitory effects on pro-inflammatory cells, expecially in the chronic phase of the inflammatory process.

Herbal drugs rich in EFAs are borage oil, blackcurrant oil and evening primrose oil. Clinical data suggest that their use have a potential role in alleviating the symptoms of rheumatic diseases; moreover, these herbal medicines are well tolerated with negligible adverse effects.

Borage oil is obtained from the seeds of *Borago officinalis* L. (Fam. *Boraginaceae*), an annual plant indigenous to the near East and common in all neglected lands (Plate 17.1). The plant is currently cultivated to produce seeds, which are a source of oil-containing unsaturated fatty acids. The seed pod typically has about 25% oil content, which is particularly rich in GLA. To date two randomized, placebo-controlled, double-blind clinical trials have been performed. The main results of both studies show significant improvement of symptoms of chronic rheumatoid arthritis in patients receiving borage seed oil. Borage oil was given as oral capsules for 4 or 12 months (1.4 g gamma-linolenic acid daily). Borage contains hepatotoxic (pyrrolizidine) alkaloids.

Blackcurrant oil is obtained from the seeds of *Ribes nigrum* L. (Fam. *Grossulariaceae*), a bushy shrub cultivated in Europe. The oil contains high concentration of GLA but also high concentration of alpha-linolenic acid (ALA), and both are thought to have additive anti-inflammatory properties. ALA alone does not appear to improve symptoms in chronic inflammation. The only randomized, placebo-controlled, double-blind clinical trial yet performed suggest that blackcurrant oil (10.5 g daily subdivided in 15 capsules) reduced disease in patients with chronic rheumatoid arthritis, but many patients dislike taking 15 capsules per day. The European Scientific Cooperative of Phytotherapy (ESCOP) suggests the dosage of 20–50 g/l infused for 15 minutes up to 500 ml/daily.

Evening primrose oil is obtained from the seeds of the plants of the *Oenothera* species including *Oenothera biennis* L. (Fam. *Onagraceae*). The oil contains high concentration of GLA. The only randomized, placebo-controlled, double-blind clinical trial yet performed suggest that the evening primrose oil (540 mg of GLA per day for 15 months) may reduce the concomitant use of non-steroidal anti-inflammatory drugs. Adverse effects may include gastrointestinal symptoms and headache.

Table 17.2

Herbal medicines traditionally used to treat headache migraine

Common name	Latin name	Part(s) of plant used	Key constituents	Daily dose
Butterbur	*Petasites hybridus*	Leaves	Sesquiterpenes, pyrrolizidine alkaloids, volatile oil	4.5–7 g
Catnip	*Nepeta cataria*	Aerial parts	Volatile oil	1 g
Cola	*Kola acuminata*	Seeds	Purine alkaloids, catechin, tannins, oligomeric proanthocyanidins	2–6 g
European peony	*Paeonia officinalis*	Roots	Monoterpenes (paeoniflorin)	1 g
Feverfew	*Tanacetum parthenium*	Aerial parts	Volatile oil, sesquiterpenes lactones (parthenolide), flavonoids	0.12–0.25 g
Lemon balm	*Melissa officinalis*	Leaves	Volatile oil, glycosides, caffeic acid derivatives, flavonoids	1.5–4.5 g
Pasque flower	*Pulsatilla pratensis*	Whole fresh plant	Protoanemonine forming agents, triterpene saponins	0.2–0.6 g
Sweet marjoram	*Origanum majorana*	Aerial parts	Volatile oil, flavonoids	a
Sweet violet	*Viola odorata*	Rhizome	Volatile oil, saponins, alkaloids	1 g
Tansy	*Tanacetum vulgare*	Aerial parts	Volatile oil, sequiterpenes, flavonoids, coumarins	a

a. reliable data not available

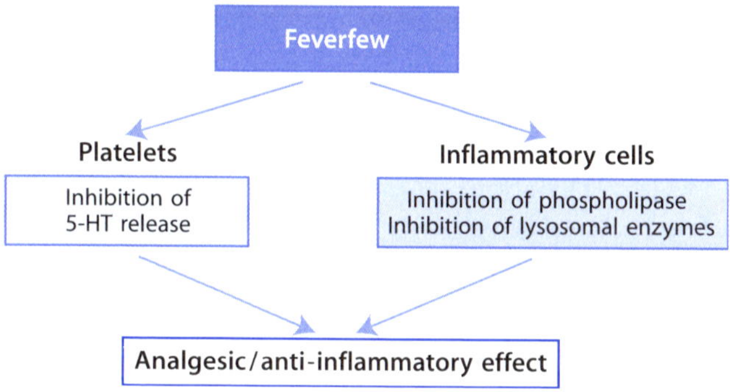

Figure 17.4 ▲ **Scheme of the possible analgesic/anti-inflammatory action of feverfew**

► *See Chapter 20 for the use of evening primrose oil in the treatment of premenstrual syndrome*
► *See Chapter 23 for the dermatological use of evening primrose*

Migraine

Clinical Picture

- Migraine is a common syndrome characterized by recurrent paroxysmal attacks of headache, often throbbing in character and sometimes, but not invariably, unilateral in distribution. The attacks, which often last for hours and less commonly for several days, are often preceded by visual or sensory phenomena accompanied by nausea or vomiting and photophobia. The aura or warning is due to arterial constriction, the headache is due to extracranial and intracranial dilatation. Often the headache occurs without an aura, less commonly the aura is not followed by headache.
- Migraine headaches are usually preceded by an asymptomatic phase where no symptoms or pathological features are evident. The acute attack is divided into a prodromal phase (characterized by visual disturbance and associated with arterial vasoconstriction, and release of serotonin) and a headache phase (characterized by pain, nausea, vomiting associated with cerebral vasodilation and below normal levels of serotonin).
- Drugs useful in the treatment and prophylaxis of migraine headaches include: (i) β-adrenergic blockers (e.g. propranolol) and methysergide, which are used in prophylaxis and (ii) ergotamine and anti-inflammatory/analgesic (e.g. aspirin or opioids such as codeine for the more severe pain), which are used to treat an acute attack.

Phytotherapy of Migraine

Plant remedies traditionally used as analgesic for the treatment of migraine are listed in Table 17.2. None of these is supported by German Commission E. Nevertheless, clinical evidence suggests a promising efficacy for feverfew and, to a small extent, for butterbut.

Feverfew

Botany/Key constituents ▸ Feverfew consists of the dried leaves (or aerial parts) of *Tanacetum parthenium* (Fam. *Asteraceae*), a perennial herb (grows up to 70 cm), indigenous to Asia Minor, and common in the neglected fields of Europe (expecially the Balkans) (Plate 17.2). The name stems from the Latin *febrifugia*, "fever reducer". The drug contains sesquiterpene lactones (e.g. parthenolide), a volatile oil, pyrethrin and flavonoids.

Mode of action ▸ Feverfew extracts inhibit the release of 5-HT from blood platelets and this could explain, at least in part, the antimigraine activity of the drug. Parthenolide is believed to be the chemical constituent responsible of this activity. Furthermore, feverfew inhibits eicosanoid synthesis by interfering with phospholipase A_2 and inhibits the release of enzymes involved in inflammatory processes (Figure 17.4).

Clinical efficacy ▸ Clinical data indicate that feverfew preparations might be efficacious for migraine prophylaxis, yet the evidence is far from compelling. A recent systematic review retrieved four controlled clinical studies (randomized, double-blind with placebo) with a total of 196 patients suffering of migraine. Compared to placebo, three studies reported positive results in favor of feverfew, while one reported negative results.

Adverse events/Contraindications ▸ Adverse events associated with feverfew use are generally mild and reversible. Mouth ulceration and gastrointestinal upset are the most frequent side effects experienced when using feverfew for a long time. Sudden discontinuation can precipitate rebound headaches (post-feverfew syndrome). Nervousness, tension, fatigue and joint ache can occasionally occur. Allergic contact dermatitis has been noted in many cases after contact with feverfew. The sesquiterpene lactones are responsible. Feverfew is contraindicated in individuals with a known hypersensitivity to other members of the family of *Compositae/Asteraceae* (e.g. chamomile) or in patients with coagulation problems (feverfew can alter platelet activity). Feverfew should be not used during pregnancy or breast-feeding.

Preparations/Dosage

Feverfew can be consumed simply by chewing the fresh leaves of the plant (or those freeze-dried or heat-dried at 37°C). Feverfew is also used either as tablets or capsules, each containing at least 125 mg dried drug (containing at least 0.2% parthenolide). One or two tablets daily are considered useful in the prophylactic treatment of migraines. A tincture (1:5, 25% ethanol; 5–20 drops daily) is also available. If chewed, feverfew may cause mouth ulceration, swelling of the lips and gastrointestinal upset.

Butterbur (Petasites)

Botany/Key constituents ▶ *Petasites hybridus* is a perennial European shrub which grows to a height of 1–1.5 meter and is usually found in wet, marshy ground, in damp forests, and adjacent to rivers or streams. Its downy leaves can attain a diameter of 1–1.5 m, making it the largest of all indigenous flora, and their unique characteristics are responsible for the plant's common name. The roots and leaves are used medicinally. The key constituents present both in the leaves and in the roots include sesquiterpenes (e.g. petasin and isopetasin), a volatile oil and pyrrolizidine alkaloids (e.g. senecionine and integerrimine).

Mode of action ▶ The current theory suggests that migraine is the result of vascular changes that lead to neurogenic inflammation, which is the immediate cause of pain. The sesquiterpene alcohol ester petasine and isopetasine are strong vasodilating substances, exerting a highly potent anti-inflammatory/analgesic effect through inhibition of leukotriene synthesis.

Clinical studies ▶ There is a paucity of clinical studies dealing with the efficacy of butterbur in treating or preventing migraine. In recent placebo-controlled, double-blind clinical trials it was found that two capsules twice daily of 25 mg extract of *P. hybridus* rhyzome for 12 weeks prevented the number, intensity and duration of migraine attacks and the accompanying symptoms. Petasites roots (but not leaves) are supported by German Commission E for kidney and bladder stones.

Adverse effects/Contraindication ▶ No adverse reactions have been reported in clinical studies. It should be noted that pyrrolizidine alkaloids possess hepatotoxic and carcinogenic effects; hence, the administration of the drug during pregnancy or by nursing mothers is strongly discouraged. The maximum daily dose of pyrrolizidine alkaloids is 0.1 mm. Alkaloid-free varieties of *Petasites* are now being cultivated.

Preparations/Dosage

Preparations equivalent to 4.5–7 g of subterranean organs may be used. Extract from petasites roots obtained with ethanol or lipophilic solvents are standardized to contain a minimum of 7.5 mg of petasin and isopetasin. The adult dosage ranges from 50–100 mg twice daily. From petasites leaves it could be prepared as an infusion (pour boiling water over 1.2–2 g drug, strain after 10 min, drink 2–3 cups of infusion per day).

► *See Chapter 18 for the use of butterbur in the treatment of allergic rhinitis*

Further Reading

Barre DE (2001) Potential of evening primrose, borage, blackcurrant, and fungal oils in human health. Ann Nutr Metab 45:47–57

Ernst E (1999) The efficacy of Phytodolor® for the treatment of musculoskeletal pain. A systematic review of randomized clinical trials. Nat Med J 2:14–17

Ernst E (2003) Complementary medicine. Curr Opin Rheumatol 5:151–155

Ernst E, Chrubasik S (2000) Phyto-anti-inflammatories. A systematic review of randomized, placebo-controlled, double-blind trials. Rheumatic disease clinics of North America 26:13–27

Ernst E, Pittler MH (2000) The efficacy and safety of feverfew (Tanacetum parthenium L.): an update of a systematic review. Public Health Nutr 3:509–514

Grossmann M, Schmidrals H (2000) An extract of *Petasites hybridus* is effective in the prophylaxis of migraine. Int J Clin Pharmacol Ther 38:430–435

Long L, Soeken K, Ernst E (2001) Herbal medicines for the treatment of osteoarthritis: a systematic review. Rheumatology 40:779–793

Pinn G (2001) Herbal therapy in rheumatology. Aust Fam Physician 30:878–883

Pittler MH, Vogler BK, Ernst E (2000) Feverfew for preventing migraine. The Cochrane Library 3:1–10

Schempp H, Weiser D, Elstner EF (2000) Biochemical model reactions indicative of inflammatory processes. Activities of extracts from *Fraxinus excelsior* and *Populus tremula*. Arzneim-Forsch/Drug Res 50:362–371

Thomet OA, Simon HU (2002) Petasins in the treatment of allergic diseases: results of preclinical and clinical studies. Int Arch Allergy Immunol 129:108–112

Thomet OA, Wiesmann UN, Schapowal A, Bizer C, Simon H (2001) Role of petasin in the potential anti-inflammatory activity of a plant extract of *Petasites hibridus*. Biochem Pharmacol 15:1041–1047

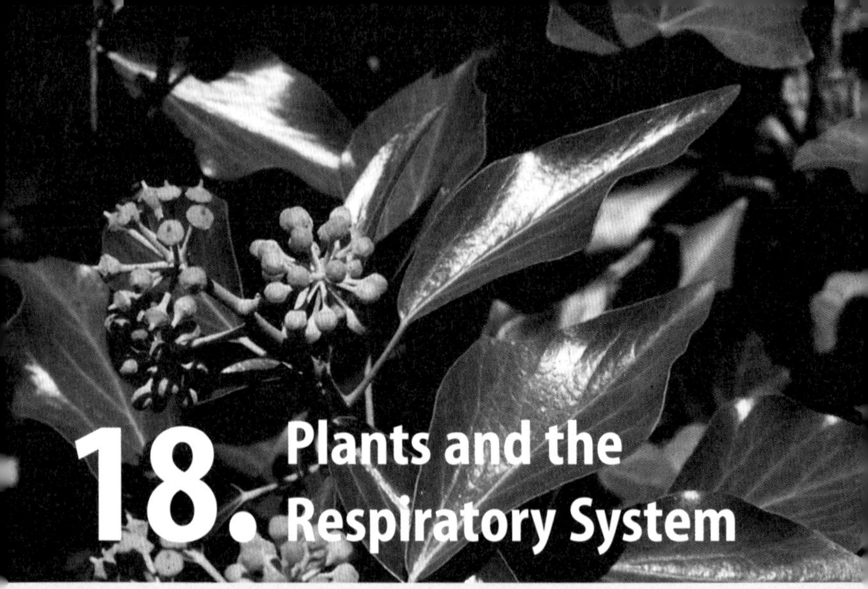

18. Plants and the Respiratory System

Introduction

The respiratory system is comprised of the lungs, bronchi and bronchioles. The major role of the respiratory system is to provide adequate oxygen for cellular metabolism, through which oxygen is consumed in favor of production of adenosine triphosphate (ATP) and carbon dioxide. The metabolic "waste" carbon dioxide is excreted through the lungs in the exhaled air, thus preventing an accumulation of harmful hydrogen ions in body fluids. Gas exchange occurs across the lung alveoli: being globular and extremely numerous (about 300 million in total) alveoli provide a huge surface area (about 70 m^2) for gas exchange with the blood.

Bronchial smooth muscle tone is produced by parasympathetic and non-adrenergic, non-cholinergic (NANC) excitatory nerves, which cause bronchoconstriction, and NANC inhibitory nerves and circulating epinephrine, which cause bronchodilation.

The most common diseases of the respiratory tract are asthma, allergic rhinitis, bronchitis and cystic fibrosis. These diseases can cause coughing, wheezing, shortness of breath and abnormal gas exchange. All these conditions can result from changes in the smooth muscle tone of the airways (e.g. bronchial asthma), mucous plugging (e.g. bronchitis) or vascular congestion of the upper respiratory tract (e.g. rhinitis).

Bronchial Asthma

Clinical Picture

- Bronchial asthma is a common disease affecting up to 20% of the population in some countries. It is characterized by difficulty in breathing caused by bronchospasm and dyspnea. The clinical features of asthma are believed to result from an inflammatory response in the airways involving local inflammatory cell accumulation (Figure 18.1). Inflammatory cells release cytotoxic mediators (including leukotrienes, free radicals, eosinophil peroxidase, eosinophil cationic protein, major basic protein) which damage the respiratory ciliated epithelial layer. The tissue damage contributes to increased airway irritability which causes coughing and wheez-

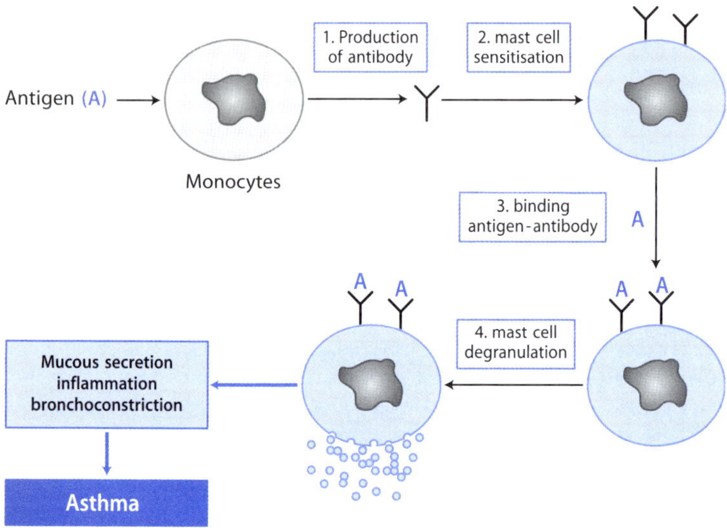

Figure 18.1 ▲ **Schematic representation of asthmatic attack**

1. First exposure to antigen causes production of specific antibodies
2. Antibodies attach to surface of mast cells (mast cell sensitization)
3. Subsequent exposure to antigen results in binding to surface-bound antibody molecules
4. Sensitized mast cells release granules containing preformed pro-inflammatory molecules, synthesize prostaglandins, leukotrienes and PAF within a few minutes, and synthesize cytokines within 30 min. Inflammatory mediators produce mucous secretion, inflammation and bronchoconstriction, the typical features of asthma

ing in response to stimuli that do not normally cause such responses (climatic modifications, inhalation of dust, physical effort, irritant gas, infection of respiratory tree, etc.).

- Standard pharmacological treatment involves the use of:
  - bronchodilators like β_2-adrenoceptor agonists (e.g. salbuterol)
  - anticholinergic (ipratropium bromide)
  - xanthines (theophylline)
  - anti-inflammatory drugs such as glucocorticoids and cromolyn sodium.

Phytotherapy of Asthma

The historical importance of herbal medicine in the treatment of asthma is indisputable. Four of the five classes of drugs currently used to treat asthma,

Table 18.1

Randomized clinical studies of plants used in traditional chinese, indian (Ayurvedic) and japanese (Kampo) herbal medicine to threat asthma. Data extracted from Huntley and Ernst, Torax 2000;55:925-929)

Plant	Part used	Preparation	Dose	Duration	Number of trials	Result
Chinese Medicine						
Ginkgo biloba (Ginkgo)	Leaf	Ginkgo liquor	15 g tid	8 weeks	1	Positive
Ligusticum wallichii (Sichuan lovage)	Mixture	Tea	10 ml tid	1 month	1	Positive (trend)
Ayurvedic Medicine						
Picrorhiza kurroa (Picrorhiza)	Root	Powder	300 mg tid	14 weeks	1	Negative
Solanum xanthocarpum, S. trilobatum (Kantakari)	Whole plant	Powder	N.R.	2 hours	1	Positive
Tylophora indica (Indian ipecac)	Leaf	Various*	Various	2–12 weeks	5	Inconclusive
Boswellia serrata (Indian olibaum)	Gum resin	Powder	N.R.	6 weeks	1	Positive
Kampo Medicine						
*Tsumura saiboku-to***	Various	N.R.	N.R.	12 weeks	1	Positive
Hedera helix (English ivy)	Leaf	Dried extract	35 mg daily	3 days	1	Partially positive

tid = three times daily
N.R. = not reported
* powder, leaves chewed and swallowed
** *Tsumura saiboku-to* is a combination of two herbal preparations containing 10 herbs

namely β_2 agonists, anticholinergics, methylxanthines and cromones, have origins in herbal treatments going back as far as 5000 years. There is a large archive of information on herbal medicine from many cultures for the treatment of asthma. Table 18.1 lists randomized clinical trials of plants used in traditional Chinese, and in Indian and Japanese herbal medicine. Phytotherapy of asthma includes the use of bronchial spasmolytics (see Table 18.2) or anti-inflammatory (e.g. ginkgo) drugs. Although some trials with herbal drugs for asthma have yielded positive results, further careful investigations are required before positive recommendations can be made.

Table 18.2
Bronchial spasmolytics traditionally used to treat asthma

Common name	Latin name	Part(s) of plant used	Key constituents	Daily dose
Argy wormwood	*Artemisia argyi*	Oil from the leaves	Trans-carveol, alpha-terpineol, canphene, carvone	0.1-0.2 ml oil
Belladonna	*Atropa belladonna*	Leaves	Tropane alkaloids (atropine, scopolamine), flavonoids	0.2-0.4 g
Bishop's weed	*Ammi visnaga*	Fruits	Furochromones, pyranocoumarins, flavonoids	a
Datura (jimson weed)	*Datura stramonium*	Leaves	Tropane alkaloids, flavonoids	0.05-0.1 g
Elecampane	*Inula helenium*	Rhizome	Volatile oil, polyynes, polysaccharides	1 g
Gingko	*Ginkgo biloba*	Leaves	Flavonoids, ginkgolides	3-6 g
Gumweed	*Grindelia camporum*	Aerial parts	Diterpene acids, saponins, tannins, volatile oil, flavonoids	4-6 g
Henbane	*Hyoscyamus niger*	Leaves	Tropane alkaloids, flavonoids	0.5-1 g
Horehound	*Marrubium vulgare*	Aerial pats	Marrubiin, flavonoids, caffeic acid derivatives	4.5 g
Ma-huang	*Ephedra sinica*	Aerial parts	Alkaloids (ephedrine, pseudoephedrine)	b
Pill-bearing spurge	*Euphorbia hirta*	Fresh branches	Flavonoids, terpenoids, phenolic acids	1 g
Sundew	*Drosera rotundifolia*	Whole plant	Naphtaquinone derivatives	3 g
Thyme	*Thymus vulgaris*	Leaves, flowering tops	Volatile oil, flavonoids, caffeic acid derivatives	10 g

a. no reliable information is available
b. 60–90 mg of total alkaloids, calculated as ephedrine

Ephedra (Ma-huang)

Botany/Key constituents ▶ There are many varieties of *Ephedra*. The Chinese variety is very common and is known by the name **ma-huang**. It consists of the dried aerial parts (or the entire plant) of *Ephedra sinica* Stapf. (Fam. *Ephedraceae*), a shrub, 60–90 cm high, native to Southern China and today largely diffused also in North-western India and Pakistan. The stem is green, erect, slender and channeled. The leaves appear as whitish, triangular, scarious sheaths; small blossoms appear in the summer. *Ma* means an astringent and *huang* means yellow, referring to the taste and color of the drug. *Ephedra* is collected in the autumn, when the alkaloid content is very high (about 2%). Ephedrine was isolated from the herb in 1887. Other constituents identified in ephedra are pseudoephedrine, norephedrine, norpseudoephedrine.

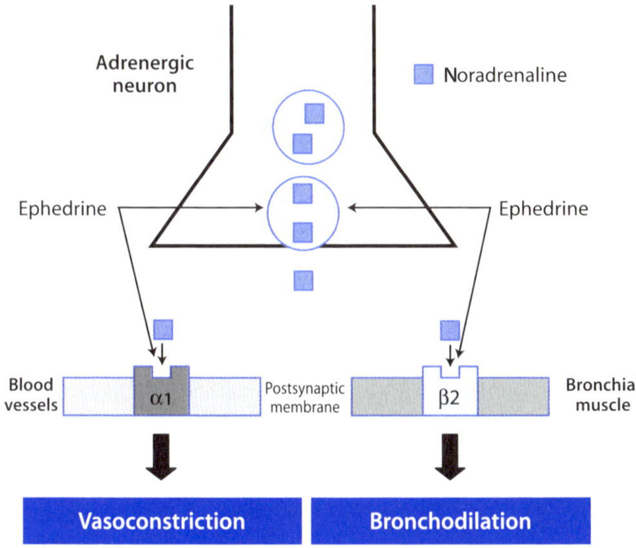

Figure 18.2 ▲ **Site of action of ephedrine, the main active ingredient of ephedra**
Ephedrine is a mixed-action adrenergic agent. It not only releases stored noradrenaline from nerve endings but also directly activates both α and β adrenergic receptors. Through its action on α_1 receptors ephedrine produces vasoconstriction in mucous membrane, thus relieving nasal congestion; through β_2 receptors, it relaxes bronchial smooth muscle

Mode of action ▸ Ephedrine is a mixed-action sympathomimetic; it not only releases stored norephedrine from nerve endings, but also directly stimulates α and β adrenergic receptors (Figure 18.2). Through its action on α_1 adrenergic receptors, ephedrine produces vasoconstriction in mucous membranes, thus relieving to some degree congestion in the nasal passages. Moreover, ephedrine relaxes bronchial smooth muscle by stimulation of β_2-adrenergic receptors; there is also an increase in ciliary activity and liquefaction of tenacious means resulting in a mild expectorant action. Pseudroephedrine possesses similar action (more selective for α than β receptors), but it is less potent than ephedrine.

Clinical efficacy ▸ *Ma huang* has been used as a medicine in China for thousands of years. However, there is a lack of randomized clinical trials which confirm the traditional use. Ephedrine is a clinically effective antiasthmatic drug, but its use has declined after the introduction of β_2 adrenergic agonists. Both pseudoephedrine and ephedrine are used to treat nasal congestion of various origins.

Adverse events/Contraindications ► Common side effect include irritability, headache, tremor and palpitations, nausea, vomiting and sleep disturbances. Higher dosages may result in blood pressure and cardiac rhythm disorders. The drug is contraindicated in patients suffering from heart conditions, hypertension, diabetes, thyroid disease or with benign prostatic hypertrophy (BPH). Due to its relative selectivity for α- over β-adrenergic receptors, psuedoephedrine tends to be free of side effects such as CNS stimulation or tachycardia.

Preparations/Dosage

Ephedra is traditionally given in the form of a tea (infusion) prepared by steeping 2 g drug in a cup of boiling water (150 ml) for 10 min: one cup 2–3 times a day. Such a preparation may contain up to 30 mg ephedrine which represents the usual dose of the alkaloid. Because of the risk of tachyphylaxis and dependence, drug preparations should be administered for short periods.

► *See Chapter 15 for the anti-obesity properties of ephedra*

Other Antiasthmatic Drugs

Ginkgo Ginkgolides are diterpenes with a unique structure and are characteristic constituents of the leaves of *Ginkgo biloba*, the only living representative of a family (*Ginkgoaceae*), which once contained at least 6 genera. *Ginkgo biloba* is a tree with an average height of 20 m, native from China. The ginkgolides in the extract are competitive antagonists of the platelet-activating factor, a well-known lipid mediator of inflammation and anaphylaxis. Animal studies have shown that ginkgolides exert a protective effect on PAF-induced bronchoconstriction and airway hyperactivity in immuno-anaphylaxis and in antigen-induced bronchial provocation tests. The possible mode of action of ginkgo is illustrated in Figure 18.3. Ginkgo has been extensively used to treat asthmatic patients in traditional chinese herbal medicine. In a randomized clinical study carried out on 61 patients, concentrated ginkgo leaf liquor (15 g three times daily) was superior to placebo after eight weeks treatment. Overall, ginkgo reduces the airways' hyperresponsiveness and bronchospasm by acting mainly as an anti-inflammatory agent. The concentrated ginkgo leaf liquor (15 g three times daily) is a well-known traditional preparation used to treat asthmatic patients.

► *See Chapter 14 for the use of ginkgo in the treatment of arterial occlusive disease*

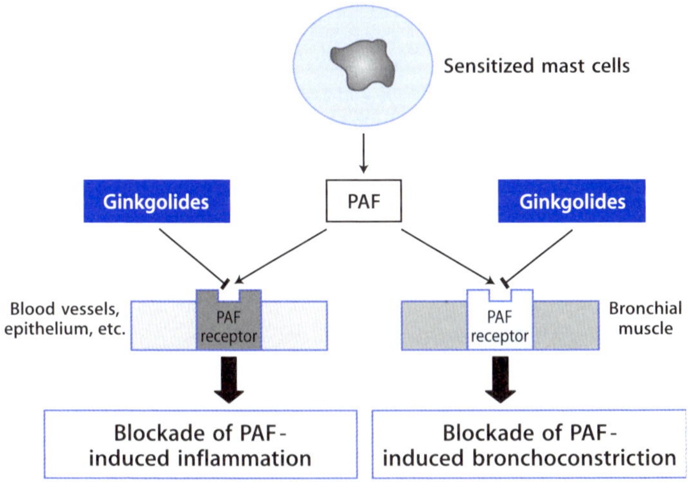

Figure 18.3 ▲ **Site of action of ginkgolides, active ingredients of Ginkgo biloba**
Ginkgolides competitively block the action of PAF on its receptor

Argy wormwood The oil extracted from the leaves of *Artemisia argyi* Levl. Et Vant (Fam. *Asteraceae*) shows anti-asthmatic, antitussive and expectorant effects. It antagonizes the bronchial constriction induced by acetylcholine or histamine, and relaxes isolated smooth muscle like isoprotenerol. The effect is relatively long-lasting. Constituents of the oil include trans-carveol, α-terpineol, 4-terpineol, canphene and carvone. The drug is given in the form of capsules, containing 0.075 ml oil, 2–3 times a day, to treat asthma and chronic bronchitis.

Sundew is obtained from the aerial parts of *Drosera rotundifolia* L. (Fam. *Droseraceae*), which are reported to prevent histamine or acetylcholine-induced bronchospasm. The antispasmodic action has been attributed to naphthoquinone constituents. Sundew also possesses antitussive and antimicrobial properties. It is used for asthma, chronic bronchitis and tracheitis. The drug is given in the form of tea prepared by steeping 1–2 g sundew in a cup (150–200 ml) boiling water for about 5 min (one cup three times daily) as tincture (1:5 in 60% alcohol three times daily or as liquid extract (1:1 in 25% alcohol; 0.5–2.0 ml three times daily). Tinctures and extracts are ingredients of proprietary syrups promoted as a treatment for spasmodic cough. Excessive use of sundew preparations should be avoided because of its content of plumbagin, an irritant principle.

Pill-bearing spurge is obtained from the aerial part of *Euphorbia hirta* L. or *E. pilulifera* L. (Fam. *Euphorbiaceae*), a herb containing flavonoids, terpenoids (amyrins), phenolic acids (shikimic acid) and choline. It is a bronchial antispasmodic and hence used for respiratory disorders including asthma, bronchitis, catarrh and laryngeal spasm. Antispasmodic and antibacterial properties are attributed, at least in part, to choline and shikimic acid. The drug is given in the form of tea prepared by steeping 300–400 mg herb in a cup of boiling water (150 ml), to be consumed three times daily. The drug does not contain known toxic principles; nevertheless, a prolonged use should probably be avoided.

Bronchitis

Clinical Picture

- Bronchitis is a general term indicating inflammation of the tracheobronchial tree. **Acute bronchitis** is infectious and most often occurs during the winter months following the symptoms of upper respiratory infection. It presents with the typical symptoms of malaise, slight temperature, sore throat, chills, dyspnea, back pain and muscular soreness or pain. **Chronic bronchitis** usually occurs in patients older than 40 years of age and is more common in women than in men. Typically, chronic bronchitis causes alveolar hypoventilation, hypercapnia, and hypoxia. Patients typically have a productive cough, sputum production, breathlessness on exertion, and airways obstruction. Respiratory infection is common and can worsen the progress of the disease.
- Treatment of bronchitis include the use of bronchodilators (to reduce airways obstruction), expectorants (to reduce mucus viscosity), antitussives (to relieve cough that accompanies bronchitis), antibiotics (to combat bacterial infections colonising the sputum), and antipyretics (to reduce fever).

Phytotherapy of Bronchitis

Herbal medicines used in the treatment of bronchitis include expectorants and antitussives (Tables 18.3-18.5).

Expectorants

Bronchial and tracheal mucus covers and keeps the respiratory tract moist, and aids in warming and purifying inhaled air. However, in the case of respiratory tract inflammation or irritation, this secretion can be transformed into an exudate which impedes air circulation and induces coughing. Expectorants are therefore useful when it is desirable to reduce mucus viscosity. This will facilitate removal of the secretions through coughing (expectoration). Indications for reflex expectorants include cough linked to bronchial congestion and bronchitis.

Expectorants can be divided into at least two main categories:

- **Reflex expectorants.** This class includes saponin-containing drugs and drug containing emetic, acid tasting or bitter compounds (Table 18.3). These expectorants evoke a reflex stimulation of respiratory secretion by activating an afferent mechanism upon contact with the gastric or duodenal mucosa (Figure 18.4). These drugs can stimulate the emetic center and will induce vomiting unless administered in small quantities.
- **Direct-acting expectorants.** This class includes essential oil-containing drugs (Table 18.4). In contrast to reflex expectorants, the essential oils are well absorbed after oral administration and are partially excreted via the lung where they stimulate the serous glandular cells and ciliated epithelium (Figure 18.5).

Reflex Expectorants

Horehound consists of the dried leaves and flowers of *Marrubium vulgare* L. (Fam. *Labiate*), a herbaceous plant 30–60 cm high, growing in Europe. It contains alkaloids, flavonoids, terpenoids including marrubiin, volatile oil and other minor constituents. Marrubiin seems to be an artefact formed from premarrubiin, during extraction. Horehound possesses expectorant and antispasmodic properties. The main expectorant principle is marrubiin. It also possesses bitter properties (twice as bitter as gentian). The drug is used for acute and chronic

Table 18.3
Herbal midicines acting as reflex expectorants

Common name	Latin name	Part(s) of plant used	Key constituents	Daily dose
Cowslip*	*Primula veris*	Flowers	Flavonoids, triterpene saponins	3 g
English ivy*	*Hedera helix*	Leaves	Triterpene saponins, volatile oil	0.3–0.8 g
Horehound	*Marrubium vulgare*	Aerial parts	Marrubiin, flavonoids, volatile oil	4.5 g
Ipecac*	*Cephaelis ipecacuanha*	Roots	Tetrahydroisoquinoline alkaloids (emetine, cephaelin)	a
Liquorice*	*Glycyrrhiza glabra*	Roots	Triterpene saponins, flavonoids	5–15 g
Quillaja	*Quillaja saponaria*	Inner bark	Tannins, triterpene saponins	0.4–0.6 g
Snakeroot*	*Polygala senega*	Roots	Triterpene saponins	1.5–3.0 g
Soapwort *	*Saponaria officinalis*	Roots	Triterpene saponins	0.03–0.15 g
White nettle*	*Lamium album*	Flowers	Iridoide monoterpenes, saponins	3 g
Wild daisy	*Bellis perennis*	Flowering plant	Triterpene saponins, polyynes, flavonoids	b

* supported by German Commission E for the treatment of cough and bronchitis
a. 10 ml of a 0.5% infusion
b. Infusion: 1 teaspoon drug in 1 cup water; 2-4 cups daily

Table 18.4

Essential oil-containing expectorants. Most of these herbal medicines are used in inhalants

Common name	Latin name	Part(s) of plant used	Key constituents of the oil
Anise*	*Pimpinella anisum*	Oil from fruits	Anethole
Cajuput	*Maleleuca leucadendra*	Oil from leaves and twigs	Eucalyptol
Citronella	*Cymbopogon nardus*	Oil from leaves	Citronellal, geraniol, geranyl acetate
Eucalyptus *	*Eucalyptus globulus*	Oil from leaves	Cineole (eucalyptol)
Niaouli*	*Melaleuca viridiflora*	Oil from leaves	Cineole, nerolidol, linalool, α- and β-pinene
Scotch pine*	*Pinus spp.*	Oil from needles	(-)-α-pinene, limonene, camphene
Spruce*	*Picea spp.*	Oil from needles	Bornyl acetate, limonene, camphene
Star anise*	*Illicium verum*	Oil from fruits	Trans-anethol, limonene, d-fenchone, d-pinene
Thyme *	*Thymus vulgaris*	Oil from herb	Thymol, carvacrol
Wild thyme*	*Thymus serpyllum*	Oil from leaves and flowering top	Carvacrol

* supported by German Commission E for the treatment of cough and bronchitis

bronchitis, whooping cough, bronchial catarrh, but also for the treatment of dyspepsia and loss of appetite. It may be consumed as a tea (infusion) prepared by steeping 1–2 g crude drug in boiling water (200 ml): two to four cups may be consumed daily. The drug is also available in the form of liquid extract (1:1 in 20% alcohol; 2–4 ml three times daily). Large doses of horehound are purgatives and may alter the menstrual cycle. Therefore, it should not be taken in excessive doses during pregnancy or lactation.

Snakeroot (seneca) is the dried root of *Polygala senega* L. var. *senega* and/or var. *latifolia* Torrey et A. Gray (Fam. *Polygalaceae*), perennial herbs about 20–30 cm in height, growing in North America and Canada and also cultivated in Japan. The drug has a particular smell due to its methylsalicylate content. Snakeroot contains triterpenoid saponins (5–10%) including senegins, acids (caffeic, ferulic, salicylic, etc.), fat, resin and sterols. Snakeroot has been used for chronic bronchitis and also for bronchitis asthma and pharyngitis. It has been shown that senegin, the main constituent of snakeroot, also known as polygalic acid, is an irritant to the gastrointestinal mucosa and causes a reflex secretion of mucus in the bronchioles. Senegin may also directly reduce the viscosity of thickened bronchial secretions. The drug is given in the form of a decoction prepared from 0.5 g crude drug in a cup of water (150 ml). The daily dose should not exceed 3 g because snakeroot may cause nausea, vomiting and exacerbate existing gastrointestinal inflammation. Excessive use should be avoided because the presence of free saponins in the intestinal lumen may cause a transient increase in

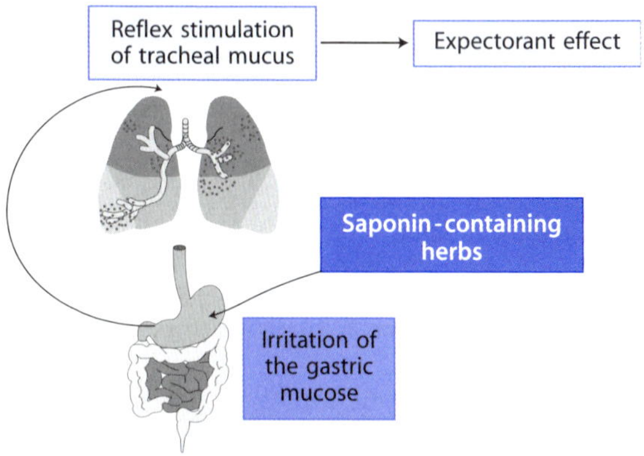

Figure 18.4 ▲ **Expectorant action of saponin-containing herbs**
Saponins are poorly absorbed from the gastrointestinal tract so they usually produce no systemic effects when administered orally. However, they can irritate the mucous membrane of the stomach and intestines. The small irritation activates a reflex pathway which leads to stimulation of mucous glands in the bronchi via parasympathetic pathways

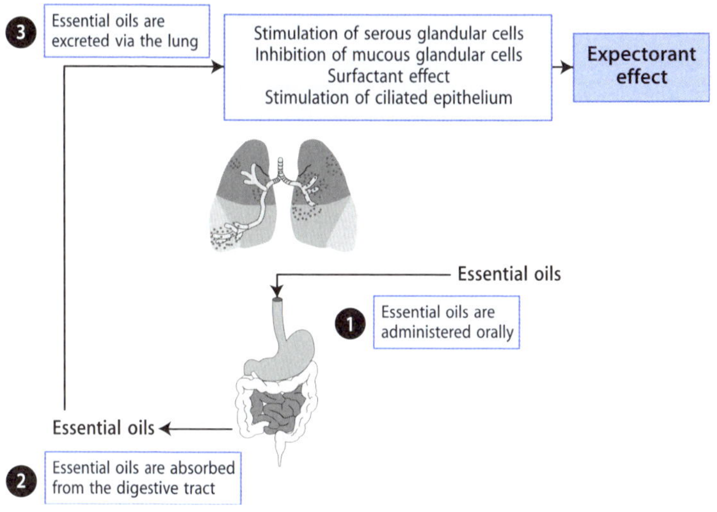

Figure 18.5 ▲ **Expectorant action of essential oils**
Following oral administration essential oils are absorbed from the gastrointestinal tract into the blood and partially eliminated through the lungs. As the exhaled molecules pass through the bronchial tree, they (i) can stimulate serous bronchial gland function, (ii) suppress mucous glandular cell activity, (iii) reduce surface tension (surfactant effect) and (iv) improve mucociliary activity

the permeability of gut mucosa and consequently facilitate the entry of antigens into the blood. Chronic exposure of the intestinal mucosa to saponins may also inhibit active nutrient absorption.

English ivy consists of the dried leaves of *Hedera helix* L. (Fam. *Araliaceae*), an evergreen climber plant that grows over the greater part of Europe and Northern and Central Asia (Plate18.1). The leaves contain sterols, saponins (5–8%) including hedera saponin B and C, caffeic esters of quinic acid, flavonoids (rutin), alkaloids (emetine), polyalcohols (falcarinol, falcarinone, II-dehydrofalcarinol), etc. Ivy extract is spasmolytic *in vitro* and α-hederin seems the constituent responsible for the activity. Ivy preparations are mostly used orally for the symptomatic treatment of cough and to treat acute benign bronchial disease. Ivy can be taken as a tea (infusion) prepared from 6 g crude drug in boiling water (1000 ml) for 10 min: one cup three to four times daily. Both ivy leaves and wood are instead used in the form of extract (30% ethanol): a daily dose must be equal to 0.3–0.8 g crude drug. The frequent use of ivy-based products can cause allergic reactions and nausea. Side effects are due mainly to to falcarinol.

Liquorice consists or the root of *Glycyrrhiza glabra* L. (Fam. *Fabaceae*) and contains at least 4% glycyrrhizin, which is a mixture of the potassium and calcium salt of glycyrrhizinic acid, a terpenoid compound. Liquorice is reported to be very useful as expectorant and antitussive. The expectorant activities of liquorice have been shown in animals. However, its mode of action in facilitating the dissolution and elimination of bronchial secretions requires further clarification. It has been postulated that glycyrrhizin (the main active ingredient of liquorice) increases the bronchial secretion and transport of mucus via a reflex pathway originating in the stomach. However, this mechanism seem to be in contrast with the antiulcer effect of glycyrrhizin. Used in appropriate dosage, liquorice is a safe herb. The daily therapeutic dose is 5–15 g dried root. Excessive consumption of liquorice can lead to sodium retention and hypertension.

► *See Chapter 21 for the antiulcer properties of liquorice*
► *See Chapter 22 for the hepato-protective effect of glycyrrhizin*

Ipecac (or ipecacuanha) consists of the roots and rhizome of *Cephaelis ipecacuanha* (Brot.) A., Rich. (Fam. *Rubiaceae*) (Mato Grosso ipecacuanha) or *C. acuminata* Karsten, known as Costa Rica ipecacuanha. The plant is a small perennial shrub (20–40 cm) native to Brazil (Mato Grosso) and Central America (Costa Rica). Cultivation has been attempted in several tropical areas but only with limited success. The drug contains isoquinoline alkaloids (2–2.5% for Rio ipecac; 2–3.5% for Cartagena) including emetine and cepheline. Emetine is the major constituent of Rio ipecac (60–75% the total alkaloids) whereas it represents only 30–50% of total alkaloids of Cartagena ipecac. The drug also contains starch (30–40%), an allergenic glycoprotein and isoquinoline glycosides like ipecoside.

Ipecac is still used in the form of syrup as an emetic in the treatment of intoxication (except if the poisonings are acids, bases, convulsants or volatile hydrocarbons). It is prepared from powdered ipecac titrated to contain 2.0+0.1% total alkaloids or from fluid extract ipecac (14 ml) added to glycerin (20 ml) and simple syrup 500 ml. The dose used is 15 ml (in adult) with tepid water, with the option of a second dose after 15 min. The syrup must be used as soon as the intoxication is diagnosed. Other components of ipecac, tannins and anthraquinones may modulate the emetic effect of the drug. However, ipecac is present in small amounts in several commercial expectorant mixtures. As noted above, by virtue of their active principles (essential oils, saponins) most expectorants tend to have an irritant effect on the gastric mucosa after oral administration, and reflexively increase bronchial secretions.

Direct-acting Expectorants (Essential Oil-containing Drugs)

Eucalyptus is the dried leaves of *Eucaliptus globulus* Labill. (Fam. *Myrtaceae*), a tree native to Australia and introduced into Southern Europe, North America and many other subtropical and tropical countries. The leaves contain volatile oil (0.5–3.5%) located in special oil glands, phenolics, flavonoids (rutin, hyperin, etc.), tannins and associated acids, caffeic acid, waxes, etc. Eucalyptus oil consists of up to about 85% eucalyptol (cineole). Eucalyptus leaves and oil have been used as mucolytic expectorant, antiseptic, and febrifuge. All these properties have been attributed to eucalyptol. Eucalyptus is used in the form of tea prepared from 2 g leaves in about 150 ml hot water: a cup three times daily. Such a preparation is used to ease the discomfort of colds and as a cough remedy. A prolonged use of the drug can lead to myopathies. Frequent contact with the drug can trigger allergic reactions of the skin and the mucous membrane. The oil is present in a variety of nasal inhalers and sprays, ointments and mouthwashes. It should be diluted before internal and external use. Externally, eucalyptus oil is nontoxic, non-sensitizing and non-phototoxic. Undiluted eucalyptus is toxic and should not be taken internally. A dose of 3.5 ml could be fatal. Symptoms of poisoning with eucalyptus oil include epigastric burning, nausea and vomiting, dizziness, muscular weakness, miosis, a feeling of suffocation, cyanosis, delirium, and convulsion. In some cases eucalyptol could be preferable to the oil, because the latter contains aldehydes which irritate mucous membranes.

Thyme consists of the dried leaves and flowering top of *Thymus vulgaris* L. (Fam. *Lamiaceae*), a small perennial herb from the Mediterranean region. The plant has glandular hairs on the leaves and stems which contain a volatile oil (0.4–3%). The main components of the oil are thymol (31–71%) and carvacrol (2.5–15%). Flavonoids, tannins, saponins, caffeic acid, oleic acid and ursolic acid are also present. Thyme is stated to possess expectorant, mucolytic, antitussive and antispasmodic properties. Such actions have been associated with the volatile oil and flavonoid constituents. Thyme oil also possesses antibacterial, antifungal and hypotensive actions and respiratory stimulant effects. Thyme is used for the treatment of the symptoms of bronchitis and catarrh of the upper respiratory tract in the form of tea (infusion) prepared from 1–4 g drug for cup of water (150 ml). One cup is drunk up to three times daily. Thyme is reputed to affect the menstrual cycle and therefore high doses should not be ingested. The drug also possesses a low potential for sensitization. Thyme oil is toxic: it should not be taken internally and only externally if opportunely diluted. Both thyme and thyme oil are ingredients of various proprietary drugs: syrups for the treatment of respiratory disorders, antiseptic and healing ointments, preparations for inhalation.

Cough

Clinical Picture

- Cough is a reflex triggered by mechanical or chemical stimulation of the upper respiratory tract, or by central stimuli (Figure 18.6). It is a protective mechanism that serves to expel foreign bodies and unwanted material from the airways. However, coughing is sometimes both useless and distressing and can exhaust the patient psychologically and physically. Cough suppression is then indicated.
- Drugs to suppress cough can reduce
  - local throat irritation (e.g. mucilaginous herbs)
  - peripheral suppression of the cough reflex (e.g. essential oils)
  - the sensitivity of the "cough center" (e.g. opiates).

Phytotherapy of Cough

Mucilaginous drugs are demulcent remedies traditionally used to relieve "dry" coughs (Table 18.5). The effect is due to formation of a protective coating that shields the mucosal surface from irritants. The long-stranded molecules that comprise mucilages are too large to be absorbed and transported to the tracheobronchial mucosa when given orally. Nevertheless, some studies carried out on an extract of marshmallow (root of *Althea officinalis* L.) have demonstrated that the effect is not limited to the pharynx but involves the tracheo-bronchial mucosa and musculature, through a vagal reflex. However, marshmallow is not the only mucilaginous drug. Other mucilaginous herbs potentially used to soothe cough include Iceland moss (thallus of *Cetraria islandica*), mullein (flowers of *Verbascum densiflorum*), mallow (flowers and leaves of *Malva sylvestris*) and plantain (leaves and flowers of *Plantago lanceolata*). Most of these drugs may be employed interchangeably. Since mucilages are water-soluble, and often given in the form of tea.

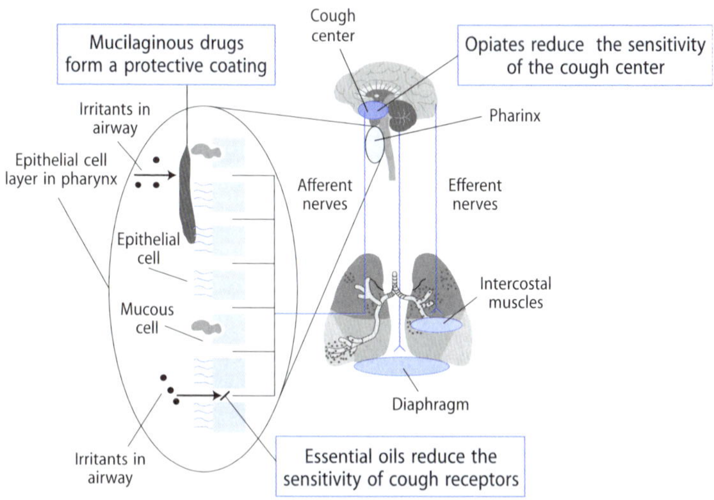

Figure 18.6 ▲ **Cough reflex arc and site of action of botanical antitussives**
Cough is a reflex mechanism and hence involves an arc with sensor (afferent), central and efferent components. Mechanical or chemical stimuli activate receptors on afferent nerves (which extend from the larynx to the division of the segmental bronchi). Afferent nerves carry the information to the cough center. Efferent nerves starting from the cough center produce contraction of the respiratory muscles which leads to a rise in intrathoracic pressure, forcing air out of the alveoli and through the airways.
Mucilaginous drugs form a protective coating that shields the mucosal surface from irritants.
Essential oils reduce the sensitivity of peripheral afferent receptors.
Opiates reduce the sensitivity of the cough center

Essential oils are very complex, aromatic-smelling, volatile mixtures containing many different compounds. The plants, rich in essential oils (0.01–10% dry weight), are found in about 30% of plant families. High contents of essential oils are especially common in members of the *Apiaceae*, *Laminaceae*, *Lauraceae*, *Mirtaceare* and *Rutaceae*. Essential oils occur in plants in specially developed organs of various kinds, e.g. glandular hair of leaves, stems and flowers. Essential oils possess different pharmacological activities; with regard to the respiratory system, they possess expectorant and antiseptic activity. The antitussive effect of essential oils is believed to lead to a reduction of the sensitivity of the peripheral cough receptors. Most of the essential oil-containing drugs used to treat cough also have expectorant properties (Table 18.4).

Table 18.5

Some mucillaginous herbs supported by German Commission E for the treatment of cough and bronchitis

Common name	Latin name	Part(s) of plant used	% mucilage in the drug	Constituents of mucilage	Daily dose
Coltsfoot	*Tussilago farfara*	Inflorescence, leaves	6-10 %	Acidic polysaccharides	4.5-6 g
English plantain	*Plantago lanceolata*	Aerial parts	2-6%	Ramnogalacturonane, arabinogalactans, glucomannane	3-6 g
Iceland moss	*Cetraria islandica*	Thallus	50%	lichenin, isolichenin	4-6 g
Mallow	*Malva sylvestris*	Leaves, flowers	5-8% leaf, 10% flower	Galacturonorhamane, arabinogalactans	5 g
Marsh-mallow	*Althaea officinalis*	Roots	5-10%	Galacturonic and glucuronic acids, ramnose, galactose	6 g
Mullein	*Verbascum densiflorum*	Flowers	3%	Xyloglucane, arabinogalactans	3-4 g

Opiates are constituent of opium poppy (*Papaverum somniferum*). Constituents of poppy with antitussive activity include morphine and codeine. Both compounds possess central antitussive actions by virtue of their agonist actions on opiate receptors in the cough center. Codeine is usually used therapeutically in proprietary "cough mixtures".

Rhinitis

Clinical Picture

- Allergic rhinitis is characterized by a sensitization of the upper respiratory tract to one or more allergens and may be seasonal or perennial. In the first case rhinitis is triggered by inhaled allergens: common inhalation allergens are pollen from various plants. In the second case, rhinitis may be evoked by common household moulds or dust.
- Rhinitis is characterized by nasal congestion, discharge, sneezing and itching. Non-allergic (or vasomotor) rhinitis has no identifiable cause, although it is believed to be caused (or exacerbated) by the consumption of certain berries and fruit, shellfish, eggs, milk, chocolate, spices and so on. Rhinitis may also be caused by overuse of nasal sprays containing decongestants. Sometimes rhinitis is associated to asthma.
- The therapeutic approach to rhinitis is to control symptoms and remove causes. Therefore it is important to identify whether or not inhaled aller-

gens are involved. Measures able to reduce exposure to pollen should be part of this treatment. Antihistamines and anti-inflammatories are the most widely prescribed drugs for the treatment of rhinitis and are available by inhalation as well as orally. Antibiotics are also prescribed in the case of infections.

Phytotherapy of Rhinitis

There are several vegetable drugs able to solve, although in part only, nasal obstruction associated to rhinitis and other manifestations like lachrymation and sneezing. The volatile oil of Niaouli instilled into the nasal cavity or oral administration of butterbur (*vide infra*) may relieve nasal obstruction. Antiallergic herbs potentially useful in the treatment of rhinitis also include immune-enhancing herbs.

Butterbur (Petasites)

Botany/Key constituents ▶ *Petasites hybridus* is a perennial European shrub which grows to a height of 1–1.5 m and is usually found in wet, marshy ground, in damp forests, and adjacent to rivers or streams (Plate 18.2). Its downy leaves can attain a diameter of 1–1.5 m, making it the largest of all indigenous flora, and their unique characteristics are responsible for the plant's common name. The roots and leaves are used medicinally. Key constituents present both in the leaves and in the roots include sesquiterpenes (e.g. petasin and isopetasin), a volatile oil and pyrrolizidine alkaloids (e.g. senecionine and integerrimine).

Mode of action ▶ The main active consituents are petasin and isopetasin. Petasin is responsible for the antispasmodic/vasoactive properties of the plants by reducing spasms in smooth muscle and vascular walls, in addition to providing an anti-inflammatory effect by inhibiting leukotriene synthesis (inhibition of the enzyme lipoxygenase).

Clinical efficacy ▶ Butterbur is traditionally used for respiratory disorders, particularly for coughs, whooping cough and bronchial asthma. Recent studies suggest the use of butterbur for treating allergic rhinitis when the sedative effects of antihistamines need to be avoided. A recent well-performed randomized clinical study (n = 131 patients) compared the efficacy and tolerability of butterbur with the antihistamine drug cetirizine in patients with seasonal allergic rhinitis (hay fever). After two weeks treatment, the effects of butterbur and cetirizine were comparable.

Adverse events/Contraindications ▶ Side effects from butterbur have been not reported. The plant's pyrrolizidine alkaloids are thought to cause liver damage and to be carcinogenic in animals; however, extracts are commercially available in which the pyrrolizidine alkaloids have been removed. Alkaloid-free varietis of *Petasites* are also cultivated. Butterbur produced fewer sedating effect than antihistamines. The administration of the drug during pregnancy or lactation is stated to be completely ruled out.

Preparations/Dosage

Typically, petasites extracts are standardized to contain a minimum content of petasin and isopetasin. Tablets containing *Petasites* carbon dioxide extract are standardized to contain 8.0 mg petasin (one tablet, four times daily). The herb should be not used unless the pyrrolizidine alkaloids content is known. The maximum daily dose of pyrrolizidine alkaloids is 0.1 µg.

► *See Chapter 17 for the use of butterbur for migraine headache*

Niaouli The leaves of *Melaleuca viridiflora* Solander [or *M. quinquenervia* (Cav.) (Fam. *Myrtaceae*)] yield an essential oil named Niaouli. The plant is a small tree native to the Moluceas but widespread in Australia, Southern Asia, New Caledonia and Madagascar. The oil contains cineole (= eucalyptol) (50–69%) as the most common major compound and terpinenol (15%); other compounds are nerolidol, linalool. It is an antiseptic known as petroleum jelly after purification with lead oxide. Niaouli oil is an ingredient of proprietary preparations used for the treatment of rhinitis and bronchial infections. The preparations containing Niaouli oil (2–3 drops three times daily) are mixtures for inhalations used only for the nasal route. The oil is well tolerated; in rare cases use of the drug can lead to nausea, vomiting and diarrhea. Cineole causes the induction of liver enzymes and thus can theoretically reduce the effect of concomitantly used drugs.

Cold and Flu

Clinical Picture

During the Winter season one is often likely to contract an acute viral infection of the upper respiratory tract, commonly called a "cold". The most common symptoms of this contagious condition are nasal congestion, sneezing, sore throat, cough, laryngitis, bronchial congestion, headache, and sometimes fever. If the infection is severe and results in joint and muscle pain and gastrointestinal disturbances, the condition is called "flu". Both cold and flu are self-limiting (five to seven days) but may become complicated by bacterial infections. Vaccination can prevent flu but we do have not a really effective vaccine for all conditions.

Phytotherapy of Cold and Flu

The treatment of cold and flu is in general symptomatic (antipyretic, anti-inflammatory drugs). However, immunostimulant drugs (echinacea, andrographis) may be beneficial in reducing the severity of symptoms associated with colds.

Echinacea

Botany/key constituents ► Echinacea (cone flower or purple cone flower) consists of the dried roots and rhizomes (as well as aerial parts) of several species of *Echinacea* (Fam. *Compositae*) (Plate 18.3). Three species of echinacea are used medicinally (*E. angustifolia* DC, *E. pallida* Nutt. and *E. purpurea* Moench.). These plants are perennial herbs native to America, west of Ohio, and cultivated in Britain. The composition of each species of herb is similar, with slight variations in the amount of each active component. The drug contains high molecular-weight polysaccharides (echinacin), phenolic compounds derived from caffeic acid (cynarin, specific to *E. angustifolia*), cichoric acid (abundant in *E. purpurea*), echinacoside (absent in *E. purpura*), sesquiterpene lactone esters, alkaloids pyrrolizidine-type (isotussilagine and tussilagine), and alkylamides (echinacein). Other constituents are betaine, fatty acids, phytosterol, resin and volatile oil.

Mode of action ► Active components of echinacea include caffeic and ferulic acid derivatives (such as cichoric acid and echinacoside) and complex polysaccharides (such as arabinogalactan, rhamnoarabinogalactans). However, echinacea's pharmacological effects appear to result from a combination of active ingredients rather than from a single agent. The immunostimulant properties of echinacea are believed to be due to actions on the non-specific branch of immunity, the phagocytic cell (Figure 18.7), rather than the specifically acquired branch. Echinacea does not stimulate all immune cells. B-cells (which produces antibodies) are not activated; T-cell proliferation is increased, but with no changes in immunostimulant cytokines.

Clinical efficacy ► The German Commission E recommends the oral use of *E. purpurea* herb for colds and respiratory tract infections. The *E. pallida* root is supported for use in the treatment of influenza-like infections. Evidence from published trials suggests that echinacea may be beneficial for the early treatment of acute upper respiratory infection. However, there is very little evidence supporting the prolonged use of echinacea for the prevention of upper respiratory infection. A recent systematic review retrieved 13 (4 prevention trials and 9 trials on treatment of upper respiratory infections) blinded placebo-controlled randomized trials of any *Echinacea* formulation. Eight of the 9 treatment trials ($n = 1264$ subjects) reported benefit, while 4 prevention trials ($n = 1152$ subjects) showed

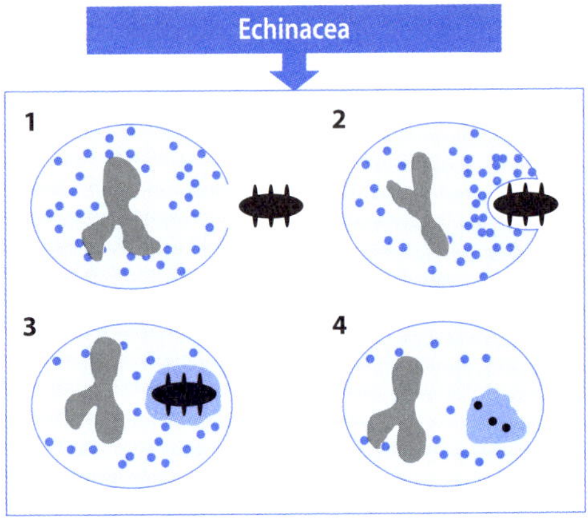

Figure 18.7 ▲ **Echinacea enhances phagocytosis**

Neutrophils and mononuclear phagocytes enter inflammatory foci with the express purpose of ingesting and disposing of unwanted particulate material, such as bacteria or broken-down cells. This process is called phagocytosis which can be enhanced by echinacea.

Phases of phagocytosis:

1. Attachment of neutrophil to opsonized bacterium
2. Engulfment of bacterium (and convergence of granules toward phagosome)
3. Discharge of granule content into phagosome (degranulation)
4. Killing and digestion of bacterium inside phagocytic vacuole

negative or a small beneficial effect. On the basis of these studies, *E. purpurea*, *E. angustifolia*, and *E. pallida* roots, leaves, and flowers cannot at this point be distinguished from each other in terms of their apparent beneficial activity.

Adverse events/Contraindications ► The safety data on echinacea are strong. Despite many reputed contraindications in the literature, the herb is unlikely to cause adverse effects. However, serious allergic or anaphylactic events have been reported, so some caution is in order. An open-label trial with more than 1000 patients found the following side effects: unpleasant taste (1.7%), nausea or vomiting (0.5%), abdominal pain (0.3%) and diarrhea (0.3%). It is generally stated that echinacea should not be administered in the presence of tubercolosis, AIDS, multiple sclerosis or collagen diseases.

Preparations/Dosage

The recommended dose of root extract is equivalent to 900 mg crude drug daily. The following preparations are described: liquid extract of *E. angustifolia* root (2–6 ml per day of 1:2 liquid extract), liquid extract of *E. purpurea* dried root (3–9 ml per day of 1:2 liquid extract), tincture of *E. angustifolia* root (5–15 ml per day of 1:5 tincture), tincture of *E. purpurea* dried root (7–22 ml per day of 1:5 tincture). A dose of 8–9 mg/day is recommended for echinacea juice (stabilized juice of the flowering top). Four preparations of echinacea are not supported by the German Commission E. These preparations are *E. angustifolia* and *E. pallida* herbs and the *E. angustifolia* and *E. purpurea* roots.

► *See Chapter 23 for the use of echinacea in dermatology*

Andrographis

Botany/Key constituents ► Andrographis, commonly known as kalmegh (meaning king of bitters) consists of the aerial part of *Andrographis paniculata* L. (Fam. *Acanthaceae*), an annual shrub native of India which grows to a height of 1 m with branches that are sharply quadrangular, often narrowly winged towards the apical region. The drug in the dried state looks more like a bundle of broom tops. Key constituents include diterpenoid lactones, collectively referred to as andrographolides, diterpenes and flavonoids.

Mode of action ► Andrographis is an immunostimulant. Andrographis extract enhances phagocytosis, and stimulates both antigen-specific and non-specific immune responses. Andrographolide is, at least in part, responsible of such activity.

Clinical efficacy ► The efficacy of andrographis in shortening the course and duration of the common cold is promising, although not fully conclusive. A non-randomized and two randomized clinical trials (n = 208 subjects) have shown that andrographics taken at the first stages of cold reduce the severity and duration of symptoms compared to placebo.

Adverse events ► Andrographis is stated to be a safe herb. No significant adverse effects from ingestion of andrographis are expected. High doses may cause gastric complaints.

Preparations/Dosage

The daily dose of andrographis is 2–3 g dried herb if formulated as liquid extract (4–6 ml per day of 1:2 liquid extract) or 5–6 g if ingested as a decoction or infusion. Andrographis extract (standardized to 4% andrographolides) formulated into tablets (1020 mg per day, about 6 g herb) has been used in most clinical studies.

Further Reading

Barrett B (2003) Medicinal properties of Echinacea: a critical review. Phytomedicine 10:66–86

Barrett B, Vohmann M, Calabrese C (1999) Echinacea for upper respiratory infection. J Fam Pract 48:628–635

Bieroly L (2001) Complementary medicine for the allergist. Allergy Asthma Proc 22:33–37

Bieroly L, Lupoli K (1999) Herbal interventions in asthma and allergy. J Asthma 36:1–65

Chichon PG (2000) Herbs and the common cold. Adv Nurse Pract 8:31–32

Ernst E (2002) The risk-benefit profile of commonly used herbal therapies: Ginkgo, St. John's Wort, Ginseng, Echinacea, Saw Palmetto, and Kava. Ann Intern Med 136:42–53

Giles GT, Palat CT, Chien SH, Chang ZG, Kennedy DT (2000) Evaluation of echinacea for treatment of the common cold. Pharmacotherapy 20:690–697

Haller CA, Benowitz NL (2000) Adverse cardiovascular and central nervous system events associated with dietary supplements containing ephedra alkaloids. N Engl J Med 343:1833–1838

Huntley A, Ernst E (2000) Herbal medicines for asthma: a systematic review. Thorax 55:925–929

Jaber R (2002) Respiratory and allergic diseases: from upper respiratory tract infections to asthma. Prim Care 29:231–261

Liu C, Douglas RM (1998) Chinese herbal medicines in the treatment of acute respiratory infections: a review of randomized and controlled clinical trials. Med J Aust 169:579–582

Mckenna DJ, Jones K, Hughes K (2001) Efficacy, safety, and use of *Ginkgo biloba* in clinical and preclinical applications. Altern Ther Health Med 7:70–86, 88–90

Melchart D, Linde K, Fischer P, Kaesmayr J (2000) Echinacea for preventing and treating the common cold. Cochrane Database 2:CD000530

Percival SS (2000) Use of echinacea in medicine. Biochem Pharmacol 60:155–158

Pinn G (2001) Herbal therapy in respiratory disease. Aust Fam Physician 30:775–779

Schapowal A (2002) Randomized controlled trial of butterbur and cetirizine for treating seasonal allergic rhinitis. Br Med Journal 324:1–4

Thomet CA, Wiesmann UN, Schapowal A, Bizer C, Simon H (2001) Role of petasin in the potential anti-inflammatory activity of a plant extract of *Petasites hybridus*. Biochem Pharmacol 61:1041–1047

Thornhill SM, Kelly AM (2000) Natural treatment of perennial allergic rhinitis. Altern Med Rev 5:448–454

Ziment I (2000) Recent advances in alternative therapies. Curr Opin Pulm Med 6:71–78

Ziment I (2002) Herbal antitussives. Pulm Pharmacol Ther 15:327–333

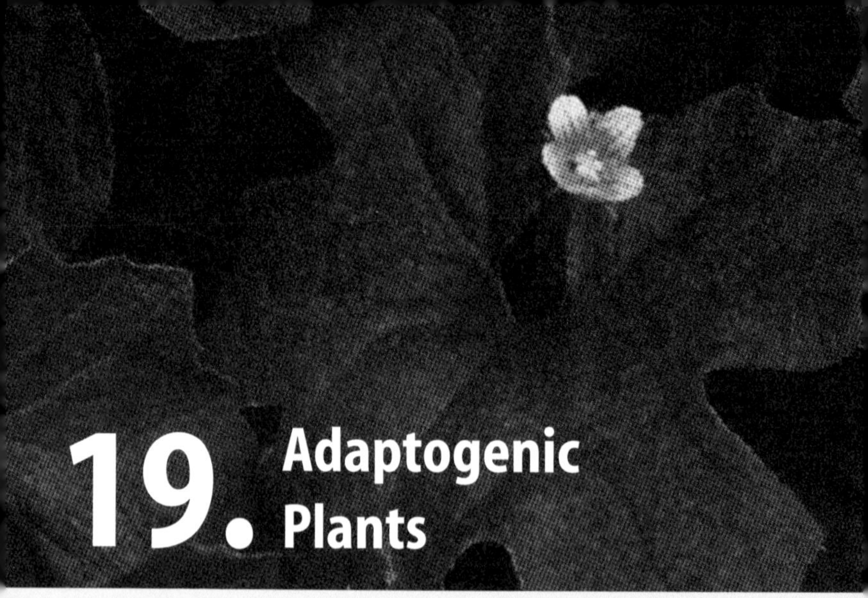

19. Adaptogenic Plants

Introduction

The term adaptogen was originally coined in 1947 by the pharmacologist N.V. Lazarev to describe the unexpected effect of dibazol (2-benzylbenzimidazol), an arterial dilator developed in France. Dibazol was found to increase the resistance of organisms to stress in experimental studies. Adaptogen derives from the Latin *adaptare* meaning to adjust or fit, and 'gen' from the Greek word *genes* meaning born of, or produced by. Incidentally, it is generally regarded as a barbarism to combine Greek and Latin roots in a single word.

The definition of adaptogens is as follow: (i) the adaptogenic effect is non-specific in that the adaptogen increases resistance to a very broad spectrum of harmful factors of different physical, chemical and biological natures; (ii) an adaptogen has a normalizing effect, that is, it counteracts or prevents disturbance brought about by stressor; (iii) an adaptogen must be innocuous to have a broad range of therapeutic effects without causing disturbances to the normal functioning of the organism.

Adaptogens, thus defined, constitute a new class of metabolic regulators (of natural origin) which have been shown to increase the ability of the organism to adapt to envirомental factors and to avoid damage from such factors. Table 19.1 lists some of these plants. Adaptogen as a new concept has become more generally recognized during the last 10 years and has recently been used as a functional term by health authorities such as the FDA. Box 19.1 illustrates the difference between adaptogens and stimulants.

Table 19.1
Herbal medicines promoted as adaptogenic

Common name	Latin name	Part(s) of plant used	Key constituents	Daily dose
Ashwagandha	*Withania somnifera*	Roots	Alkaloids, steroidal lactones	3–6 g
Astragalus	*Astragalus spp.*	Roots	Flavonoids, polysaccharides	2–6 g
Cat's claw	*Uncaria tomentosa*	Root bark	Triterpenes, organic acids, glycosides, procyanidins, alkaloids	0.3–1 g
Cordyceps #	*Cordyceps sinensis*	Fruiting body#	Polysaccharides, nucleoside fractions	3–9 g

continued on page 220

Table 19.1
Herbal medicines promoted as adaptogenic (*continued*)

Common name	Latin name	Part(s) of plant used	Key constituents	Daily dose
Ginseng*	*Panax ginseng*	Roots	Triterpene saponins	1–2 g
Golden root	*Rhodiola rosea*	Roots	Organic acids, flavonoids, tannins, phenolic glycosides	a
Gotu kola	*Centella asiatica*	Leaves	Triterpenes, flavonoids, volatile oil	1.8 g
Sarsaparilla	*Smilax spp*	Roots	Steroid saponins	0.3–1.5 g
Schizandra	*Schizandra chinensis*	Fruits	Volatile oil, ascorbic acid, lignans	1.5–6 g
Siberian ginseng (eleuthero)*	*Eleutherococcus senticosus*	Roots, rhizome	Eleutherosides, carbohydrates, caffeic acid derivatives	2–3 g
White bryony	*Bryonia alba*	Roots	Terpenoids, steroids, fatty acids	0.3–0.5 g

* supported by German Commission E for lack of stamina

\# *C. sinensis* is a fungus

a. an extract standardised to contain 1% of the glycosides rosavin is generally used (100–170 mg/daily)

Table 19.2
True ginseng (Panax ginseng) and various succedaneous

Common name	Botanical name
Korean or Chinese or Asian ginseng	*Panax ginseng*
Japanese ginseng	*Panax japonicus*
American ginseng	*Panax quinquefolium*
San-chi or Tien-chan ginseng	*Panax notoginseng*
Vietnamese ginseng	*Panax vietnamensis*
Alaskan ginseng	*Echinopanax horridum*
Siberian ginseng (eleuthero)	*Eleutherococcus senticosus*
Indian ginseng (ashwagandha)	*Withania somnifera*
Brazilian ginseng (suma)	*Pfaffia paniculata*
Peruvian ginseng (maca)	*Lepidium meyenii*
Wild ginseng	*Aralia nudicaulis*
Red wild ginseng	*Rumex hymenosepalu*

Adaptogenic Plants

Ginseng

Botany/Key constituents ▶ Ginseng is the root of the perennial herb of a plant of the genus *Panax* (Fam. *Araliaceae*). Three medicinal species of ginseng are currently recognized: *P. ginseng* C.A: Meyer (Chinese or Korean ginseng, a perennial herb indigenous to the mountainous forests of Eastern Asia); *P. japonicus* C.A:

Box 19.1

Differences between stimulants and adaptogens

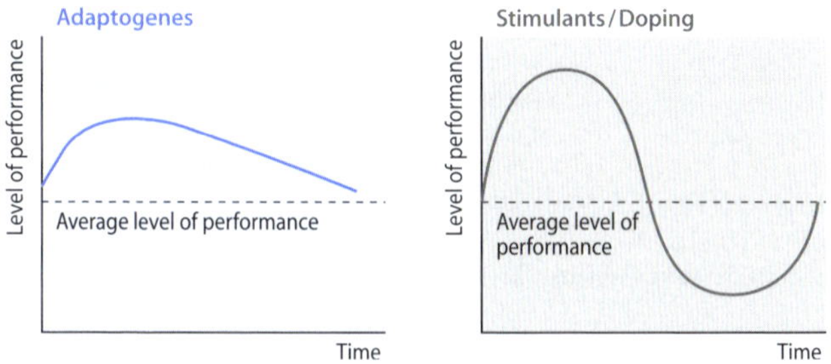

The differences between stimulants and adaptogens are illustrated in these qualitative pictures. Stimulants like phenteramine give a temporary increase in work capacity. However, after the initial increase there follows a period of marked decrease (with respect to an average level of performance) of the work capacity. In humans, a number of unpleasant side effects appear at this state. Moreover, a repeated application of central stimulants leads to a decrease in conditioned reflexes, due partly to an exhaustion of brain catecholamines. As a contrast, adaptogens are believed to display a completely different kind of pharmacodynamic action. In particular the level of performance after reaching its maximum is not followed by a corresponding minimum of the average work capacity.

A series of experiments, designed to demonstrate this difference at a more basic biochemical level was undertaken in the late 1960s. The general assumption behind the experiments was the hypothesis that the adaptogenic action was dependent on the cellular synthesis of nucleic acids (increased synthesis of RNA), an effect which is in sharp contrast to central stimulants.

In contrast to central stimulants, neither the International Olympic Committee nor the US Olympic Committee include ginseng on their lists of banned substances. According to the US Olympic Committee on Substance Abuse Research and Education, there is no scientific evidence available to support the claim of performance enhancement or efficacy of ginseng.

Meyer (Japanese ginseng from Vietnam, Southern China and Japan); and *P. quinquefolius* (American ginseng, found growing in rich woodland in the Eastern and Central USA and Canada). The most commonly used is *Panax ginseng* (true ginseng, se also Table 19.2), a perennial slow-growing herb (Plate 19.1). The main active constituents of the *Panax* species are recognized to be triterpenoid glycosides or saponins, termed ginsenosides, whose structures and distribution vary with species and variety. There are twenty-five ginsenosides that have been separated and detected based on the sugar unit sequences and aglycone moieties.

Mode of action ► Experimental studies have confirmed the adaptogenic properties of ginseng in several stress models used to establish an adaptogenic effect. Ginseng may enhance resistance to X-irradiation, viral and tumor load, temperature stress, hyperbaric hypoxia, and physical exercise. Some studies report that ginseng augments work capacity and increases swimming time in rats. Many of these activities have been attributed to a corticosteroid-like action and endocrinological studies have suggested that ginsenosides may augment adrenal steroidogenesis via an indirect action on the adenohypophysis (Figure 19.1).

Clinical studies ► German Commission E monograph on ginseng states that the herb is used "as a tonic to counteract weakness and fatigue, as a restorative for declining stamina and impaired concentration, and as an aid to convalescence". Ginseng is promoted to increase physical performance, psychomotor performance and cognitive function, immunomodulation, diabetes, and erectile dysfunctions. However, the evidence for ginseng's efficacy is not compelling for any of these indications (Box 19.2).

Adverse events/Contraindications ► When used appropriately, ginseng appears to be relatively safe. Nevertheless, documented side effects include hypertension, diarrhea, insomnia, mastalgia, and vaginal bleeding. The long-term use of ginseng could cause central nervous system excitation and arousal (referred to as ginseng abuse syndrome). A dose of 15 g/daily has been associated with depersonalization, confusion and in some cases depression. There is also evidence that ginseng could cause Steven-Johnson syndrome. The German Commission E recommends that the use should be limited to 3 months. Documented herb/drug interactions include maniac symptoms, headaches, hallucinations and insomina when ginseng is co-administered with the antidepressant phenelzine and over-anticoagulation when given together with the anticoagulant warfarin.

Preparations/Dosage

Ginseng can be administered as an infusion, powder and galenic preparation for internal uses. According to German Commission E the recommended daily dosage is 1–2 g crude drug. Many clinical studies have used a daily dose of 200 mg of a concentrated aqueous standardized extract (extract G115 standardized to 4% ginsenosides; each capsule is equivalent to 500 mg of *P. ginseng* root). It is supplied as capsules, liquid extract (1:2) and tablets.

► *See Chapter 14 for the use of ginseng in the treatment of angina*
► *See Chapter 15 for the use of ginseng in the treatment of diabetes mellitus*
► *See Appendix B for the use of ginseng in cancer prevention*

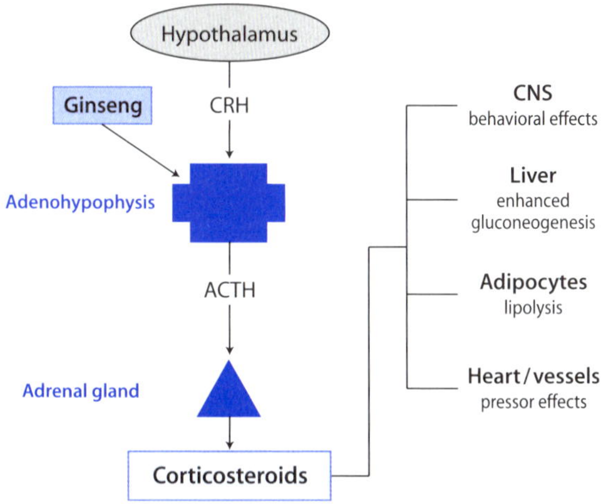

Figure 19.1 ▲ **Possible mechanism of ginseng in experimental studies**
Ginseng may augment adrenal synthesis of corticosteroids via an action on the hypothalamus/adenohypophysis axis. Corticosteroids are known to play a significant role in the adaptation capabilities of the body to stress. Corticosteroids have several targets including the central nervous system, adipocytes, liver, heart and vasculature. CRH, corticotrophin-releasing hormone; ACTH, adrenocorticotropic hormone; CNS, central nervous system

Eleuthero (Siberian ginseng)

Botany/Key constituents ▸ Eleuthero (also named Siberian ginseng) consists of the dried roots and/or rhizome of *Eleutherococcus senticosus* (Fam. *Araliaceae*). *Eleutherococcus* (from the Greek *eleutheros* meaning "free", and *kokkos* meaning 'pip' or 'seed') *senticosus* is a thorny shrub that grows in the Russian Far East, the Amur Region, Primorksy Krai, Sakhalin, and also in North-east China, Korea and Japan. The thorniness, reflected by the specific epithet senticosus, an adjective meaning in Latin 'full of briers or thorns' has led to the common name in Russian of 'thorny Eleutherococcus' (*eleutherokokk koljuchii*). Key constituents include eleutherosides A-M (an heterogenous group of compounds including sterols, phenylpropanoids, coumarins, monosaccharides and lignans), carbohydrates and caffeic acid derivatives (including chlorogenic acid).

Mode of action ▸ The adaptogenic properties of eleuthero has been extensively investigated in the ex-Soviet Union and pharmacological studies started in the 1950s. Nevertheless, eleuthero is reported to have immune-stimulating, antiviral, antioxidant, anticancer and hypocholesterolemic activities. In various stress models, the endurance of rodents was enhanced. In healthy volunteers, the lym-

Box 19.2

Ginseng and eleuthero: randomized clinical studies[1]

Physical performance

Seven trials investigated the effect of ginseng on physical performance in young, active volunteers during submaximal and maximal exercises on cycle ergometers. The four most recent studies found no improvement of physical performance after ingestion of *Panax ginseng*, *Panax quinquefolium* or *Eleutherococcus senticosus*. Other studies found a significant decrease in heart rate and an increase in maximal oxygen uptake compared with placebo, which persisted for three weeks after the treatment.

Psychomotor performance and cognitive function

Five studies investigated the effects of ginseng on psychological functions. Four of these were conducted on young, healthy volunteers while the only non-placebo-controlled trial was performed on elderly people. Three studies reported significant improvements in mental arithmetic and abstraction tests with *Panax ginseng* and in selective memory tests with *Eleutherococcus*. Four studies investigated whether ginseng may alter psychological functions and improve tolerability to exercise-induced stress. None of these studies confirmed this hypothesis. The results suggest no significant effects on the ratings of perceived exertion during cycle ergometer tests.

Immunomodulation

Two studies assessed the effects of ginseng on the immune system in healthy volunteers. One study reported a significant increase of the total number of T-lymphocytes and of the activity of leukocytes compared with baseline after the ingestion of *Panax ginseng*. A more recent study, however, found no effects on total and differential leukocyte counts and lymphocyte subpopulations.

Diabetes

One study investigated the effect of ginseng on Type-II diabetes mellitus. Patients received either 100 mg or 200 mg ginseng daily. At the end of an 8-week treatment period, psychophysical performance, mood and vigor were significantly improved compared with baseline in both ginseng groups. HbA_{1C} was significantly reduced in patients who received 200 mg ginseng extract, while a reduction of the fasting blood glucose level was observed in both ginseng groups compared with baseline.

Herpes infection

One study investigated the effect of *Eleutherococcus senticosus* on herpes simplex Type-II infection. Administration of 400 mg standardized *Eleutherococcus* extract once daily for 6 months produced a beneficial effect on the severity and duration of infections.

[1] From Vogler et al. 1999

phocyte count, expecially that of T-lymphocytes, increased after eleuthero administration. Hypoglycemic effects have been also demonstrated in the herb along with enhancement of a platelet aggregation-inhibiting effect. The exact mechanisms responsible are not known.

Clinical efficacy ▸ Eleuthero is traditionally used as a tonic for invigoration and fortification in times of fatigue and debility or declining capacity for work and concentration, and during convalescence. It has been used as an inexpensive substitute for the ginseng roots of *Panax ginseng* in the republic of the former Soviet Union and other countries. The German Commission E monograph on eleuthero recommends its use "as a tonic to counteract weakness and fatigue, as a restorative for declining stamina and impaired concentration, and as an aid to convalescence". However, clinical evidence for randomized clinical studies is scarse (Box 19.2).

Adverse events/Contraindications ▸ Health risks or side effects following the proper administration of designated therapeutic dosages are not recorded. As with ginseng, the German Commission E recommends that the use should be limited to 3 months. It is stated that eleuthero should be avoided by individuals who are highly energetic, nervous, tense, hysteric, manic or schizophrenia, and that it should not be taken with stimulants, including coffee, antipsychotic drugs or during treatment with hormones. In view of documented pharmacological actions eleuthero may theoretically interfere with a number of therapies including, cardiac, anihypertensive, anticoagulant and hypoglycemic therapy. The German Commission E notes hypertension as a contraindication. Eleuthero may interfere with plasma digoxin assay.

Preparations/Dosage

The recommended daily dose is 2–3 g crude root or an equivalent dose of an extract-based preparation. Extracts are normally standardized to contain more than 1% eleutheroside E. The extract is prepared from root powder and 75% ethanol (1:7) with back flow to which is added a 10% alpha-naphthol solution until there is no reaction. It is then evaporated to a paste.

Ashwagandha

Botany/Key constituents ▸ Ashwagandha is the root of *Withania somnifera* (Fam. *Solanaceae*) and is sometimes erroneously referred to as Indian ginseng because of its popular use similar to that of ginseng. *Withania somnifera* is a small shrub widely distributed throughout the drier regions of India. The chemistry of Ashwagandha has been extensively studied and over 35 chemical constituents have been identified. The biologically active chemical constituents are alkaloids (isopelletierine, anaferine), steroidal lactones (withanolides, withaferins) and terpenoids with a tetracyclic skeleton like cortisol (sitoindosides I-IV). Ashwagandha is also rich in iron.

Mode of action ▸ Many pharmacological studies have been conducted to investigate the properties of ashwagandha in an attempt to authenticate its use as a multi-purpose medical agent. Experimental studies have shown that ashwagandha possesses anti-inflammatory, antitumour, antioxidant, hemopoietic and immunomodulant properties. It also appears to exert a positive influence on the endocrine, cardiopulmonary, and central nervous systems. Moreover, ashwagandha induces a state of non-specific increased resistance during stress, sitoindosides being the active ingredients. The mechanisms of action for these properties are not fully understood.

Clinical efficacy ▸ Aswagandha is widely used in Ayurvedic medicine, the traditional medical system of India. It is an ingredient in many formulations prescribed for a variety of musculoskeletal conditions (e.g. arthritis, rheumatism), and as a general tonic to increase energy, improve overall health and longevity, and prevent disease in athletes, the elderly and during pregnancy. However, there is a lack of randomized clinical studies to support the adaptogenic use. One double-blind clinical trial in 141 healthy male volunteers (aged 50–59), showed that ashwagandha, given for a period of one year, improved the hematological profile, lowered serum cholesterol and had other positive effects.

Adverse events/Contraindications ▸ No health hazards or side effects are known in conjunction with the proper administration of designated therapeutic dosages. However, high doses of the root in mice (750 mg/kg daily for 15 days) caused serious side effects, including diarrhea, weight loss, and death.

Preparations/Dosage

The usual daily dose of the dried powdered root is 3–6 g. It may be consumed in the form of decoction (2 g in 150 ml water for 5 min, about half an hour before meal time), liquid extract or tablets. A liquid extract (1:2, 6–12 ml) preparation is also available.

Other Adaptogenic Plants

Schizandra (Wu-Wei-Zi). Schizandra fruit is the dried, ripe fruit of *Schizandra chinensis* (Turez.) Baillon (Fam. *Schizandraceae*), a liana plant indigenous to North-Eastern China and Korea. The fruit is harvested in Autumn, then steamed before being dried in the sun. Key constituents include a volatile oil, vitamin C and lignans (schizandrine A to C, schizandrol A and B). Schizandra fruit and seeds are believed to bring about a non-specific increase in physical performance ability. Schizandra fruit activate formation of both nitric oxide and cortisol in blood plasma and saliva and this activation is believed to "strengthen" the organism. Lignans are believed to be active principles with adaptogenic properties. Schizandrine and schizandrol possess liver-protective effect, have anti-inflammatory and antitumor activity in animal studies. Despite claims of efficacy, there are no clinical studies to support the adaptogenic properties of schizandra. No specific side effects are known in conjunction with the proper administration of schizandra fruit. Schizandra fruit is generally administered as whole and powdered drug for internal use. The daily dose is 1.5–6 g.

► *See Chapter 22 for the hepato-protecting properties of shizandra*

White bryony. Bryony consists of the dried tap-root of *Bryonia alba* L. (Fam. *Cucurbitaceae*), a plant indigenous from North-Eastern and South-Eastern Europe and also Iran (Plate 19.2). *Bryonia alba* is an extremely fast-growing perennial plant. It has a thick, tuberous root. The root is fleshy, wrinkled horizontally, yellowish-grey on the outside and white and slimy on the inside. Key constituents include terpenoids with a tetracyclic skeleton like cortisol (cucurbitacins), steroids and polyhydroxy fatty acids. White bryony has been used prophylactically and therapeutically for metabolic disorders, liver diseases, acute and chronic infectious diseases and to increase stress resistance. Like lignans of schizandra, cucurbitacins activate formation of both nitric oxide and cortisol and this activation is believed to adapt the organism to physical stress. Moreover, white bryony root has been used as a strong purgative and emetic. The drug is highly toxic when freshly harvested. The toxicity of the drug declines rapidly with dehydration and storage because of the instability of the cucurbitacins. Due to the cucurbitacin content, the drug has a severely irritating effect on skin and mucous membranes. The daily dosage is 0.3–0.5 g. The intake of high dosage can lead to vomiting, bloody diarrhea, colic, kidney complaints, paralysis and, under certain conditions, to death.

Cat's claw is the root bark of *Uncaria tomentosa* L. (Fam. *Rubiaceae*), a large woody vine that sometimes reaches heights of 30 m, indigenous to the rain forest areas of Central and South America. A less common *U. guaianensis* is also used. Key constituents include alkaloids (rynchophyllin, 5-carboxystrictosidine, isopteropodine), triterpenes, organic acids, sterols and procyanidins. Cat's claw possesses several pharmacological actions including anti-inflammatory/immunostimulating effects, inhibitory effect on platelet aggregation, contraceptive effects, antihypertensive and anticancer effects. Moreover, rhynchophylline increases the level of neurotransmitters such as serotonin and dopamine in several brain areas. Cat's claw has been used in folk medicine for rheumatic complaints, diarrhea, gastritis, treatment of wounds, as an adjunct to cancer treatment, menstrual irregularity and as a contraceptive. A case report of a cancer patient in Austria who underwent a miraculous recovery helped bring attention to cat's claw in the 1970s. There are European reports that it is useful in the treatment of AIDS when used in combination with zidovudine. However, cat's claw is probably now best classified as an adaptogen, although randomized clinical trials are lacking. Despite its extreme popularity in Hispanic communities, cat's claw cannot presently be viewed as a safe and effective phytomedicine. Serum estradiol and progesterone levels may be reduced after long-term cat's claw use and its use has been associated to acute renal failure. The daily dosage is up to 1000 mg (the total alkaloid equivalent should be 10–30 mg). Cat's claw is available in 300 mg capsules to be taken three times daily, liquid concentrate (8:1 in 20% alcohol) to be diluted in water and taken 1–3 times daily, and as a crude drug to be used for tea.

Golden root. The root of *Rhodiola rosea* (golden root or arctic root), is a plant widely distributed at high altitudes in Arctic and mountainous regions throughout Europe and Asia. It contains a range of biologically active substances including organic acids, flavonoids, tannins, and phenolic glycosides. It is a popular herbal drug in traditional medical systems in Eastern Europe and Asia, with a reputation for stimulating the nervous system, decreasing depression, enhancing work performance, eliminating fatigue, and preventing high altitude sickness. Golden root has been categorized as an adaptogen by Russian researchers due to its observed ability to increase resistance to a variety of chemical, biological, and physical stressors. The adaptogenic properties of golden roots have been attributed to p-tyrosol and the phenolic glycoside rhodioloside, which influence levels and activity of monoamines and opioid peptides in the brain and in peripheral tissues such as the cardiovasular and respiratory systems. Golden root is stated to be safe; however, some individuals might experience an increase in irritability and insomnia within several days. An extract standardized to contain 1% of the glycoside rosavin is generally used (100–170 mg/daily).

Further Reading

Bahrke MS, Morgan WP (2000) Evaluation of the ergogenic properties of Ginseng. Sports Med 29:113–133

Bucci LR (2000) Selected herbals and human exercise performance. Am J Clin Nutr 72:624S–636S

Davydov M, Krikorian AD (2000) *Eleutherococcus senticosus* (Rupr. & Maxim.) Maxim. (*Arialiaceae*) as a adaptogen a closer look. J Ethnopharmacol 72:345–393

Kelly GS (2001) Rhodiola rosea: a possible plant adaptogen. Altern Med Rev 6:293–302

Kitts D, Hu C (2000) Efficacy and safety of ginseng. Public health Nutr 3:473–485

Mishra LC, Singh BB, Dagenais S (2000) Scientific basis for therapeutic use of *Withania somnifera* (ashwagandha): a review. Altern Med Rev 5:334–346

Murphy LL, Lee TJ (2002) Ginseng, sex behavior, and nitric oxide. Ann N Y Acad Sci 962:372–377

Nocerino E, Amato M, Izzo AA (2000) The aphrodisiac and adaptogenic properties of ginseng. Fitoterapia 71:1–5

Panossian A, Wikman G, Wagner H (1999) Plant adaptogens III. Earlier and more recent aspects and concepts on their mode of action. Phytomedicine 6:287–300

Rege NN, Thatte UM, Dahanukar SA (1999) Adaptogenic properties of six rasayana herbs used in Ayurvedic medicine. Phytother Res 13:275–291

Thomson Coon J, Ernst E (2002) Panax ginseng: a systematic review of adverse effects and drug interactions. Drug Saf 25:323–344

Vogler BK, Pittler MH, Ernst E (1999) The efficacy of ginseng. A systematic review of randomized clinical trials. Eur J Clin Pharmacol 55:567–575

20. Plants and the Reproductive System

Introduction

The human reproductive system may be considered "silent" until puberty, when a trigger activates the genetic code responsible for the production and secretion of hormones responsible for the initiation and continuation of this developmental stage. The reproductive system consists of primary sex organs, the male testes and the female ovaries, collectively called the gonads. Male sexual organs include the testes (which produce sperm and sex hormones), vas deferens and urethra (which carry sperm out of the body), prostate and glands seminal vesicles (which contribute to the majority of fluid within the semen), penis (which is an organ of copulation and excretion) and scrotum (housing the testes outside the pelvic cavity which is essential for viable sperm production). Female sexual organs include the ovaries (which produce ova and sex hormones), the uterine tubes (which carry ova from the ovary to the uterus), the uterus (which represents the house and nourishes developing embryo), the vagina (which receives sperm during intercourse and which also represents the exit point for menstrual flow), the vulva (which serves as a protection) and mammary glands (which produce milk). As with any organ system failure, imbalances include a wide number of conditions, both for male and female. This chapter will focus on menopausal symptoms, premenstrual syndrome and benign prostatic hyperplasia.

Menopausal Symptoms

Clinical Picture

- In humans the maturity of the reproductive system is signalled by an eruption of hormones that determine the secondary sexual characteristics of young men and women. A considerable number of botanicals have been used over the centuries to treat ailments of the reproductive system. The majority of these were used in women with conditions such as menstrual disorders and complications of childbirth.

- More modern applications have been focused on alleviating the vasomotor symptoms ("sweats/hot flushes") of the menopause and "mood swings" associated with cyclic fluctuations in female hormones. About 75–85% of premenopausal and menopausal women complain of "hot flushes" – sudden feelings of warmth, flushing and perspiration occurring mostly on the upper body and face and for which about 33% of affected women seek medical attention. These episodes can last seconds to 20 min, and may occur infrequently or more than 10 times a day. Some women suddenly awake, drenched in perspiration, and suffering from insomnia. On average, these symptoms last about 2–3 years in the absence of any pharmacotherapy. Triggers include a warm environment, alcohol, spicy foods, caffeine, hot drinks, stress, embarrassment, and exercise.
- The mechanism may involve interference with the central temperature-regulating and/or peripheral autonomic control mechanism(s). Vaginal dryness and changes in sexual desire are other major consequences of the decrease in estrogen that occurs at this time in a woman's life. Symptoms associated with diminished cirulating levels of estrogen are treated by replacing the hormone with synthetic or plant-derived estrogenic molecules.

Premenstrual Syndrome

Clinical Picture

- Premenstrual syndrome is a complex combination of psychological symptoms, including irritability, aggression, tension, anxiety, depression, and somatic changes such as fluid retention, breast tenderness, headache, feeling of bloating, and weight increase which occur during the luteal phase of the menstrual cycle and disappear within a few days of the onset of menstruation. Although it has been estimated that 30–80% of women report premenstrual symptoms, when strict diagnostic criteria are applied, the prevalence of severe premenstrual syndrome is estimated to be about 2.5% in women of reproductive age.
- The etiology of premenstrual syndrome has not been firmly established and suggestions have included hormonal imbalances, sodium retention, nutritional deficiencies, and abnormal neurotransmitter responses to normal ovarian function, and abnormal hypothalamic-pituitary-adrenal axis function. Pharmacological treatments have included antidepressants, diuretics, progesterone, estrogen implants, combined contraceptives and gonadotrophin-releasing hormone agonists.

Herbal Medicines used to Treat Menopausal Symptoms and/or Premenstrual Syndrome

Phytotherapy is often recommended for alleviating symptoms of premenstrual syndrome as well as for menopausal symptoms. Figure 20.1 shows some herbal drugs used to treat symptoms of the female reproductive system according to German Commission E. Table 20.1 shows herbal medicines used to treat premenstrual syndrome and/or menopausal symptoms.

Black cohosh

Botany/Key constituents ► The drug consists of the dried rhizome and roots of *Cimicifuga racemosa* (L.) Nuttor or *Actaea recemosa* L. (Fam. *Ranunculaceae*), a perennial 1–1.5 m high herb native to the temperate climates of North America and also cultivated in Europe (Plate 20.1). This herb, commonly known as "woman's herb" contains triterpene glycosides (e.g. actein, 27-deoxyactein, cimifugoside), isoflavones (formononetin), quinolizidine alkaloids (cytisine, methylcytisine), caffeic and isoferulic acids and 15–20% resins (cimicifugin).

Mode of action ► Experiments and clinical studies have shown that a methanol extract of black cohosh caused a selective reduction of luteinizing hormone (LH) from the anterior pituitary gland. In human studies, it has decreased elevated levels of LH associated with hot flushes. The triterpene glycosides are believed to work together, at least in part, to suppress the hormone. Follicle-stimulating hormone (FSH) and prolactin levels were unchanged. Clinical and experimental investigations indicated that black cohosh does not show hormone-like activity, as was originally postulated.

Mastodynia	Chasteberry
Menorrhagia and metrorrhagia	Sheperd's purse
Dysmenorrheic complaints	Black cohosh, potentilla
Breast pain and tension	Bugleweed
Premenstrual syndrome	Black cohosh, chasteberry, bugleweed, potentilla

◄ Figure 20.1
Main herbal medicines used to treat symptoms of the female reproductive system according to German Commission E

Table 20.1

Herbal medicines used for the treatment of premenstural syndrome and/or menopausal complaints

Common name	Latin name	Part(s) of plant used	Key constituents	Daily dose
Black cohosh**	*Cimicifuga racemosa*	Roots, rhizome	Triterpenes, quinolizidine derivatives, flavonoids	0.04 g
Bugleweed *	*Lycopus virginicus*	Aerial parts	Caffeic acid derivatives, flavonoids, diterpenes	1–2 g
Chasteberry**	*Vitex agnus castus*	Fruits	Iridoid glycosides, flavonoids, volatile oil, fatty oils	0.03–0.04 g
Dong quai	*Angelica sinensis*	Roots	Phytosterols, flavonoids, polysaccharides	3–15 g
Evening primrose*	*Oenothera biennis*	Fixed oil from the seeds	Linoleic acid, gamma-linolenic acid	3–6 g
Ginseng	*Panax ginseng*	Roots	Triterpene saponins	1–2 g
Hops	*Humulus lupulus*	Glandular hairs	Bitter acids, volatile oil, resins, phenolic acid, flavonoids	5 g
Kava	*Piper methysticum*	Rhizome	Kava lactones, flavonoids	1.5–3 g
Potentilla (silverweed)*	*Potentilla anserina*	Leaves, flowers	Tannins, flavonoids, coumarins	4–6 g
Rhapontic rhubarb	*Rheum rhaponticum*	Roots	Stilbene derivatives (rhapontin), antrhaquinones	1–2 g
Red clover	*Trifolium pratense*	Flower heads	Volatile oil, flavonoids, coumarin derivatives, cyanogenic glycosides	4 g
Shepherd's purse*	*Capsella bursa-pastoris*	Aerial parts	Glucosilonates, sinigrin, flavonoids	10–15 g
St John's wort	*Hypericum perforatum*	Aerial parts	Anthracene derivatives, flavonoids, phloroglucinol derivatives	2–4 g
Wild yam	*Dioscorea villosa*	Roots	Steroid saponins (dioscin, aglycone diosgenin), alkaloids (dioscorin, dioscorine)	
Yarrow	*Achillea millefolium*	Aerial parts	Volatile oil (chamazulene, camphor), sesquiterpene lactones, flavonoids, alkamids	3–4.5 g

* supported by German Commission E for the treatment of premenstrual syndrome

** supported by German Commission E for the treatment of premenstrual syndrome and menopausal complaints

Clinical efficacy ▶ The German Commission E has found black cohosh to be effective in the treatment of nervous conditions associated with the menopause. However, in 1986 the U.S. Food and Drug Administration found no pharmacological evidence of therapeutic value in black cohosh and cautioned against its overuse. A recent systematic review retrieved four randomized clinical trials (n = 226 subjects) and three of these studies reported positive results in menopausal symptoms. However, two studies reporting positive results were without placebo. Overall, black cohosh seem to have a little beneficial effects on menopausal symptoms. Further studies are needed to fully define its efficacy.

Adverse events/Contraindications ▶ No adverse effects from ingestion of black cohosh are expected when used at the recommended dosage. High doses cause a frontal headache, with a dull, full or bursting feeling. This headache is the most characteristic effect observed when given even therapeutic doses. Stomach complaints have occasionally been observed in clinical trials. It is stated that black cohosh may potentiate the effect of antihypertensive medicines; however, no clinical evidence support this statement.

Preparations/Dosage

The German Commission E recommends daily doses of 40 mg dried rhizome and root, with its use not to exceed 6 months. An ethanolic extract of the rhizome standardized to contain 1 mg triterpenes calculated as 27-deoxyacteine per 20 mg tablets (Remifemin®) is commonly prescribed in European phytotherapy for the relief of climacteric (menopausal) disorders including hot flushes and profuse sweating. Black cohosh can also be prepared as a tincture (1:10, 60% ethanol). The dose is 0.4–2 ml/day. The onset of action of these preparations can take up to two weeks to occur.

Chasteberry

Botany/Key constituents ▶ Chasteberry (chaste tree, Monk's pepper) is the fruit of *Vitex agnus castus* L. (Fam. *Verbenaceae*), a 3–5 m high shrub indigenous to Southern Europe as far as Western Asia (Plate 20.2). The black spherical berries are about 5 mm in size and contain four seeds. The name is supposedly derived from the belief that it would suppress libido. In fact a tincture of the fresh berries was traditionally used by the Eclectis and was said to 'repress the sexual passions'. Key constituents include iridoid glycosides (e.g. aucubin, agnoside), flavonoids (e.g. casticin) and a volatile oil with cineole and sesquiterpenoid hydrocarbons.

Mode of action ▶ Many patients with premenstrual syndrome show latent hyperprolactinemia associated with corpus luteum insufficiency. Experimental studies have shown that chasteberry inhibits basal and TRH-stimulated prolactin secretion in isolated rat pituitary cells and this effect is counteracted by dopamine antagonists (Figure 20.2). Chasteberry does not affect LH or FSH. Although a single active constituent has not been identified, iridoid glycosides, flavonoids and the essential oil are believed to be responsible for the action of chasteberry. Dopaminergic substances in chasteberry extract may have a catechol structure and therefore easily undergo auto-oxidation after isolation. It is possible that

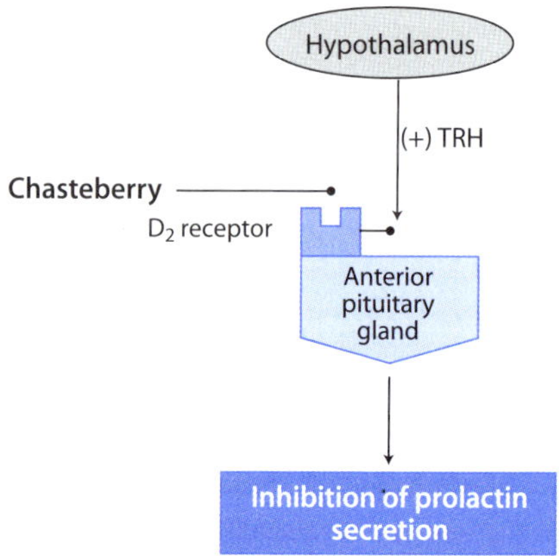

Figure 20.2 ▲ **Mode of action of chasteberry**
Hyperprolactinemia is one of the most frequent causes for cyclical disorders, from corpus luteal insufficiency to secondary amenorrhea, and premenstrual mastalgia. Prolactin secretion from the anterior pituitary gland is inhibited by dopamine and stimulated by thyroxin-releasing hormone (THR) released from the hypothalamus. Chasteberry inhibited basal and TRH-stimulated prolactin secretion by blocking the stimulatory (D_2 receptor mediated) effect of dopamine on anterior pituitary gland

chasteberry protects dopaminergic substances by an endogenous production of antioxidants.

Clinical efficacy ► The German Commission E recommends chasteberry for a number of disorders including premenstrual syndrome, mastalgia and menopausal symptoms. Controlled clinical trials have demonstrated the efficacy of chasteberry in the treatment of premenstrual syndrome. Notably, a recent randomized, placebo-controlled study, carried out on 178 women, indicated that chasteberry (ethanol extract Ze 440, 20 mg/daily over a period three menstrual cycles) is effective treatment for the relief of symptoms (irritability, mood alteration, anger, headache, bloating, breast fullness) of the premenstrual syndrome.

Adverse events/Contraindications ► Chasteberry is considered a safe herb although allergic reactions, which resolved following discontinuation of the herb, have been reported. In clinical studies patient acceptance is high and side effects are few and mild (acne, multiple abscesses, intermenstrual bleeding, urticaria). Chasteberry may cause sleep disturbance, tachycardia, nausea, vomiting, sensation of epigastric pressure and headache.

Preparations/Dosage

The usual dose of chasteberry is 30–40 mg per day of herb. Chasteberry can be prepared as a tincture or a decoction. Ethanolic extracts standardized to casticin (one 20 mg tablet once daily) have been used in most clinical trials. A solid extract equivalent of the tincture has been developed for those who are sensitive to alcohol.

Minor Herbs

Evening primrose. Evening primrose oil is the fixed oil obtained from the seeds of *Oenothera species* including *Oenothera biennis* L. (Fam. *Onagraceae*). The fixed oil (14%) contain cis-linoleic acid (72%), cis-gammalinolenic acid (2–16%), oleic acid, palmitic acid and stearic acid. The presence of essential fatty acids (which play a role in the structure of cell membranes, modulate the behaviour of membrane-bound proteins and are precursors of prostaglandins, leukotrienes and thromboxanes) could contribute to the therapeutic effects; however, the exact mode of action is not known. There is no convincing evidence about the efficacy of evening primrose oil. Four small randomized clinical trials of the oil of evening primrose failed to show any difference in overall symptoms of premenstrual syndrome between evening primrose oil and the placebo with doses from 3–6 g per day. Moreover, one double-blind randomized clinical trial (n = 56 subjects) showed no benefit for evening primose in reducing the frequency of hot flushes. Daily doses for primrose oil are specific to the condition being treated. In premestrual syndrome, a daily dose of 3–4 g is recommended. These doses are based on a standardized gammalinolenic acid content of 8%. Evening primrose oil is very well tolerated, with few side effects.

► *See Chapter 17 for the anti-inflammatory action of evening primrose oil*
► *See Chapter 23 for the use of evening primrose oil for the treatment of inflammatory skin diseases*

Dong quai (Chinese angelica) is the root of *Angelica sinesis* (Oliv.) Diels (Fam. *Umbelliferae*). It has a 2000 year history as a treatment for dysmenorrhea, amenorrhea or excessive menstrual flow. The actions of dong quai is said to be due to the presence of coumarins, phytosterols, flavonoids and polysaccharides. Curiously, different components of dong quai can have opposite effects on uterine contractions; a volatile fraction inhibits contraction and non-volatile substances stimulate the uterus to contract. It seems most probable that the estrogenic effects of dong quai are indirect rather than through a constituent binding to estrogen receptors. Preparations of dong quai can enhance metabolism, lower blood pressure, inhibit platelet aggregation, and suppress inflammation. A double-blind randomized clinical trial (n = 71 subjects) failed to show any beneficial effect of dong quai in relieving menopausal symptoms. Dong quai may be taken for long time at the dosage of 3–15 g per day of the dried root by decoction. No adverse effects are expected, except for photosensitization leading to dermatitis. According to traditional Chinese medicine, contraindications include diarrhea caused by weak digestion, hemorrhagic disease, bleeding tendency, tendency to spontaneous abortion and acute viral infections such as colds and influenza. Dong quai contains anticoagulant coumarins and clinical reports suggest interaction with warfarin leading to an increased anticoagulant effect and widespread bruising.

Red clover consists of the flower heads of *Trifolium pratense* (Fam. *Fabaceae*), a plant indigenous to Europe, Central Asia, Northern Africa and naturalized in many other parts of the world. It contains a volatile oil, flavonoids, coumarin derivatives and cyanogenic glycosides. Red clover is often promoted as a phytoestrogen source similar to soybeans and traditionally has not been used long-term. A recent systematic review retrieved two double blind placebo-controlled trials and both studies found no beneficial effects of red clover extracts on hot flushes or other menopausal symptoms. No side effects have been associated with the proper administration of red clover. The presence of anticoagulant coumarins should be taken into account. The daily dosage is 4 g drug, taken as infusion, up to 3 times a day.

Benign Prostatic Hyperplasia

Clinical Picture

- The prostate gland is susceptible to infection, enlargement and benign or malignant tumors. Enlargement of the prostate is common in men over 50 years of age. By the age of 65–70 most men will develop benign prostatic hyperplasia (BPH).
- Pathological BPH is characterized by an increased number of stromal and epithelial cells. Since the prostate surrounds the urethra, the resulting prostate enlargement can obstruct the flow of urine, resulting in difficult urination but with greater urinary frequency and urgency. There are two components to these symptoms: (i) static obstruction as a consequence of the enlargement of the gland and (ii) dynamic obstruction due to the activation of bladder smooth muscles. Correction involves partial or total removal of the prostatic gland.

Treatment of Benign Prostatic Hyperplasia

- Approaches to the treatment of BPH include the use of drugs that alter the action and concentration of testosterone, which address static obstruction reducing the prostate size, and α_1 adrenoceptor antagonists, which influence dynamic obstruction by diminishing prostatic smooth muscle tone.

- Testosterone stimulates the growth of the prostatic gland; it is converted in the prostatic cell by the enzyme 5α-reductase to its prostate-activating derivative, dihydrotestosterone (DHT), which is the active form of testosterone. The DHT binds to a specific receptor and this complex promotes protein synthesis, cell metabolism and division. DHT increases 4–6 times in hyperplastic prostate. The action of testosterone on the prostate may be prevented by 5α-reductase inhibitors or testosterone antagonists. Alternatively, testosterone synthesis may be inhibited by estrogens, probably secondary to inhibition of the release of gonadotropin releasing hormone (GnRH) from the hypothalamus and/or luteinizing hormone releasing hormone (LHRH). Analogs of LHRH stimulate the formation of testosterone in the testis.
- A second pharmacological approach is to use α_1 adrenoceptor antagonists that improve the dynamic component of urination and reduce the symptoms of BPH. Adrenoceptor activation of the trigone muscle and urethra increases the resistance to urine flow. α_1-adrenoceptor antagonists remove such activation and lower the resistance to urine flow, thereby quickly relieving symptoms.

Phytotherapy of Benign Prostatic Hyperplasia

Phytotherapy for treating BPH symptoms was first described in Egypt in the 15th century BC. Currently, phytotherapy is common in Europe and is increasing in the Western hemisphere. Phytotherapeutic agents represent nearly half the medications dispensed for treatment of BPH in Italy, compared with 5% for α-adrenergic antagonists and 5% for 5α-reductase inhibitors. In Germany and Austria, phytotherapy is the first-line treatment for mild-to-moderate lower urinary tract symptoms and represents more than 90% of all drugs prescribed for the treatment of BPH. In the United States, phytotherapies for BPH are readily available as non-prescription dietary supplements.

Among the herbal medicines recommended in BPH (Table 20.2) saw palmetto, pygeum, urtica, phytosterols from African potato (*Hypoxis rooperi*), rye grass pollen and pumpkin seed (oil) are perhaps the most important. Overall, randomized studies indicate a strong evidence for the efficacy of saw palmetto, moderate evidence for pygeum and phytosterols and rye grass pollen, while preliminary evidence supports the use of nettle or pumpkin for the treatment of BPH.

Table 20.2
Herbal medicines used for the treatment of benign prostatic hyperplasia

Common name	Latin name	Part(s) of plant used	Key constituents	Daily dose
African potato	*Hypoxis rooperi*	Rhizome	Phytosterols, lignans, polysaccharides	6–10 g
Heather	*Calluna vulgaris*	Aerial parts	Flavonoids, catechins, tannins, phenols, triterpenes	1.5–3 g
Stinging nettle*	*Urtica dioica*	Roots	Steroids, lectins, polysaccharides, coumarins, lignans	4–6 g
Pygeum (African plum)	*Pygeum africanum*	Bark	Phytosterols, triterpenoids, fatty acids	10–20 g
Pumpkin*	*Cucurbita pepo*	Seeds	Steroids, fatty oil, proteic substances, γ-tocopherol	10 g
Saw palmetto*	*Serenoa repens*	Fruits	Steroids, flavonoids, fatty oil, polysaccharides	1–2 g

* supported by German Commission E

Saw palmetto

Botany/Key constituents ▸ Saw palmetto consists of the dried ripe fruit of *Serenoa repens* (Bartram) Small (= *Sabal serrulata*) (Fam. *Arecaceae*), a dwarf palm native to the West Indies and the South-Eastern United States (Florida, South Carolina) (Plate 20.3). The fruits are globular (2–3 x 1.5 cm), monoseeded and bluish to black at maturity. They contain fatty acids (20%) and their glycerides (oleic, caprilic, myristic, lauric, stearic, palmitic, etc.), phytosterols (sitosterol, campesterol, cycloartenol) and sitosterol derivatives. Other constituents are organic acids (caffeic, chlorogenic, anthranilic, etc.) polysaccharides, tannin, sugars, volatile oil (1.5%) and flavonoids.

Mode of action ▸ Although the antiandrogenic components seem to reside in the acidic lipophilic fraction of the fruit they remain unidentified. The phytosterols, and fatty acids (lauric, oleic, myristic and palmitic acid) are believed to be the pharmacologically active agents. Like finasteride, saw palmetto inhibits enzyme 5α-reductase (*in vitro*) blocking the conversion of testosterone to dihydrotestosterone (Figure 20.3), a major growth stimulator of the prostate gland; saw palmetto also inhibits dihydrotestosterone binding to its receptor (Figure 20.3). In addition, its anti-inflammatory (inhibition of cycloxygenase and 5-lipoxygenase enzymes) and spasmolytic activities on bladder muscle (blockade of calcium channels, α-adrenergic antagonistic properties) are thought to be important in decreasing the edematous component of BPH (Figure 20.4).

Clinical efficacy ▸ There can be little doubt about the efficacy of saw palmetto. A recent systematic review evaluated 18 studies (16 were double-blind) lasting 4–48

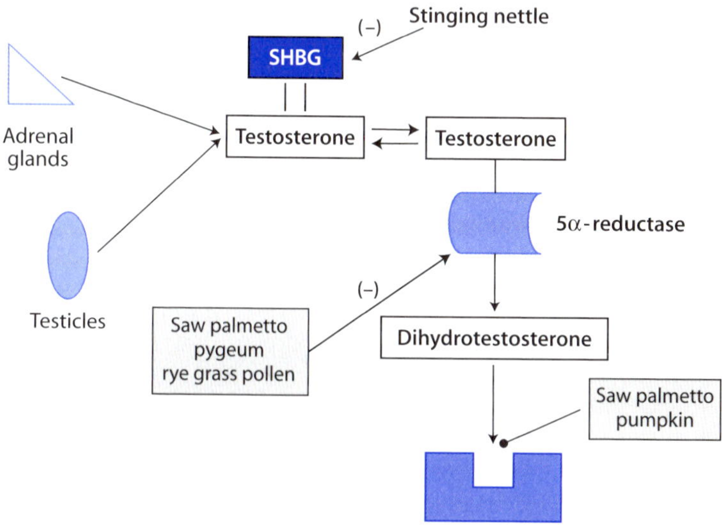

Figure 20.3 ▲ **Conversion of testosterone to dihydrotestosterone and site of action of herbal medicines**
Saw palmetto, **pygeum** and **rye grass pollen** block the enzyme 5α-reductase, which catalyzes the conversion of testosterone to dihydrotestosterone, a major growth stimulator of the prostate gland. There are two isoforms of 5α-reductase: Type 1 and Type 2, the latter is mainly found in the prostate gland. Several lignans from **stinging nettle** root reduced binding activity of sex hormone-binding globulin (SHBG) to testosterone. **Saw palmetto** and **pumpkin** reduce the binding of dihydrotestosterone to its receptor

weeks including a total of 2939 men. These selected studies were randomized, placebo-controlled and included clinical outcomes such as urological symptoms or urodynamic measurements. Data suggest that saw palmetto is superior to placebo and as effective as finasteride in improving urinary symptom scores and urinary flow in patients with benign prostatic hyperplasia. Saw palmetto is supported by German Commission E for the treatment of prostate complaints and irritable bladder.

Adverse events/Contraindications ▸ Adverse effects due to saw palmetto are mild (e.g. gastrointestinal upset) and it is better tolerated than finasteride. Other evidence indicates that, unlike finasteride, saw palmetto did not cause impotence, decrease libido, or alter prostate-specific antigen levels. Saw palmetto might interact, theoretically, with existing hormonal therapy (contraceptive pills, hormone replacement therapy); however, no clinical report of herb-drug interactions has so far been reported.

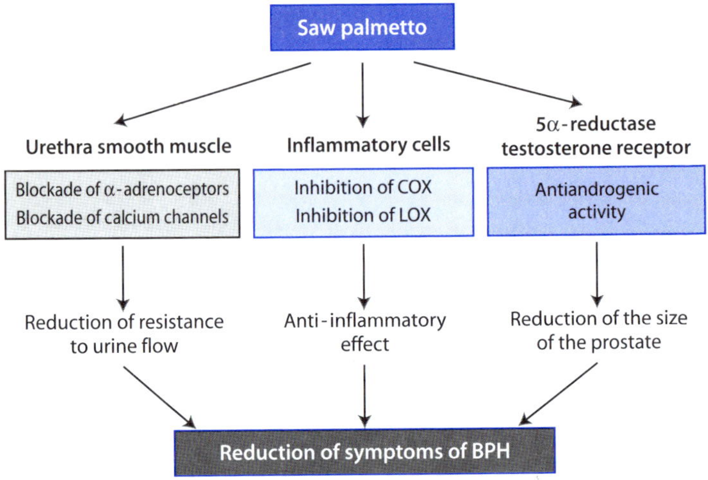

Figure 20.4 ▲ **Possible mode of action of saw palmetto**
(see text for details) COX = cyclooxygenase, LOX = lipoxygenase

Preparations/Dosage

The German Commission E recommends a daily dose of 1–2 g crude drug or 360 mg lipo-sterolic extract containing 85–95% fatty acids and sterols. Aqueous beverages will not contain the water-insoluble active constituents, so it will have little value.

Pygeum (African plum)

Botany/Key constituents ► Pygeum consists of the bark of *Pygeum africanum* (Fam. *Rosaceae*), a tall tree (30 m) native to Africa, with elliptic, weakly acuminate and coriaceous leaves. The bark is dark brown or red and smells weakly of hydrocyanic acid. The bark contains phytosterols (beta-sitosterol, beta-sitosteryl glucoside, beta-sitostenone) and other sterols and steroid intermediates; triterpenoid pentacyclic acids (ursolic, oleanolic, and their homologs sometimes acylated by ferulic acid); alcohols especially docasanol, and C12–C22 fatty acids of which palmitic acid is the most predominant.

Mode of action ► The mechanism of action of pygeum has not been elucidated completely. Several mechanisms could contribute to the therapeutic effect (Figure 20.5). These include (i) inhibition of prostatic fibroblast proliferation in response to growth factors, (ii) anti-inflammatory activity (inhibition of the

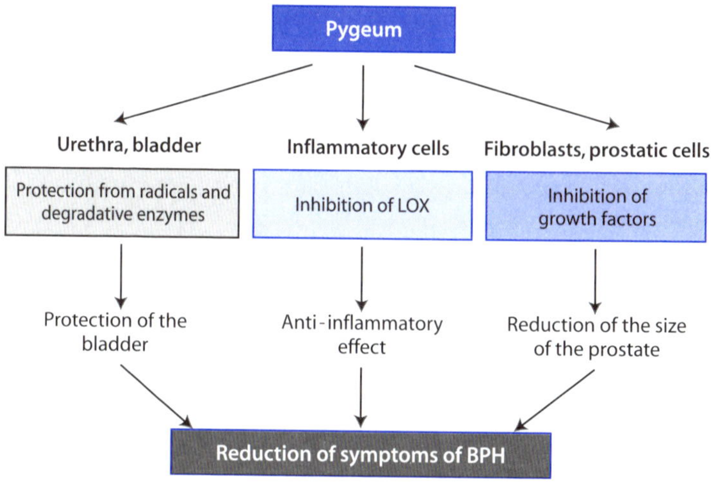

Figure 20.5 ▲ **Possible mode of action of pygeum** (see text for details) LOX = lipoxygenase

enzyme lipoxygenase) and (iii) weak inhibition of 5α-reductase. Pygeum has a positive effect not only on the prostate, but also on the bladder by protecting it by destructive effects of free radicals and degradative enzymes.

Clinical efficacy ▶ The literature on pygeum for the treatment of BPH is limited by the short duration of studies (30–122 days, mean duration 64 days) and the variability in study design, the use of phytotherapeutic preparations, and the types of reported outcome. In a meta-analysis of 18 randomized controlled trials involving 1562 men with treatment period of at least 30 days, pygeum provided a moderately large improvement in urologic symptoms and flow measures. Nocturia was reduced by 19% and residual volume by 24%, peak urine flow was increased by 23%. It has no effect on the volume of the adenoma.

Adverse events ▶ The extract appears devoid of serious side effects; headache, and gastrointestinal problems have been observed in some patients.

Preparations/Dosage

The product most commonly used is a lipid and sterol extract; the component concentrations in this extract are 6.2% fatty acids, 10.7% sitosterol, 2% sitostenone, 2.9% ursolic acid, 0.7% oleanolic acid and 0.39–0.64% docasanol. The extract may also reach concentrations as high as 15.7% for beta-sitosterol. The usual dose of a lipophilic extract of pygeum is 100–200 mg daily (in 6–8 weeks cycles). Tadenan® is a product commonly prescribed in France and other European countries; each capsule contains an extract prepared with 10 g dry bark.

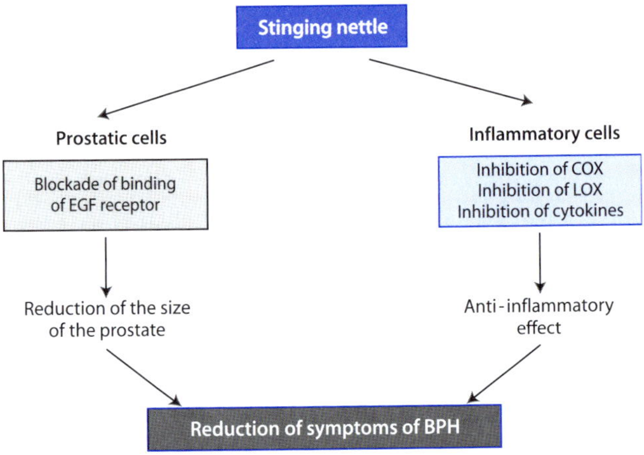

Figure 20.6 ▲ **Possible mode of action of stinging nettle**
(see text for details) EGF = epidermal growth factor, COX = cyclooxygenase, LOX = lipoxygenase

Stinging nettle (root)

Botany/Key constituents ▸ Nettle root derives from *Urtica dioica* L. (Fam. *Urticaceae*), an herbaceous plant which grows wild around rural houses, in piles of rubble and in ditches (Plate 20.4). The stem bears opposite and dark green leaves with long triangular teeth. The roots are ramified and yellowish. The leaves contain sterols (sitosterol), glycoproteins, acids (salicylic, malic, carbonic and formic), flavonoids (rutin, kaempferol, quercetin, etc.), minerals (calcium, potassium) amines (histamine, etc.), tannins, etc. The roots contain polysaccharides, lectins, sterols and their glucosides (3-beta-sitosterol,sitosterol-3-D-glucoside, etc.), lignans, fatty acids and scopoletin.

Mode of action ▸ The identity of the active substances is not completely known and several mechanisms of action have been proposed (Figure 20.6). A number of lignans from nettle root reduced binding of testosterone to human sex hormone-binding globulin (SHBG) (Figure 20.3) and also nettle extracts inhibit prostatic aromatase (the enzyme which converst testosterone to estogens). This is in line with the observation that BPH is characterized by an increase in the estrogen:androgen ratio. Polysaccharides and the lectin *Urtica dioica* agglutin (UDA) can block the binding of the epidermal growth factor (EGF) secreted by the prostatic tissue to its receptor with suppression of prostate-cell metabolism and growth. Moreover, nettle displays anti-inflammatory activity (inhibition of cycloxygenase and lipoxygenase and inhibition of cytokine production) and also inhibits proteolytic enzyme (human leukocyte elastase, HLE) which is involved in genitourinary tract infection/inflammation. Nettle is a very weak inhibitor of 5α-reductase, and does not influence the binding of dihydrotestosterone to the receptor.

Clinical efficacy ▸ The German Commission E monograph states that the herb is indicated for "micturition difficulties associated with Stage I-II prostatic adenoma". This drug only relieves the symptoms of an enlarged prostate without eliminating the enlargement itself. However, the evidence supporting the use of nettle for the treatment of BPH is not as convincing as other phytotherapeutics, namely saw palmetto, pygeum and African potato (*Hypoxis rooperi*). Controlled studies are limited although nettle may be effective combined with other plant extracts such as saw palmetto and pygeum. Nevertheless, four double-blind, placebo-controlled randomized clinical trials (n = 210 subjects) reported doubtful beneficial effects.

Adverse events/Contraindications ▸ Nettle root preparations are well tolerated in humans: instances of scanty urination, skin irritation and gastric distress have been noted. It is stated that nettle may interact with conventional antihypertensive, diabetes and diuretic drugs.

Preparations/Dosage

The German Commission E recommends a daily dose of 4–6 g crude drug. Nettle can be administered in the form of tea, fluid extract (1:1, 45% of ethanol, 1.5–7.5 ml) or tincture (1:5, 40% of ethanol, 5 ml).

▸ *See Chapter 17 for the anti-inflammatory effect of nettle top*

Rye grass pollen

Preparation/Composition ▸ Rye grass pollen extract is prepared from the pollen of *Secale cereale* (Fam. *Graminaceae*). This preparation is obtained by microbial digestion of the pollen followed by extraction with water and an organic solvent. The total extract consists of a water-soluble and acetone-soluble fraction. The last fraction contains sterols.

Mode of action ▸ Several mechanisms could be contributed to the clinical efficacy (Figure 20.7). These include (i) anti-inflammatory activity (inhibition of cytokine production, (ii) inhibition of 5α-reductase and (iii) blockade of α-adrenergic receptors. The active ingredient is not known.

Clinical efficacy ▸ The German Commission E states that pollen extract is useful in the treatment of "micturition difficulties associated with Stage I-II benign prostatic enlargement". A recent systematic review retrieved four randomized

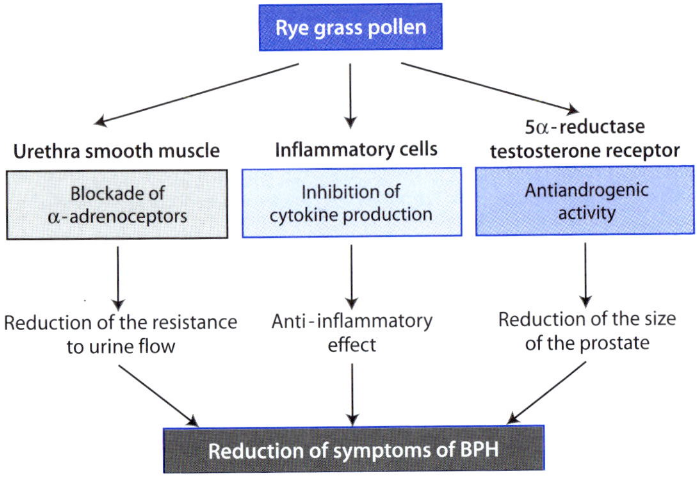

Figure 20.7 ▲ **Possible mode of action of rye grass pollen**
(see text for details)

clinical studies involving a total of 444 men with treatment ranging from 12 to 24 weeks. It was found that rye grass pollen improved self-rated urinary symptoms. However, rye grass pollen did not improve urinary flow rates, residual volume or prostate size. Overall, the available evidence suggests that rye grass pollen modestly improves urological symptoms including nocturia.

Adverse events ▸ Rye grass pollen is well tolerated. Adverse events are rare and mild. Rare gastrointestinal symptoms or allergic skin reactions have been reported.

Preparations/Dosage

The recommended daily dose is 80–120 mg extract taken in 2 or 3 divided doses. Cernilton® is a well-known preparation obtained from the rye grass pollen and used in most clinical studies.

Pumpkin

Botany/Key constituents ▸ The oil of pumpkin (*Cucurbita pepo* L., Fam. *Cucurbitaceae*) seeds has been used for many years for the treatment of an enlarged prostate gland. The pumpkin seeds yield 49% oil, mostly linoleic acid (43–55%) and oleic acid, along with tocopherol, but it is the sterol composition that has retained the attention of researchers. The main constituents are Δ^7-sterols (avenasterol, spinasterol) and Δ^5-sterols (sitosterol, stigmasterol, etc.), to which the positive effect of the oil in BPH is attributed.

Mode of action ▶ The active ingredients and the mode of action are not known. The benefit of pumpkin seed oil appears to be due to its tonic effect on the bladder and relaxation of sphincter at the neck of the bladder. Δ^7-sterols displace dihydrotestosterone from its receptors.

Clinical efficacy ▶ The German Commission E states that pumpkin seeds are indicated for "micturition difficulties associated with Stage I-II prostatic adenoma and irritable bladder". Pumpkin relieves the difficulties associated with an enlarged prostate but does not reduce the enlargment itself. Clinical studies involving pumpkin are limited although this drug may be effectively combined with other plant extracts such as saw palmetto and pygeum.

Adverse events/Contraindications ▶ No side-effects are noted with pumpkin seed extract.

Preparations/Dosage

The daily dose recommended by Commission E is 10 g ground seeds.

Further Reading

Cristoni A, Di Pierro F, Bombardelli E (2000) Botanical derivatives for the prostate. Fitoterapia 71:S21–S28

Borrelli F, Ernst E (2003) Cimicifuga racemosa: a systemati review of its clinical and pharmacological effects. Eur J Clin Pharmacol 58:235–241

Borrelli F, Izzo AA, Ernst E (2003) Pharmacological effects of Cimicifuga racemosa. Life Sci in press

Dvorkin L, Song KY (2002) Herbs for benign prostatic hyperplasia. Ann Pharmacother 36:1443–1452

Fugh-Berman A, Kronenberg F (2001) Red clover (Trifolium pratense) for menopausal women: current state of knowledge. Menopause 8:333–337

Ishani A, MacDonald R, Nelson D, Rutks I, Wilt TJ (2000) *Pygeum africanum* for the treatment of patients with benign prostatic hyperplasia: a systematic review and quantitative meta-analysis. Am J Med 1:654–664

Kang HJ, Ansbacher R, Hammoud MM (2002) Use of alternative and complementary medicine in menopause. Int J Gynaecol Obstet 79:195–207

Liske E (1998) Therapeutic efficacy and safety of *Cimicifuga racemosa* for gynecological disorders. Adv Ther 15: 45–53

Levin RM, Das AK (2000) A scientific basis for the therapeutic effects of *Pygeum africanum* and *Serenoa repens*. Urol Res 28:201–209

Lowe FC, Fagelman E (2002) Phytotherapy in the treatment of benign prostatic hyperplasia. Curr Opin Urol 12:15–18

McKenna DJ, Jones K, Humphrey S, Hughes K (2001) Black cohosh: efficacy, safety, and use in clinical and preclinical applications. Altern Ther Health Med 7:93–100

McQueen CE, Bryant PJ (2001) Pygeum. Am J Health Syst Pharm 58:120–123

Schellenberg R (2001) Treatment for the premenstrual syndrome with agnus castus fruit extract: prospective, randomised, placebo controlled study. Br Med J 322:134–137

Stevinson C, Ernst E (2001) Complementary/alternative therapies for premenstrual syndrome: a systemic review of randomized controlled trials. Am J Obstet Gynecol 185:227–35

Tesch BJ (2002) Herbs commonly used by women: an evidence-based review. Dis Mon 48:671–696

Wilt TJ, Ishani A, Stark G, MacDonald R, Lau J, Mulrow C (1998) Saw palmetto extracts for treatment of benign prostatic hyperplasia. JAMA 280:1604–1609

Wilt TJ, Ishani A, Rutks I, MacDonald R (2000) Phytotherapy for benign prostatic hyperplasia. Public Health Nutr 3:459–72

Wilt TJ, MacDonald R, Ishani A, Rutks I, Stark G (2000) Cernilton for benign prostatic hyperplasia. Cochrane Database Syst Rev. 2:CD001042

Wilt TJ, Ishani A, Stark G, MacDonald R, Lau J, Mulrow C (2000) Serenoa repens for benign prostatic hyperplasia. Cochrane Database Syst Rev. 2:CD001423

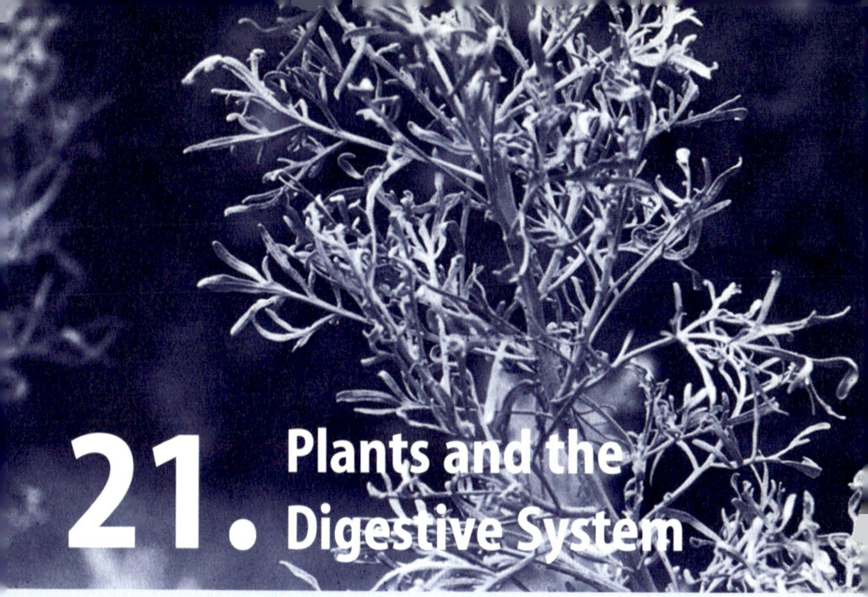

21. Plants and the Digestive System

Introduction

Digestion takes place in the alimentary canal by means of enzymes secreted mostly by the stomach, pancreas and small intestine. Mechanical movements such as chewing initially break down food before mixing it in the stomach and intestine. Besides enzymes, some glands in the intestine produce a mucus which lubricates and protects the digestive tract, but which can also interact with and reduce the absorption of herbal medicines. Digestion is facilitated by peristalsis, a wave of muscle contractions that begins in the duodenum and spreads towards the colon.

In the mouth, chewing initiates digestion through the action of ptylin (to digest starch). The stomach stores ingested food and subjects it to further digestion through the action of hydrochloric acid secreted by parietal cells and pepsin (a protease) secreted by the chief cells. In the small intestine proteases, lipases and amylases complete the digestion of most foods. The stomach lining is well protected by a layer of mucus against the corrosive action of gastric juice. In the small intestine most drugs, sugars and minerals are absorbed, while in the large intestine mostly water and mineral salts are absorbed.

Transit of intralumenal contents depends upon the coordination of intestinal longitudinal and circular muscle contractions. Contrary to common belief, transit through the intestinal tract may be decreased when circular muscle contractions increase, as this narrows the lumen and restricts the flow of its contents. This can be the case in constipated patients and is the major pharmacological effect of morphine and other opiates on the bowel.

Botanical drugs may act in a variety of ways on the digestive tract. In this chapter herbal stomatics, antikinetosics, eupeptics, antacids (ulcer healing), laxatives, antidiarrheals as well as herbal medicines useful in the treatment of irritable bowel syndrome will be discussed.

Stomatits, Gingivitis, Glossitis

Clinical Picture

- A component of salivary secretion is mucus which has a trophic and protective function in the mouth. Diminished saliva secretion (due to fever, excessive perspiration, mild diabetes, belladonna intoxication) causes difficulty in speaking and swallowing and often leads to infections like stomatitis, gingivitis, and glossitis.
- Stomatics are medicines which treat infection and irritation in the oral cavity.

Stomatic Plants

There are a number of herbal medicines that may be useful against oral infections and ulcers. Essential oils have demonstrated antimicrobial effects *in vitro* and an efficacy towards oral bacteria. Drugs containing tannins (especially tannic acid and propyl gallate) have shown anti-inflammatory and antimicrobial effects. Suspension of decoctions of high-tannin herbs in gum tragacanth or gum Arabic produce healing effects in mouth ulcers.

Herbal medicines to be considered for this role include tannin-containing plants (rhatany root, oak bark, tormentil root and witch hazel bark). Other botanicals possess topical anti-inflammatory effects, in addition to their astringent and demulcent properties. Herbal medicines with high mucilage content (*Althaea officinalis*, *Linum usitatissimum*, etc.) have notably soothing effects. Stomatic plants are listed in Table 21.1.

Table 21.1

Main herbal stomatits supported by German Commission E for inflammatory states of the mouth and pharynx

Common name	Latin name	Part(s) of plant used	Key constituents
Agrimony	*Agrimonia eupatoria*	Flowering plant	Tannins
Anise	*Pimpinella anisum*	Fruit	Volatile oil, caffeic acid derivatives, flavonoids
Arnica	*Arnica montana*	Flowers	Sesquiterpene lactones (helenalin), volatile oil, flavonids
Bilberry	*Vaccinium myrtillus*	Fruit	Fruit acids, tannins, anthocyanosides, flavonoids, iridoids
Blackberry	*Rubus fruticosus*	Leaves	Fruit acids, flavonoids, tannins

continued on page 257

Table 21.1

Main herbal stomatits supported by German Commission E for inflammatory states of the mouth and pharynx (*continued*)

Common name	Latin name	Part(s) of plant used	Key constituents
Cinquefoil	*Pontentilla erecta*	Rhizome	Tannins, flavonoids, triterpenes
Clove	*Syzygium aromaticum*	Flower buds	Volatile oil, flavonoids, tannins, triterpenes, steroids
Coffee charcoal	*Coffea arabica*	Seeds	Purine alkaloids, hemicellulose derivatives
Coltsfoot	*Tussilago farfara*	Leaves, Inflorescences	Mucilages, tannins, flavonoids, steroids
Echinacea	*Echinacea purpurea*	Aerial parts	Polysaccharides, flavonoids, caffeic acid derivatives
English plantain	*Plantago lanceolata*	Aerial parts	Iridoide monoterpenes, caffeic acid derivatives, tannins, mucilages, flavonoids
German chamomile	*Matricaria recutita*	Flower heads	Volatile oil, flavonoids, coumarins, mucilages
Iceland moss	*Cetraria islandica*	Thallus	Mucilages, lichen acids
Jambolan	*Syzygium cumini*	Bark	Tannins, steroids, triterpenes, flavonoids
Japanese mint	*Mentha arvensis piperascens*	Aerial parts	Menthol, menthone, limonene, α- and β-pinene
Knotweed	*Polygonum aviculare*	Aerial parts	Flavonoids, silicic acid, tannins, lignans
Mallow (high mallow)	*Malva sylvestris*	Flowers, leaves	Flavonoids, mucilages
Marigold	*Calendula officinalis*	Flowers	Triterpene saponins, triterpene alcohols, flavonoids, volatile oil
Marshmallow	*Althea officinalis*	Roots	Mucilages, pectins
Myrrh	*Commiphora myrrha*	Resin from bark	Volatile oil, triterpenes, mucilages
Oak	*Quercus robur*	Bark	Tannins
Peppermint	*Mentha piperita*	Oil from aerial parts	Menthol, menthone, menthyl acetate, neomenthol, isomenthone
Potentilla	*Potentilla anserina*	Aerial parts	Tannins, flavonoids, coumarins
Rhatany	*Krameria triandra*	Roots	Tannins, neolignans
Rose	*Rosa centifolia*	Petals	Tannins, volatile oil
Sage	*Salvia officinalis*	Aerial parts	Volatile oil, caffeic acid derivatives, diterpenes, flavonoids
Sloe	*Prunus spinosa*	Fruits	Cyanogenic glycosides, fruit acids, tannins
Spruce	*Picea spp.*	Oil from needles	Bornyl acetate, limonene, camphene, α-pinene
White nettle	*Lamium album*	Flowers	Iridoide monoterpenes, triterpene saponins, flavonoids

Marshmallow

Botany/Key constituents ▶ Marshmallow is the dried root of *Althaea officinalis* L. (Fam. *Malvaceae*), a perennial herb (1–2 m tall) with erect woody stems, which grows in Central Europe and which has been naturalized in the United States. Frequently the root (crude drug) is cut into small cubes (5 mm in diameter) to facilitate production of a starch-free mucilage: the starch present on the surface of small cubes is easily washed away and the washed crude drug gives a clear mucilage. It contains mucilage (25–35%), the enzyme asparagine, starch (30–35%) and pectin (7–10%).

Mode of action ▶ Althea does not possess anti-inflammatory action. However, the mucilage content supports the reputed demulcent action. Drugs containing mucilages have a property of covering and protecting mucosa and may be used in the treatment of inflammatory conditions.

Clinical efficacy ▶ The demulcent properties of marshmallow have a strong tradition in the treatment of stomatitis, gingivitis and glossitis. Efficacy has been demonstrated when used as a gargle for inflammation of the mucous membrane of the mouth and throat. However, the German Commission E recommends its use only for the treatment of cough.

Adverse events/Contraindications ▶ No adverse effects are expected in conjunction with the proper administration of designated therapeutic dose. However, the absorption of concomitantly used drugs may be delayed.

Preparations/Dosage

As a demulcent marshmallow is used in the form of infusion (3%) to make mouthwashes in the case of stomatitis, gingivitis, glossitis. The daily dose is 6 g dry root.

Propolis

Origin ▶ Propolis (bee pollen) is a resinous material, dark-colored which is collected by honeybees from the buds of living plants mixed with bee wax and salivary secretions. In the temperate zone, the main sources of propolis are the bud exudate of *Populus* species; in the tropical zone the leaf exudate of *Cistus* spp. (Tunisia), and the flower exudate of *Clusia* spp. (Venezuela). Other plant sources of propolis are *Ambrosia deltoidea* (Sonoran desert), *Arancharia* spp. and *Baccharis* spp. (Brazil), *Xanthorrhoea* spp. (Australia). Bees apply propolis in a thin layer on the internal wall of their hive and use it to block holes and cracks, to repair combs to strengthen the thin borders of the combs and for making the entrance of the hive weather-tight or easier to defend.

Composition ► The chemical composition of propolis is a complex mixture of about 150 compounds including flavonoids, coumaric acids, lignans, terpenoids, aromatic compounds, sugars, hydrocarbons, mineral elements, etc. The main problem is the extraordinary variability of these compounds depending on the site of collection of propolis: samples from different geographic origin may possess totally different chemical composition. This is why the chemical standardization of propolis based on its active compounds has not been realized.

Mode of action ► Propolis possesses several biological activities such as anti-inflammatory, antifungal, antiviral, antibacterial and tissue regenerative among others. Caffeic acid methyl ester (CAPE) and flavonoids such as galangin are considered to be the main active ingredients. CAPE is an inhibitor quite selective of cycloxygenase II (COX II, which produces inflammatory prostaglandins) and also potently inhibits nuclear factor kB (NF-kB, an intracellular molecule which plays a key role in inflammatory processes). Propolis, like myrrh, also promotes a local leukocytosis.

Clinical efficacy ► Propolis has been used for thousands of years in folk medicine for several purposes (laryngitis and gastric disturbances, dermatitis, duodenal and oral ulcers). Propolis is used in oral infections and aphthous ulceration because it accelerates the healing of the ulcers and corrects any underlying imbalances. For topical treatment of accessible mucosae, mouthwashes and gargles can be made with propolis, combined or not with fluid extract of liquorice and of other drugs (echinacea, calendula). Non-controlled clinical studies have indicated the efficacy of propolis-containing mouth rinse in reducing plaque formation. However, there is a lack of randomized clinical trials.

Adverse events ► Propolis seems relatively safe, but it is contraindicated in case of allergic predisposition to bee sting. Propolis is a potent sensitizer and is well recognized as a cause of occupational allergic eczematous contact dermatitis in apiarists. Cases of allergic contact dermatitis have been described in patients using propolis. Case reports have also revealed acute oral mucositis with ulceration as a result of using propolis-containing lozenges.

Preparations/Dosage

The drug is used internally in the form of liquid extracts and tinctures. It is also used externally. The daily dose is 3 g crude drug, divided into three doses.

Other Stomatic Drugs

Myrrh (gum myrrh) is an oleo-gum resin collected from the bark of *Commiphora myrrha*, (Fam. *Burseraceae*), a short thorny tree which grows in Kenya, Somalia, Ethiopia, Arabia (Plate 21.1). The name myrrh is from the Arabic *murr* and means bitter; *commiphora* is from the Greek, meaning gum-hearing. Myrrh contains volatile oil, resin (25–40%), gum (about 60%), sesquiterpenes, (furanoeudesma-1, 3-diiene, curzarene, etc.). Related *Commiphora* species produce similar resins, and other "myrrhs" are described such as the "African myrrh" from *C. abyssinica* or guggulu resin (Indian myrrh) from *C. mukul* (see Chapter 15).

Myrrh is recommended by the German Commission E for the treatment of inflammation of the mouth and pharynx. It is used frequently in mouthwashes as an astringent to treat mouth ulcers, mouth infections, sore throat and similar conditions (tincture 20%; 5–10 gtt in 300 water; 2–4 mouthwashes/day). Topical application of a high alcoholic tincture (or extract) of myrrh can be particularly beneficial. This is because such a preparation is quite resinous. When it is painted on the ulcer mucose the alcohol dries and the resin fixes the active compounds so that they are not readily washed away by saliva. Myrrh also promotes a local leukocytosis (increase of white blood cells).

Myrrh can be used alone or in association with propolis, echinacea, marigold and liquorice. All of these drugs are beneficial when applied topically as well as when taken internally. In Germany the health authorities allow myrrh powder and tincture for the topical treatment of mild inflammation of the oral and pharyngeal mucosa. Myrrh, apart from an ingredient in several mouthwash products, is widely used also as a fragrance component in soaps, toothpaste, cosmetics and perfumes and as a flavor component in candy and other food products. It is relatively nontoxic.

Aloe gel (aloe vera) is a colorless gelatin obtained from the central portion of the leaves of several *Aloe* species (*vera*, *barbadensis*, *vulgaris*, etc.), succulent plants with strong and fibrous roots and numerous large, fleshly leaves, carrying spines at the margin. The mucilaginous parenchymal tissue is excised from fresh leaves and immediately utilized for pharmaceutical preparations or lyophilized and kept dry until use. Aloe gel is sensitive to heat and light and can quickly deteriorate when stabilized at high temperature. It contains mainly mucilage (30%); other components are: anthraquinone derivatives, polysaccharides, glycoproteins (aloctins A and B), lectins, enzymes (cyclooxygenase, bradykininase), salicylic acid and fatty acids (e.g. campesterol). Aloe gel has been used for the treatment of mouth ulcers and aphthous stomatitis. Aloe gel may simply act as a protective barrier; however, the therapeutic use of aloe gel in justified by its anti-inflammatory, immunomodulating and antibacterial activities. Aloe gel comes in a variety of forms: as pure gel, in a natural or decolorized state; as a liquid concentrated or concentrated and dried to produce spray and freeze-dried powder; as reconstituted aloe gel (that is a product prepared from powder or liquid concentrated). Aloe gel is generally well tolerated. Aloe gel is totally different from aloe latex (aloe) which possesses laxative properties.

► *See Chapter 15 for the use of aloe vera in the treatment of diabetes*
► *See Chapter 23 for the dermatological use of aloe gel*

Dyspepsia

Clinical Picture

- Functional dyspepsia (i.e. disturbed digestion) is a syndrome featuring nausea, epigastric pressure, bloating, flatulence and crampy abdominal pain. The cause of functional dyspepsia is unknown. Deficiency in gastric secretion, motility gastric disorders, deficient bile production as well as diet, alcohol, tobacco, aspirin-like drugs abuse, psychosocial factors, *Helicobacter pylori* infection, failure of fundal relaxation on meal ingestion are all possible causes, but none of these has been found to be a definitive, unique cause of the disease. Because the only certainty in dyspepsia is the presence of symptoms, such as pain or discomfort, modern therapy aims at the impairment of the genesis and transmission of nociceptive impulses in the visceral sensorial fibres before they reach the central nervous system. In this respect, the use of chili (*Capsicum annuum*) could be clinically relevant.

Phytotherapy of Dyspepsia

Traditional herbal remedies used in the treatment of dyspepsia include **bitter drugs** (e.g. quassia, gentian, holy thistle, bitter-orange peel), **cholagogues/choleretics** (e.g. artichoke, boldo, celandine, turmeric, dandelion, wormwood) or **carminatives** (e.g. caraway, fennel and anise). Herbal anti-dyspeptics which do not fall into the above three mentioned categories include chili and emblic myrobalan. Bitters and carminatives are described in this chapter, cholagogue and choleretics are described in Chapter 22.

Table 22.2 lists the main herbal medicines supported by the German Commission E for the treatment of dyspeptic complaints. Randomized clinical studies have shown preliminary positive results for celandine (*Chelidonium majus*), turmeric (*Curcuma longa*), emblic myrobalan (*Emblica officinalis*), and banana (*Musa paradisiaca sapientum*). Clearer positive evidence has been shown for the association between peppermint and caraway (*Mentha piperita* and *Carum carvi*), for the herbal formula Iberogast® and for chili. There appear to be few adverse effects associated with these remedies, although, in many cases, comprehensive safety data are not available.

Chili

Botany/Key constituents ▸ Chili (red pepper, capsicum, cayenne) is the dried fruit of *Capsicum annuum* L. var *longum* (DC) Sendter and other related species (Fam. *Solanaceae*). This is an annual herb from the tropical parts of America, now cul-

Table 21.2

Main herbal medicines supported by German Commission E for the treatment of dyspeptic complaints. Asterisk denotes that the herbal medicine is also recommended for loss of appetite

Common name	Latin name	Part(s) of plant used	Key constituents	Daily dose
Angelica*	*Angelica archangelica*	Roots	Furanocoumarins,flavonoids, volatile oil, caffeic acid derivatives	4.5 g
Anise	*Pimpinella anisum*	Fruits	Volatile oil, fatty oil, flavonoids, proteic substances, caffeic acid derivatives	3 g
Bitter orange*	*Citrus aurantium*	Fruit peel	Volatile oil, flavonoids	4–6 g
Blessed thistle*	*Cnicus benedictus*	Aerial parts	Sesquiterpene lactones (cnicin), lignans, volatile oil, triterpenes	4–6 g
Bog bean*	*Menyanthes trifoliata*	Aerial parts	Iridoide monoterpenes, flavonoids, coumarins, alkaloids	1.5–3 g
Boldo	*Peumus boldus*	Leaves	Isoquinoline alkaloids (boldine), volatile oil, flavonoids	4.5 g
Caraway	*Carum carvi*	Fruits	Volatile oil, fatty oil, polysaccharides, proteins	1.5–6 g
Centaury *	*Centaurium erythraea*	Aerial parts	Monoterpenes, pyrridine alkaloids, xantones	1–2 g
Chicory*	*Cichorium intybus*	Leaves, roots	Sesquiterpenes, caffeic acid derivatives, coumarins	3–5 g
Chinese cinnamon*	*Cinnamomum aromaticum*	Flowers	Volatile oil, diterpenes, tannins, proanthocyanidins	2–4 g
Cinnamon*	*Cinnamomum verum*	Oil from the bark, bark	Volatile oil, diterpenes, proanthocyanidins, mucilages	2–4 g
Condurango*	*Marsdenia condurango*	Bark	Pregnane- and pregnan -5-ene glycosides, caffeic acid derivatives	2–4 g
Coriander*	*Coriandrum sativum*	Fruits	Volatile oil, fatty oil, coumarins	3.0 g
Dandelion*	*Taraxacum officinale*	Leaves, root	Sesquiterpene lactones, triterpenes, sterols, flavonoids, mucilages	3–4 g
Devil's claw*	*Harpagophytum procumbens*	Secondary roots	Iridoids, triterpenes, phenols	4.5 g
Dill	*Anethum graveolens*	Fruits	Volatile oil, phtalides, fatty oil, furanocoumarins	3 g
Fennel	*Foeniculum vulgare*	Oil from the fruits	anethole, fenchone, estragole	0.1–0.6 ml oil
Gentian*	*Gentiana lutea*	Roots	Iridoid glycosides, sugars, pyrridine alkaloids	3 g
Ginger*	*Zingiber officinale*	Roots	Volatile oil, aryl alkanes, gingerols, shogaols, gingerdiols	2–4 g
Haronga	*Haronga madagascariensis*	Leaves, bark	Anthracene derivatives, volatile oil, procyanidins	0.025–0.05 g

continued on page 263

Table 21.2

Main herbal medicines supported by German Commission E for the treatment of dyspeptic complaints. Asterisk denotes that the herbal medicine is also recommended for loss of appetite (*continued*)

Common name	Latin name	Part(s) of plant used	Key constituents	Daily dose
Horehound*	*Marrubium vulgare*	Aerial parts	Marrubin, caffeic acid derivatives, flavonoids	4.5 g
Iceland moss*	*Cetraria islandica*	Thallus	Mucilages, lichen acids	4–6 g
Lavender*	*Lavandula angustifolia*	Flowers	Volatile oil, coumarins, tannins, caffeic acid derivatives	20–80 mg oil
Lesser galangal*	*Alpinia officinarum*	Rhizome	Volatile oil, diarylheptanoids, gingerole, flavonoids	2–4 g
Onion*	*Allium cepa*	Bulb	Alliins, flavonoids	20 g
Peppermint	*Mentha piperita*	Leaves, oil from leaves	Volatile oil (menthol, menthone), caffeic acid derivatives, flavonoids	3–6 g drug 6–12 drops oil
Quinine*	*Cinchona pubescens*	Bark	Quinoline alkaloids, triterpenes, tannins	1–3 g
Rosemary*	*Rosmarinus officinalis*	Leaves	Caffeic acid derivatives, diterpenes, flavonoids, triterpenes	4–6 g
Sweet orange*	*Citrus sinensis*	Fruit Peel	Volatile oil, flavonoids	10–15 g
Turmeric*	*Curcuma domestica*	Rhizome	Volatile oil, curcuminoids	1.5–3 g
Wormwood*	*Artemisia absinthium*	Aerial parts	Volatile oil, sesquiterpenes	2–3 g
Yarrow*	*Achillea millefolium*	Aerial parts	Volatile oil, sesquiterpene lactones, polyynes, flavonoids, alkilamids	3–4.5 g

tivated in all tropical and subtropical countries. It contains 0.1–0.5% pungent alkaloid capsaicin (located in the fruit wall, especially in the ridges carrying the seeds), together with a number of other structurally related pungent compounds. Strains which lack capsaicin, but which have a high content of vitamin C, are used as vegetable under the name of sweet pepper.

Mode of action ▸ Capsaicin, contained in the ingested chili, acts on gastric sensory fibers of visceral nociceptive neurones. The effect is biphasic: capsaicin first binds to capsaicin (also named vanilloid) receptors causing an increase of activity, related to the release of algic/proinflammatory neuropeptides such as substance P (sensitization); thereafter a prolonged activation causes a decrease in the activity of the sensory fibers so that the fibers become unresponsive to nociceptive stimuli (desensitization). The desensitization corresponds to an attenuation of sensitivity to pain.

Clinical studies ▶ A very relevant placebo-controlled clinical study performed on 30 patients demonstrated that red pepper powder (2.5 g red pepper powder for 5 weeks) taken before meals was significantly more effective than placebo in decreasing the symptom intensity of patients with functional dyspepsia (not associated with gastro-esophageal reflux and irritable bowel syndrome). In particular, epigastric pain, epigastric fullness and nausea showed more significant improvement after taking red pepper than after placebo. Topical chili is supported by the German Commission E for painful conditions such as muscular tensions and rheumatism.

Adverse events/Contraindications ▶ Internal administration of chili may affect gastrointestinal peristalsis, resulting in diarrhea, intestinal and gallstone colics. Chili may also produce respiratory problems (increased sensitivity to cough), allergic reactions due to its antigenic components and transient epigastric pain, which decreased after a few days of treatment. This effect is likely to be due to the transient desensitization of sensory fibers by capsaicin.

Preparations/Dosage

The clinical effective dosage of chili is 2.5 g powder/daily, administered in gelatine capsule (0.5 g powder per capsule), to be taken before meals (one capsule before continental breakfast, two before lunch and two before dinner).

Emblic myrobalan (amalik) is the pericarp of the dried fruits of *Emblica officinalis* Gaertn. (Fam. *Euphorbiaceae*), a medium to large tree found both in the wild and cultivated states; it is common on the hills in the forests of India. Key constituents include tannins (up to 28%), phyllemblic acid, lipids, gallic acid emblicol and vitamin C. The mechanism of the anti-dyspeptic action of emblic myrobalan is not known. In traditional Ayurvedic medicine, emblic myrobalan is used to treat hemorrhage, diarrhea, dysentery and, in combination with iron, it is used as a remedy for anemia, jaundice and dyspepsia. One randomized clinical trial (n = 38 subjects, 10 with peptic ulcer and 28 with non-ulcer dyspepsia) showed that both conventional antacids and emblic myrobalan reduced dyspepsia symptom scores and acid output compared with baseline values. Adverse events were reported by four patients treated with antacids (weakness and pain in the lower limbs) and three patients treated with emblic myrobalan (loose motions and vomiting). According to Ayurvedic medicine, the daily dose of emblic myrobalan is 3–6 g crude drug.

Bitter Drugs

These medicines (also known as eupeptics from *eu* = well and *pepsis* = digestion) promote gastric juice secretion and facilitate digestion. They are useful in cases of loss of appetite, anorexia, dyspepsia and gastric ailments which cause food to remain in the stomach for a long time without being sufficiently digested.

Bitter drugs (with an intense bitter taste) seem to be able to stimulate appetite and improve gastric digestion. In practice bitter drugs sensitize oral taste receptors (facilitating saliva secretion). This sensitization lasts 20–30 minutes; which is why bitter eupeptics (particularly pure bitter) must be followed by a meal within 20 minutes of administration. Bitter drugs also induce gastrin secretion, a hormone which stimulates hydrochloric acid secretion. However, according to some scientists, they are able to stimulate digestion only in patients with gastric secretion insufficiency. Bitter drugs are sometimes used to treat loss of appetite in elderly patients with gastric secretion insufficiency but not for nervous anorexia. They are administered in concentrated infusion (2–4%) or in tincture form to be swallowed slowly.

Bitter drugs are classified into pure (e.g. gentian, centaury, quassia), aromatic (e.g. wormwood, bitter orange), mucilaginous (e.g. colombo, Iceland moss), pungent (e.g. ginger) and alkaloidic (e.g. quinine). The first, also called aperients, contain mostly bitter substances. Bitter drugs combined with an essential oil have a direct stimulus on taste and olfactory receptors and gastric secretion; moreover they tend to have antibacterial action on intestinal flora, and they stimulate bile secretion. Also, since they promote the expulsion of excessive intestinal gas, they also behave as carminatives. Drugs of this group can also be used between meals as digestives provided they are used in small quantities. These drugs have low activity when used in tea form because the essential oil is not very soluble in water (only 10–15% of essence passes into the tea). Fluid extracts and tinctures prepared with 30–70% alcohol are more effective. Alkaloid bitter drugs are not used as eupeptics as they cause unpleasant side effects.

Gentian

Botany/Key constituents ▸ Gentian is the dried root of *Gentiana lutea* L. (Fam. *Gentianaceae*), a tall perennial herb (1 m) with broad, elliptic, decussate leaves and large yellow flowers (Plate 21.2). The plant grows in the mountainous areas in Central and Southern Europe. The root, which can be over 1 m long, is harvested from plants 2–5 years old. Gentian contains iridoid glycosides (bitter principles) [amarogentin (0.05–0.3%), amaroswerin (0.03–0.1%), amaropanin (0.05–0.2%) and gentiopicroside (2–3%)], sugars and alkaloids.

Mode of action ▸ Gentian stimulates the taste buds and increases by reflex action the flow of saliva and stomach secretions. The bitter taste of the drug is attributed mainly to amarogentin and amaroswerin which both have a bitterness value of 58,000,000 and to amaropanin which has a bitterness value of 20,000,000. Gentiopicroside has a bitterness value of 12,000.

Clinical efficacy ▶ The use of gentian as eupeptic and appetite stimulants is very old, especially in the elderly. The drug is also useful in the case of flatulence and bloating. It is supported by German Commission E for dyspeptic complaints and loss of appetite. A recent systematic review identified one randomized clinical trial. This study showed that gentian (alone or in combination with boldo, cascara and rhubarb) administered to 359 patients (duration of the trial: 28 days) with slight or moderate functional disorders of the gastrointestinal tract produced significant improvements in the loss of appetite and dyspepsia compared to placebo.

Adverse events/Contraindications ▶ Gentian may cause headache in some individuals; because of the drug's stimulation of gastric juice secretion, it is contraindicated in gastroduodenal ulcers. Gentian is stated to be contraindicated in individuals with high blood pressure, although no rationale is given to this statement.

Preparations/Dosage

The daily dose is 3 g crude drug, divided in three 1 g doses. It may be consumed in the form of a decoction (1 g in 150 ml water for 5 min) about 30 min before mealtime. The tea may be sweetened with honey to alleviate the bitter taste. A tincture (1:5 in 45% alcohol), 1–4 ml, three times daily is also available.

Other Bitter Drugs

Centaury consists of the dried aerial parts (leaves, stems and flowers) of *Centaurium erythraea* Rafin (Fam. *Gentianaceae*), a plant native to Europe (Mediterranean region) and naturalized in North America. It contains, like gentian, amarogentin, gentiopicroside and related bitter compounds including centapicrin, swartiamarin, sweroside. Centapicrin has a bitterness value 15 times greater than gentiopicroside. Centaury is used, like gentian, to treat indigestion and appetite loss. The drug (1–2 g) is extracted with cold water (150 ml) for 6–10 h. The macerate is warmed before use. Centaury is supported by the German Commission E for dyspeptic complaints and loss of appetite.

Quassia (Bitterwood) is the wood of *Quassia amara* L. (Surinam quassia) or *Picrasma excelsa* L. (Jamaican quassia) (Fam. *Simaroubaceae*). *Q. amara* is a shrub 2–3 m high native to Venezuela, Brazil and Guyana. *P. excelsa* is a tree (12–25 m) native to Jamaica. The bitter substances contained in quassia are quassinoids such as quassin (which has a bitterness value of 17,000,000) and canthinones. The use of the drug to stimulate appetite and promote digestion is traceable to these bitter substances which it contains. The drug is marketed in the form of chips. It has been used to treat dyspeptic complaints (2–10 ml of a 1:10 tincture). Abuse of quassia induces nausea and irritation of gastric mucosa.

Wormwood (absinth) consists of the dried aerial parts of *Artemisia absinthium* L. (Fam. *Asteraceae*). This is a perennial herb 160–120 cm tall which grows in Asia, Europe and North Africa, densely covered with hair on the leaves and stems (Plate 21.3). The plant has an aromatic smell and a very bitter taste. The bitter taste of the crude drug is due to its content of absinthin. The bitterness value is 10,000. Besides absinthin, wormwood contains a volatile oil, which is often colored blue due to the presence of chamazulene. The oil also contains thujone and the corresponding alchohol thujol. These are poisonous substances, which affect the central nervous system and cause dizziness, convulsions, and delirium. Wormwood herb was formerly used in Europe for the preparation of absinth, a liqueur whose manufacture is now prohibited because of the toxic effects due to thujone and thujol. German Commission E monograph on wormwood states that the crude drug should have a minimum content of 0.3% volatile oil and a relative bitterness of at least 15,000. The monograph cites as indications poor appetite, dyspeptic complaints, and biliary dyskinesia, recommending an average daily dose of 2–3 g crude drug.

Blessed thistle (Holy thistle) consists of the dried aerial parts of *Cnicus benedictus* L. (Fam. *Asteraceae*), an annual, thistle-like herb with sharp thorns on the leaves and yellow flower-heads. It grows spontaneously in the Mediterranean region. The bitter compound is cnicin, which is present to the extent of about 0.2%. The bitterness value is approximately 1,500. Cnicin stimulates the secretion of saliva and gastric juice. Holy thistle is supported by German Commission E for dyspeptic complaints and loss of appetite. The daily dosage is 4–6 g crude drug.

Bitter-orange peel is the dried fruit peel of the bitter orange (=Seville or Bigarade orange), *Citrus aurantium* L. (Fam. *Rutaceae*). The tree is a close relative of the orange and lemon trees. Its home country is India and it is grown in most subtropical countries. Like the peel of other *Citrus* fruits, the fresh bitter-orange peel comprises two layers: an outer, firm, yellow colored and an inner, soft, odorless layer. The yellow layer has large cavities containing a volatile oil, with up to 90% of the terpene limonene. The aroma of the oil is due essentially to geranial (2–4%). Bitter orange has a mild spasmolytic effect on the gastrointestinal tract and increases gastric juice secretion. It is supported by German Commission E for loss of appetite and dyspeptic complaints. The daily dosage is 4–6 g crude drug.

Flatulence

Clinical Picture

- Flatulence is defined as the presence of excessive amount of gas in the stomach or in the intestine. Gas in the digestive tract comes from two sources: swallowed air and normal breakdown of certain undigested foods (sugars, starches and fibers found in many foods) by colon bacteria. The most common symptoms of gas are abdominal bloating, abdominal pain, and belching. However, not everyone experiences these symptoms. Predisposing factors include biliary stasis, hypochlorhydria, pancreatic insufficiency, bacterial imbalance in the colon and food sensitivity. The most common ways to reduce the discomfort of gas are changing diet, reducing the amount of air swallowed, taking digestive enzymes (lactase supplements help to digest carbohydrates and may allow people to eat foods that would normally cause gas).

- Herbal medicines play a special role in the treatment of flatulence.

Carminatives

Carminative agents are drugs used to relieve flatulence. They prevent the formation or cause the expulsion of gas in the alimentary tract. Typical herbal carminatives include caraway (*Carum carvi*), fennel (*Foeniculum vulgare*) and anise (*Pimpinella anisum*). Other herbal medicines considered to have carminative actions are chamomile (*Matricaria recutita*), peppermint (*Mentha piperita*), lemon balm (*Melissa officinalis*) and angelica (*Angelica archangelica*). Caraway, fennel, anise, peppermint and angelica are supported by the German Commission E for the treatment of dyspeptic complaints and/or loss of appetite (Table 22.2).

Caraway

Botany/Key constituents ▶ Caraway consists of the fruits of *Carum carvi* L. (Fam. *Umbelliferae*), a biennial herb growing wild in Europe and Asia, but also cultivated for medicinal purposes. The fruit is a schizocarp that is glabrous, oblong and ellipsoid (also referred to as caraway seed). Key constituents include a volatile oil [(2–7%) main constituents: carvone (50–60%), limonene], a fatty oil (10–20%), polysaccharides and proteins. The oil is obtained from the squashed fruit when ripened by a process of aqueous steam distillation.

Mode of action ▶ Animal studies have shown that caraway alcoholic extracts inhibit gastric smooth muscle contractions and stimulate bile flow. The gastric antispasmodic activity of caraway extracts is shared by other typical carminative herbal medicines, including fennel and anise. By contrast, volatile oils of these herbal carminatives (caraway, anise and fennel) tend to stimulate intestinal motility by increasing the muscle tonus. Caraway also possesses antimicrobial activity.

Clinical efficacy ▶ Caraway is considered the most typical and effective of the carminative herbal medicines. Caraway is supported by the German Commission E for the treatment of dyspeptic complaints. A recent systematic review retrieved four randomized clinical trials of fixed combinations of caraway oil (daily dose: 60–150 mg) and **peppermint** oil (daily dose: 180–270 ml). Of these four studies, two were performed in patients with non-ulcer dyspepsia (defined as dismotility-type or essential/idiopathic dyspepsia with irritable bowel syndrome) (n = 268 subjects) and two studies were performed in patients with functional dyspepsia (n = 216 subjects). The duration of the treatment was four weeks. Overall, these studies showed that the peppermint and caraway oil were more effective than placebo and as effective as the reference drug cisapride in the treatment of dyspepsia.

Adverse events ▸ Caraway is a safe herbal medicine if administered in designated therapeutic dosages. Clinical studies have shown an encouraging safety profile. The intake of larger dosages of the volatile oil for long periods can lead to kidney and liver damage.

Preparations/Dosage

The average daily dose of the crude drug is 1.5-6 g. The comminuted fresh drug is used for infusions and other galenic preparations. Clinical studies have used caraway oil at doses ranging from 60 to 150 mg. Caraway is a component of the herbal formula Iberogast® (see below).

Other Carminative Herbs

Anise (green anice) is the fruit (a schizocarp also referred to as anise seed) of *Pimpinella anisum* L. (Fam. *Umbelliferae*), a herbaceous plant probably coming from the Near East, but today cultivated mainly in Southern Europe. Anise contains 2–6% volatile oil (94% anethole), 30% fatty oil, flavonoids, proteic substances and caffeic acid derivatives (chlorogenic acid). Anise is approved by the German Commission E for the treatment of dyspeptic complaints and loss of appetite. The average daily dose is 3 g crude drug. Sensitization has very rarely been observed.

Fennel is the fruit (a schizocarp also referred to as fennel seed) of *Foeniculum vulgare* Miller (Fam. *Umbelliferae*), a plant indigenous to the Mediterranean region, but also found in other parts of the world (Argentina, Germany, England, India, China, Australia). Two varieties are known: *F. vulgare* var *vulgare* (which generally grows spontaneously) and *F. vulgare* var *dulcis* (which is cultivated because the foliaceous sheets are edible). Fennel contains 2–7% volatile oil (50–70% anethole, 15–30% fenchone and 2–5% estragole) and about 10% fatty oil. Fennel volatile oil is supported by the German Commission E for the treatment of dyspeptic complaints. The daily dosage is 0.1–0.6 ml oil or 5–7 g crude drug. Allergic reactions following intake of fennel have only very rarely been observed.

Herbal formula (Iberogast®) Peppermint, caraway, German chamomile, liquorice, lemon balm, bitter candytuft

Iberogast® is a combination of peppermint (*Mentha piperita* L, Fam. *Labiatae*) leaves, caraway (*Carum carvi*, Fam. *Umbelliferae*) fruits, German chamomile (*Matricaria recutita* L., Fam. *Asteraceae/Compositae*) flowers, liquorice (*Glycyrrhiza glabra* L., Fam. *Fabaceae*) roots, lemon balm (*Melissa officinalis* L., Fam. *Labiatae*) leaves and bitter candytuft (*Iberis amara* L., Fam. *Brassicaceae*) seeds.

Peppermint and **caraway** are well known carminatives and are supported by the German Commission E for the treatment of dyspeptic complaints (see key data Table 21.2); **German chamomile** possesses antiulcer activity (see key data Table 21.3) as well as carminative properties; **liquorice** is supported by the German Commission E for the treatment of gastritis (see key data Table 21.3); **lemon balm** (see key data Table 13.1) possesses carminative and spasmolytic effects; it is used in folk medicine to treat lower abdominal disorders, meteorism, and nervous gastric complaints; **bitter candytuft** is obtained from *Iberis amara*, a herbal plant found in most parts of Western, Central and Southern Europe, in the Caucasus, and also in Algeria; the seeds contain cucurbitacins, glucosinolates and a fatty oil; the cucurbitacins contained in the seeds are toxic and generally irritating to the small intestine. In folk medicine bitter candytuft aerial parts are used to treat digestive problems.

The clinical efficacy of Iberogast® is very promising. A recent systematic review identified four randomized clinical trials, including a total of 372 subjects; the dose used was 60 drops daily of the Iberogast® preparation; three out of four studies showed superiority of Iberogast® over the placebo while another study showed similar activity of Iberogast® and the reference drug metaclopramide in reducing dyspeptic symptoms. A post-marketing surveillance study involving 2267 patients reported that 95% patients considered the tolerability of Iberogast® "good" or "very good".

Gastritis and Peptic Ulcer Disease

Clinical Picture

- Gastritis is a general term indicating an inflammation of the mucosal lining of the stomach often caused by a number of factors including alcohol, tobacco, spices, toxins, bacteria and drugs (e.g. aspirin). Peptic ulcer disease refers to a discrete mucosal damage of the stomach and/or duodenum affecting at least 10% of the population in developed countries. The mechanisms of mucosal injury in gastritis and peptic ulcer disease are thought to be an imbalance of aggressive factors, such as acid production or pepsin, and defensive factors, such as mucus production, bicarbonate, and blood flow. *Helicobacter pylori* (a gram-negative bacillus) is thought to infect virtually all patients with chronic active gastritis and represents the leading cause of peptic ulcer disease (with the exception of gastric ulcer induced by aspirin-like drugs). *H. pylori* colonizes the deep layers of the mucosal gel that coats the gastric mucosa and presumably disrupts its protective properties.

- Treatment goals are the relief of discomfort and protection of the gastric mucosal barrier to promote healing. Eradication of *H. pylori* infection and the use of antacids may be sufficient in mild cases. Most patients require a histamine H2-receptor antagonist (e.g. ranitidine), anticholinergic drugs (e.g. pirenzepine) or a proton pump inhibitor (e.g. omeprazole), which has been proven to provide faster and more reliable healing than antacids. Either an H2-receptor blocker or a proton pump inhibitor can be used as a first-line agent. With continued symptoms, they may be used together. In refractory cases, sucralfate also may be indicated.

Phytotherapy of Gastritis and Peptic Ulcer Disease

Plant products have produced therapeutic agents with beneficial effects in gastritis and peptic ulcer disease. The alkaloid atropine and scopolamine derived from belladonna (*Atropa belladonna*) are the prototypes of the anticholinergic drugs. Atropine, scopolamine and preparations from *A. belladonna* leaves are now infrequently (or no more) used to inhibit gastric acid secretion because the dose required often produces undesirable side effects. Nowadays a variety of botanical products have been reported to possess anti-ulcer activity (Table 21.3), but the documented literature has centred primarily on pharmacological action in experimental animals; limited clinical data are available to support the use of herbal medicine as gastroprotective agents. The main herbal medicines used for gastritis (gastric ulcer) relief include liquorice, chamomile and chili.

Ulcer-healing Plants

Antacids. These drugs have a neutralizing action on gastric secretion, reducing acidity.

The use of antacids is based on the principle that even when gastric hypersecretion is not proved the existing secretion may be harmful to the stomach lining but inhibiting the normal mucous defense system. Alternatives are plant materials that elaborate a slippery mucilage, which coats the mucosa and protects it from gastric acid and pepsin. Mucilaginous drugs include marshmallow, Iceland moss and mallow. Antacid/ulcer healing plants are listed in Table 21.3.

Table 21.3
Herbal medines with antiulcer properties

Common name	Latin name	Part(s) of plant used	Key constituents	Daily dose
Banana	*Musa paradisiaca*	Fruit	Polysaccharides, protein, ascorbic acid, amines	a
Cabbage	*Brassica oleracea*	Juice from leaves	Mustard oils, amino acids, alkyl nitriles	3 teaspoons
Chili	*Capsicum annuum*	Fruits	Capsaicin	5–10 g
German chamomille	*Matricaria recutita*	Flower heads	Volatile oil, flavonoids, coumarins	5 g
Iceland moss	*Cetraria islandica*	Thallus	Mucilages, lichen acids	4–6 g
Liquorice*	*Glycyrrhiza glabra*	Roots	Triterpene saponins, flavonoids, coumarins	2–4 g
Mallow (high mallow)	*Malva sylvestris*	Flowers, leaves	Anthocyans, mucilages	5 g
Mandrake	*Mandragora officinarum*	Roots, leaves	Tropane alkaloids (atropine, scopolamine)	6 g roots 5 g leaves
Marshmallow	*Althaea officinalis*	Roots	Mucilages, pectins	6 g
Slippery elm	*Ulmus rubra*	Inner bark and wood	Steroids, sesquiterpenes, tannins	b

* supported by German Commission E for the treatment of gastritis
a. reliable data not available
b. the dose for decoction is 4 to 16 ml per day

Liquorice

Botany/Key constituents ► Liquorice (licorice or glycyrrhiza) is the dried roots and rhizome of *Glycyrrhiza glabra* L. (Fam. *Fabaceae*), known in commerce as Spanish liquorice (Plate 21.4). The plant is a perennial herb, 1–2 m high, growing in Southern Europe (var. *typica*), in Central Russia (var. *glandulifera*) and in Iraq and Iran (var. *violacea*). Liquorice (*radix dulcis*) was recommended by the Greeks to treat stomach ulcers and by Arab physicians to treat cough and to relieve the side effects of laxatives. Liquorice contains a saponin-like glycoside, glycyrrhizin (glycyrrhizic acid) which is 50 times sweeter than that of saccharose. The content of glycyrrhizin is 6–13% in the root and 20–25% in the extract. For hydrolysis, the glycoside is converted in the aglycone glycyrrhetic acid (glycyrrhetinic acid) plus two molecules of glucuronic acid. Other constituents include flavonoid glycosides (liquiritin, liquiritoside, rhamnoliquiritin, etc.), coumarin derivatives (herniarin, umbelliferone), asparagine and starch (22%).

Mode of action ▸ Both glycyrrhizin and glycyrrhetinic acid possess anti-inflammatory properties which account for the effectiveness of liquorice in the treatment of intestinal inflammation. In recent years it has been shown that the antiulcer effects of liquorice are due to inhibition of 15-hydroxyprostaglandin dehydrogenase, and enzyme that metabolizes prostaglandin E_2 and F_2 to 15-keto-prostaglandins, an inactive compound. The block of prostaglandin metabolism causes an increase of protective prostaglandins in the stomach and consequently a secretion of protective mucous and a cell proliferation of the gastric mucosa leading to the healing of ulcers.

Clinical efficacy ▸ Liquorice has a long tradition of efficacy in the treatment of peptic ulcer. Simple derivatives of glycyrrhetinic acid such as carbenoxolone and deglycyrrhinized liquorice (DGL) have been used extensively in gastric ulcer treatment. Carbenoxolone was the first drug found to accelerate peptic ulcer healing by a mechanism not involving the inhibition of acid secretion. However, given the side effects associated to the use of liquorice and its derivatives and the availability of safe and effective synthetic drugs, its use has declined. Liquorice is supported by the Commission E for the treatment of gastritis.

Adverse events/Contraindications ▸ Glycyrrhetic acid is also a potent inhibitor of the enzyme 11-hydroxysteroid dehydrogenase (11-OHSD), which converts cortisol to cortisone. Cortisol, in contrast to cortisone, has the same binding affinity for mineral corticoid receptors as aldosterone. 11-OHSD is present in high concentrations in the kidney. Glycyrrhetic acid inhibiting the enzyme in this organ increases the renal levels of cortisol which binds to mineralcorticoid receptors promoting sodium reabsorption. This mineralcorticoid activity of liquorice and its derivatives promotes side effects including sodium and water retention, hypertension and hypokalaemia (potassium depletion). Patients with cardiac, liver and kidney problems, hypertension or potassium deficiency should avoid consumption of significant quantities of glycyrrhetic acid. Liquorice and DGL have minimal fluid retaining properties. An abuse of liquorice-based preparations can lead to abnormalities in skeletal muscle contractility (like the hypocholesterolemic agents statins).

Preparations/Dosage

In peptic ulcer therapy liquorice is consumed in the form of a beverage prepared by adding 150 ml boiling water to 2–4 g drug and simmering the mixture for 5 min. This quantity of beverage may be drunk 3 times daily after meals. Because of the mineralcorticoid-like action, the treatment must not be longer than four to six weeks and the daily dose no more than 600 mg glycyrrhizin. Liquorice is also used as flavoring agents to mask the taste of bitter drugs including aloe, ammonium chloride, quinine and other. The surfactant properties of saponins present in liquorice may also facilitate absorption of poorly absorbed drugs, such as anthraquinone glycosides.

Other anti-ulcer drugs

Chamomile consists of the dried flowers heads of *Matricaria recutita* L., known as **German chamomile** or matricaria, or *Chamaemelum nobile* (L.) All. (= *Anthemis nobilis*), known as **Roman chamomile** (Fam. *Asteraceae/Compositae*). Chamomile contains a volatile oil (0.25–1%), flavonoids (about 2.4%) and coumarin derivatives, pectin-like mucilages (5–10%). Mucilages, released during the infusion process soothe the irritation of the gastric mucosa. Chamomile is usually taken as a tea (infusion) to treat acute gastritis and peptic ulcer. This preparation contains only 10–15% volatile oil originally present in the plant material, but almost all mucilaginous substances and flavonol glycosides. Obviously, whole plant extracts or volatile oil preparations are much more effective. Chamomile may cause hypersensitivity reactions in allergic individuals: these reactions are, however, relatively infrequent.

► *See Chapter 13 for the anxiolytic properties of chamomile*
► *See Chapter 23 for the dermatological anti-inflammatory effect of chamomile*

Chili (capsicum) is the fruit of various *Capsicum* species (Fam. *Solanaceae*). Chili and its pungent ingredient, capsaicin, have a protective effect on ethanol and for aspirin-induced lesion formation in the rat gastric mucosa. Capsaicin and long-term chili intake (360 mg/day for four weeks) also protects against hemorrhagic shock-induced gastric mucosal injury in animals, an effect which may be mediated by capsaicin-sensitive afferent neurons. Epidemiological and clinical data also suggest that chili ingestion may have a beneficial effect on human peptic ulcer disease.

► *See above for the use of chili to treat dyspepsia*

Mucilages and gums. Drugs containing mucilages have a property of covering and protecting gastric mucosa and may be used in the treatment of gastric ulcer. Mucilaginous plants traditionally used to treat gastric ailments include *Althaea officinalis* (marshmallow), *Malva sylvestris* (mallow) and *Cetraria islandica* (Iceland moss). Gums decrease gastric acidity and the rate of emptying of gastric content because of their effect on viscosity and neutralization of gastric activity. Guar gum obtained from the endosperm of the seed of *Cyamopsis tetragonolobus* is an old remedy. Myrrh (*Commiphora mukul*) too shows protective effects.

Kinetosis

Clinical Picture

- Kinetosis is a malaise characterized by nausea and vertigo (though rarely). Some people are subject to excessive salivation, nausea and vomiting when traveling even when movement is slight or in more extreme conditions such as sea or air turbulance. Where kinetosis stimulus is not increased tolerance is established after 2–3 days. It is simpler to prevent this condition by administering an antikinetosic 30–60 min before departure.

Antikinetosics

Treatment of kinetosis includes the use of scopolamine, (an alkaloid found in various *Solanacae* such as *Atropa belladonna*, *Datura stramonium*, *Josciamus niger*), which is very effective although of limited use due to its side effects. The antihistamines H1, though less effective, are used more often. Their action lasts from 6–24 h and are particularly effective if associated with ephedrine. The vegetable drug used in mild cases of kinetosis is ginger.

Ginger

Botany/Key constituents ▶ Ginger is the rhizome of *Zingiber officinale* Roscoe (Fam. *Zingiberaceae*), known in commerce as African ginger, Cochin ginger or Jamaica ginger, according to its geographical origin. The plant is cultivated in most tropical countries. The rhizomes are collected in December or January, peeled, washed and dried in the sun for 5–6 days. They contain volatile oil (1–2%) in which camphene, cineole, citral and the sesquiterpenes bisabolene, zingiberone and zingiberol are present. In addition, ginger contains an oleoresin (containing gingerol homologues, shogaol homologues) and zingerone (degradation product of gingerols) and more than 50% of starch. Pungent (hot) principles include gingerols, shogaols and gingerone.

Mode of action ▶ Gingerols, in particular 6-gingerol, have been identified as the active ingredient of ginger, and also responsible for its characteristic taste. The exact mechanism responsible for the antiemetic effects of ginger and its components is not completely known. Ginger works on the gastrointestinal system to increase gastric motility, an effect which could be brought about through 5-HT_3 antagonism (6-gingerol and other constituents of ginger possess anti-5-HT action; in particular galanolacotone is a competitive antagonist at ileal 5-HT_3 receptors). An effect on the central nervous system has been also suggested.

Clinical efficacy ▸ Ginger is a promising antiemetic herbal remedy. Indications supported by the German Commission E include loss of appetite, travel sickness and dyspeptic complaints. A recent systematic review retrieved six randomized, double-blind, placebo-controlled clinical trials. Three studies on postoperative women (a total of 288 women after gynecological surgery) with nausea and vomiting were identified; two of these studies (180 women) suggested that ginger was superior to placebo and equally effective as metoclopramide. One study was found for each of the following conditions: seasickness (80 subjects), morning sickness (30 pregnant women with severe nausea) and chemotherapy-induced nausea (41 patients receiving compazine for leukemia). These studies collectively favored ginger over placebo.

Adverse events/Contraindications ▸ There are no reports of adverse reactions to ginger compared to placebo in any of the above studies. Although used in clinical studies on pregnant women, the German Commission E warns that ginger should not be taken during pregnancy. The caution is based on data in experimental studies suggesting that ginger is mutagenic. Large doses could cause exfoliation of gastric surface epithelial cells, depression of the central nervous system and cardiac arrhythmias. Ginger has an antithrombotic effect and thus it is recommended that patients taking anticoagulants or those with bleeding disorders must avoid the use of large doses of ginger.

Preparations/Dosage

Most clinical studies used a daily dose of 1 g ginger powder. Ginger is available in the form of gelatin capsules, each containing 500 mg powdered drug. Ginger is also available as liquid extract (0.7–2 ml per day of 1:2 liquid extract) and as a tincture (1.7–5 ml per day of a 1:5 tincture).

Constipation

Clinical Picture

- Constipation may be defined as the delayed transit of "less than usual" volume feces. An alternative definition includes the occcurence of straining at the time of a bowel movement, with expulsion of stool with a hard consistency.
- Constipation can be due to *systemic or local* organic causes, or can be induced by drugs. In any case a careful and objective examination of the patient must be carried out to locate the organic cause, particularly if the condition suddenly arises in a patient with previous regular bowel movement. The most common reasons for constipation are poor dietary habits (not enough fiber), intestinal motility disturbances, and lack of physical

activity. This condition is also caused by over-use of certain laxatives for many years.

Laxatives

These are medicines which induce and facilitate defecation and are used in cases of constipation.

Laxatives improve the abnormal motility patterns and/or reduce fluid absorption in the intestines, which reduces intestinal transit time and promotes the elimination of a soft stool. Laxatives of botanical origin include anthraquinones (senna, cascara, frangula, aloe, rhubarb), bulk-forming agents (bran, psyllium, agar), sugar-containing herbs such as tamarind, cassia and plum, and finally castor oil. Botanical laxatives supported by the German Commission E to treat constipation are listed in Table 21.4.

Anthraquinones

The principal anthraquinones are found in *Rhamnus frangula* (frangula), *Aloe* spp (aloe), *Rheum palmatum* and *officinale* (rhubarb) and *Cassia acutifolia* and *C. angustifolia* (senna). The anthraquinones usually occur in nature as glycosides, which behave like pro-drug, liberating the aglycone that acts as the laxative. Figure 21.1 shows the principal glycoside forms of natural anthraquinones and their metabolism to the active aglycones. The metabolism takes place in the

Table 21.4
Main botanical laxatives supported by German Commission E to treat constipation

Common name	Latin name	Part(s) of plant used	Key constituents	Daily dose
Aloe	*Aloe spp.*	Juice of the leaves	Anthraquinones, flavonoids	0.05–0.2 g
Buckthorn	*Rhamnus catharticus*	Fruit	Anthraquinones, flavonoids, tannins	2–5 g
Cascara	*Rhamnus purshiana*	Bark	Anthraquinones	1
Flax	*Linum usitatissimum*	Seeds	Mucilages, fatty oil, proteins, lignans	1–2 g
Frangula	*Rhamnus frangula*	Bark	Anthraquinones	1 g
Manna	*Fraxinus ornus*	Juice from the bark	Mannitol, oligosaccharides	20–30 g
Psyllium	*Plantago psyllium*	Seeds	Fatty oil, iridoids (aucubin), mucilages, proteins	12–40 g
Rhubarb	*Rheum palmatum*	Bark	Anthraquinones , tannins, flavonoids	1–2 g
Senna	*Cassia spp.*	Leaves, fruits	Anthraquinones (sennosides)	a

a. 20–60 mg sennosides

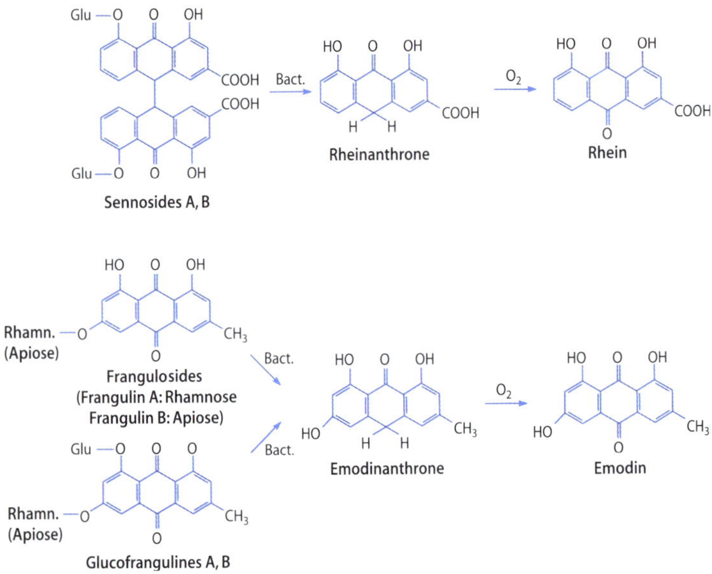

Figure 21.1 ▲ **Metabolism of sennosides, frangulosides and glucofrangulines to the aglycones rhein and emodin**

colon, where bacterial glycosidases remove sugars. The products obtained are poorly absorbed and act by evoking secretory and motility changes in the colon.

As in the case of many laxatives, the precise mode of action of anthraquinones is not known. It is generally believed that these compounds act on enteric nerves or mucosal cells to stimulate the release or synthesis of autacoids and/or neurotransmitters (i.e. prostaglandins, nitric oxide, 5-hydroxytryptamine), which are known to increase intestinal motility and stimulate fluid accumulation in the intestine (Figure 21.2). The laxative action of the anthraquinones occurs 6–12 h after oral ingestion.

Anthraquinone-containing herbal drugs are currently recommended for short-term (1–2 weeks) in case of atonic constipation, in some cases of acute constipation and before endoscopy of the gastrointestinal tract; they are not advisable for spastic constipation. Anthraquinones combined with fiber are also effective and well tolerated for chronic constipation in elderly patients.

The side effects of anthraquinones include discoloration of the urine, reversible melanosis of the colon and hemorrhoid congestion. No changes in serum electrolyte levels were found with recommended doses of anthraquinones, in particular sennosides. Contrary to what was first believed, treatment of lactating

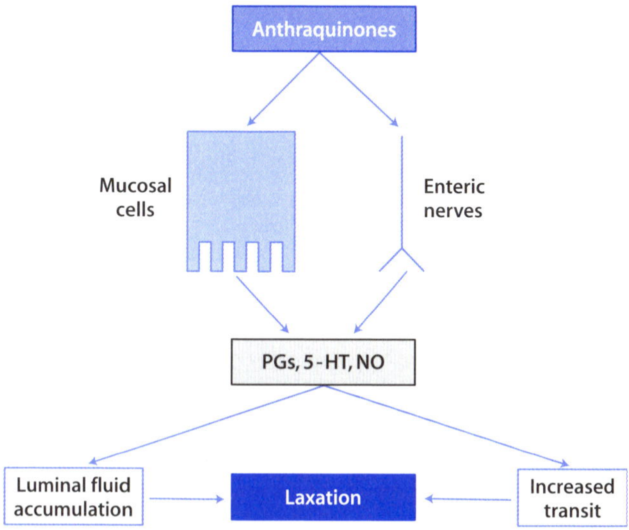

Figure 21.2 ▲ **Mode of action of anthraquinones**
Anthraquinones could act on mucosal cells and/or enteric nerves to stimulate the release/synthesis of neurotransmitters and/or autacoids such as prostaglandins (PGs), 5-hydroxytryptamine (5-HT) and nitric oxide (NO). These are able to increase intestinal transit and/or intraluminal fluid accumulation. The effect on both motility and secretion produces a laxative effect

mothers with anthroquinone drugs do not carry a risk of producing a laxative effect in the infant. Clinical studies also indicate that treatment with senna does not involve any increased risk during pregnancy or for the fetus.

Senna

Botany/Key constituents ▸ Senna consists of the dried leaves and fruits of *Cassia acutifolia* (or *C. senna*) and *C. angustifolia* referred to as Tinnevelly or Indian senna (Fam. *Leguminosae*). Taxanomists now group both of these species together under the scientific name *Senna alexandrine* Miller. These *Cassia* species (shrubs) are native to Egypt, the Middle East (Somalia, the Arabian peninsula) and India; they grow to 20–60 cm high and are characterized by paripinnate compound leaves arranged in clusters of 4–7 small leaves opposite each other, and pod-like fruits. The leaves are green-greyish in color with an elongated, pointed form. The fruit is blackish, elongated, flat and kidney-shaped. Senna is harvested in April and September. The laxative effect of leaves is greater than that of fruit. Anthraquinones contained in senna are dianthrone glycosides (1.5–3%

leaf; 2–5% fruit), primarly sennosides A and B (rhein dianthrones). Free anthraquinones including aloe-emodin and rhein are also present in small quantities.

Mode of action ▸ Sennosides A and B can be regarded as pro-drugs: they reach the large intestine without changes and are hydrolyzed by the bacteria flora to form the main active metabolites, rhein and rhein anthrone (Figure 21.3). Rhein anthrone and to a lesser extent rhein act upon both the secretion and motility to cause laxation and these actions are largely independent of one another. Sennosides or their active compound rhein and rhein anthrone have been shown to stimulate the synthesis or release of a number of intestinal secretagogues including prostaglandins, 5-hydroxytryptamine and nitric oxide.

Clinical use ▸ Of all the anthraquinone-containing laxatives, the most commonly used certainly is senna. Although senna is not as mild in its action as cascara and frangula, it is nevertheless, for its low cost, more widely recommended in atonic constipation, for short-term treatment (1–2 weeks), in cases of acute constipation and before endoscopy of the gastrointestinal tract.

Adverse events/Contraindications ▸ The use of large doses of senna is associated with abdominal complaints (meteorism, flatulence, cramping, abdominal pain), discoloration of the urine and hemorrhoid congestion. Long-term use (abuse) includes melanosis of the colon, electrolyte imbalance, dehydration and changes in muscular function. Clinical studies have shown that the treatment of lactating mothers with senna does not carry a risk of producing a laxative effect in the infant. Clinical studies also indicate that treatment with senna does not involve any increased risk during pregnancy or for the fetus. On the contrary, senna seems the laxative of choice in pregnancy and during feeding.

Preparations/Dosage

Senna is taken in the form of tea (prepared from 0.5–2 g leaves or fruit), fluid extract (2 ml) or syrup (8 ml). Such preparations usually produce a single bowel evacuation within 6 h. A beverage prepared by soaking senna in cold water for 10–12 h is also used: such a preparation is more active than hot tea as it contains more sennosides and less resinous material. Crystalline senna glycosides (sennosides) are also available (usual dose 20–60 mg); they are more stable, more reliable and safer than the preparations of crude drug. No intestinal discomfort is found with recommended doses of senna.

Other Anthraquinone-containing Laxatives

Cascara consists of the dried bark of the trunk or branches of the *Rhamnus purshiana* (Fam. *Rhamnaceae*), a shrub that grows along the Pacific coast of North America. The plant is 4–10 m high, with eliptical leaves dented at the edges, and

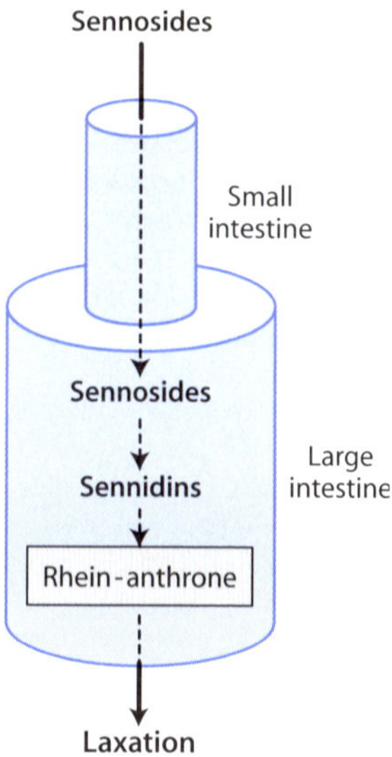

Figure 21.3 ◂ **Laxative effect of sennosides**
Sennosides are not metabolized in the small intestine; they are catabolized by the microorganisms in the colon to form rhein-anthrone. This compound act upon both the secretion and motility to cause laxation and these actions are largely independent of one another

flowers gathered in corymbs at the axil (Plate 21.5). The bark should be collected at least one year prior to use (to allow the reduced glycosides to be oxidized to monomeric forms which exhibit a milder cathartic activity) at the beginning of the spring and continuing until the rainy season starts. Once dried, the bark becomes rounded in a pipeform which is curved or almost flat, with a thickness of 1–4 mm and a variable length and width. Cascara owes its action to a mixture of cascarosides A, B, C and D, with other anthraquinone glycosides in minor amounts. Cascara must contain not less than 7% total hydroxyanthracene derivatives calculated as cascaroside A on a dried basis. The principal use of cascara is in the correction of habitual constipation where it acts as a laxative and to restore natural tone to the colon.

Cascara is used in the form of extract, fluid extract, aromatic fluid extract (a 5 ml dose usually causes a laxative effect) and powder (1 g in capsule form). The bitter taste of the drug is reduced by treating cascara extracts with magnesium oxide or alkaline earths: this treatment also reduces the activity of the extracts. The drug is an ingredient of several over-the-counter (OTC) and proprietary laxatives. In many preparations cascara is combined with one or more of the following substances: rhubarb, genziana, senna, artichoke, boldo, aloe, frangula, belladonna, chamomile. A preparation containing cascara, boldo, inositol and cyanocobalamin has been used in the treatment of constipation in geriatric patients. Preparations containing purified anthranol glycosides from cascara are also available (the adult dose is 30 mg).

Frangula (buckthorn bark) is the dried bark of *Rhamnus frangula* (Fam. *Rhamnaceae*), a shrub 3–5 m high growing in Southern Central Europe and Western Asia. Frangula means brittle, in reference to the brittle stems of this species. The dried bark appears as a single or double pipe form which is almost flat or rounded. Its thickness is 0.5–2 mm and its length and width vary. The bark has a brown-greyish surface. Like cascara, frangula should be collected one year prior to use, preferably in May and June. The laxative effect of frangula is due to the presence of anthraquinone derivatives, particularly gluco-frangulins A and B and frangulins A and B. For its mild laxative action frangula is comparable to cascara.

The drug must contain not less than 6% total hydroxyanthracene derivatives calculated as glucofrangulin A on a dried basis. It is popular in its native Europe but less so in the United States (where it is of considerable use in veterinary practice). It is used in the form of fluid extract but it is possible to consume the powdered bark (1 g) in capsule form. The laxative action occurs after about 10–12 h. Frangula is an ingredient in proprietary products (Crisolax, Fave di Fuca, Hepasil, Frangulina, Neo-heparbil, Sintobil) and in several OTC laxatives.

Rhubarb consists of the dried rhizome and root deprived of periderm tissues of *Rheum palmatum* L., and *R. officinale* Baill. (Fam. *Polygonaceae*) or of related species (*R. emodi* Wallich, *R. webbianum* Royl) or hybrids common in China (Chinese rhubarb), or in India, Pakistan or Nepal (Indian or Himalayan rhubarb). *R. palmatum* and *R. officinale* are perennial herbaceous plants, 1–3 m tall with large heart-shaped or rounded leaves. The anthraquinones are especially concentrated in the rhizome which is collected in the autumn or spring from plants 8–10 years old: it is peeled, strung on ropes and dried either in the sun or by artificial heat. The drug is of various forms (cylindrical, oval, rounded or with a convex surface) and sizes (5–15 mm in length and 4–10 mm in diameter). It contains sennosides A-F with purgative properties, tannins and other substances like isolindleyin, lindleyin, stilbenes. Its use almost always causes intestinal griping or colic. However, a laxative action without abdominal pain is caused by a dose of 0.5–2 g. The preparations most used are tinctures, infusions, and fluid extracts. Frequent use is not recommended.

▶ *See Chapter 15 for the use of rhubarb in the treatment of obesity*

Bulk-forming Laxatives

A fiber-rich diet, in conjunction with other non-pharmacological measures, is the most appropriate method for prevention and treatment of functional constipation. Dietary fiber is also of benefit for patients in whom it is desired that the feces be maintained soft, to avoid straining at the stool, and in the management of irritable bowel disease and diverticular disease of the colon. The related bulk-forming agents polysaccharides and cellulose derivatives are similar to those characterized as dietary fiber. They are useful as a supplement to dietary adjustment or when a constipating, fiber-poor diet cannot be corrected.

Dietary fiber and bulk-forming agents increase the mass of stool, its water content, and the rate of colonic transit. These effects are usually apparent within 24 hours, but the full effect during repeated use may be delayed for several days or longer. The laxative effect is commonly attributed to the hydrophilic bulk-forming properties of the component polysaccharides (Figure 21.4). However, a likely additional factor is metabolism of the polysaccharides by the intestinal microflora, with accumulation of metabolites that are osmotically active.

The bulk-forming laxatives have minimal systemic effects. Allergic reactions have been reported for several of the natural products. Flatulence may occurr, particularly if the dosage of bulk-forming agent is increased abruptly. The bulk-forming agents potentially absorb other drugs administered concurrently, thereby interfering with their intestinal absorption.

Psyllium is the cleaned, dried, ripe seeds of *Plantago psyllium* (or *P. indica*), known in commerce as French or Spanish psyllium or of *P. ovata* Forskal, known in commerce as blond psyllium or Indian plantago. These and other species in the genus *Plantago* provide laxative drugs used in pharmacy: psyllium seeds, plantago seeds, plantain seeds or ispaghula seeds and teguments. *Plantago* plants are annual, coalescent and pubescent herbs; they belong to the *Plantaginaceae* family, which are native to Asia and the Mediterranean countries and cultivated in Europe (Spain), Pakistan and India. Psyllium contains 10–30% of a substance which is hydrophilic and in water produces a mucilaginous mucoid-like substance. This drug is useful in treating atonic as well as spastic constipation and when excessive straining must be avoided following anorectal surgery. Its action is due to the swelling of the mucilaginous seed coat, thus giving bulk and lubrication.

Psyllium is used in amounts of 5–10 g, one to three times daily, usually suspended in a considerable amount of water. It is also combined with senna

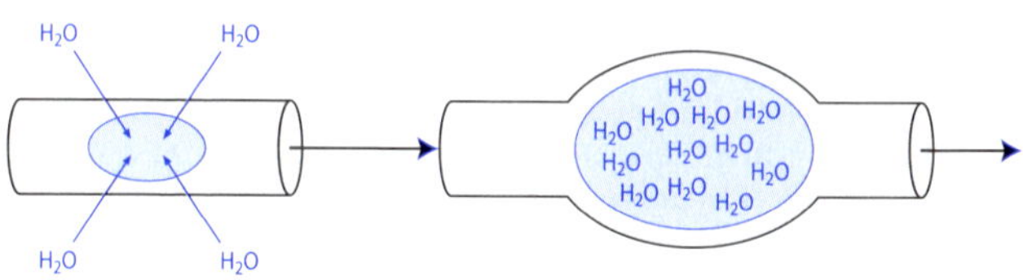

Figure 21.4 ▲ **Laxative effect of bulk-forming agents (e.g. psyllium, agar, bran, tragacanth)**
The celluloses, hemicelluloses and lignins contained in bulk-forming laxatives are resistant to human digestive enzymes so they pass unchanged through the small intestine into the colon. In the colon they can retain water and hence stimulate sensory receptor of peristalsis in the intestinal wall; this stimulation produces increased motility

(Agiolax®), or chemicals such as anhydrous dextrose, sodium bicarbonate, monobasic potassium phosphate and citric acid (Metamucil®). In this case it is used as an adjunct in the treatment of constipation. A relatively common side effect is an allergic reaction to psyllium. Sensitization (with asthmatic symptoms) after chronic inhalation of psyllium powder has been reported in atopic individuals. It may also cause renal pigmentation (if the seeds are ground or chewed).

▶ *See Chapter 15 for the use of psyllium in treating obesity*

Agar is obtained from different species of algae (*Gelidium*, *Gracilaria*, *Euchema*), which grow along the coasts of the United States, Spain, New Zealand, Australia and South Africa. Agar occurs as bundles, consisting of thin, agglutinated strips, or in granulated forms. It contains about 90% polysaccharides, comprised of agarose and agaropectin; the remaining 10% is water, nitrogen compounds and lipids. Agar swells in water and increases the moisture of the stool, thus producing a laxative effect. Sometimes it can take up to a week after initiating therapy with over 400 g agar before any benefit is realized. Agar cannot be assimilated, will not ferment and is not toxic. The cell walls of certain brown algae of the species *Fucus* (*F. vesiculosus*), *Laminaria* and *Macrocystis* (*M. pyrifera*) which grow on the rocks along the North Atlantic coast, contain polysaccharides like alginic acid, that are hydrophilic. Alginic acid is a polyuric acid composed of D-mannuronic and L-guluronic residues. It is a colorless and tasteless powder that forms a colloidal solution with a mucilaginous character.

Bran has been recognized as a laxative since 430 BC. The addition of bran to the diet softens the fecal consistency and increases transit through the intestinal tract. About 20 g bran daily is considered to be the minimum amount to produce a laxative effect. Bran is particularly useful in treating the spastic-type constipation associated with irritable bowel syndrome, although it can take several weeks before symptoms are relieved. The increased bulk produced by bran is also believed to be beneficial in diverticular disease of the colon. Patients with atonic constipation may not be responsive to treatment with bran because of neuromuscular damage associated with chronic debility, old age or chronic laxative abuse. Some patients will experience bloating due to increased production of intestinal gas related to bacterial degradation of the components of bran. This symptom will usually disappear with time. Bran must be taken with a sufficient quantity of fluids to avoid any risk of obstruction of the intestine. It should not be employed in individuals with intestinal ulceration, stenosis or adhesions.

Tragacanth. The dried gum from *Astragalus gummifer* (Fam. *Fabaceae*) and other species of *Astragalus* provides the laxative tragacanth. Related products are karaya or sterculia (*Sterculia urens* Roxb.; Fam. *Sterculiaceae*) and bassora gum. The gums are collected during the period from March to June, dried and triturated to give a fine powder with a slight smell of acetic acid. The mucilaginous substance present in gums can absorb up to 40 times its own volume of water; it also reduces the fermentative and putrefying processes. Tragacanth, karaya and bassora gum are used as bulk laxatives. Allergic reactions such as urticaria, rhinitis, atopic dermatitis and asthma have been attributed to these agents.

Other Laxative Herbs and Fruits

Certain vegetables and fruits like tamarind, cassia, plums, may have a mild laxative action when consumed in sufficient quantities. This is due to their organic acids (citrate, tartrate) and sugar content.

Tamarind pulp is obtained from the fruit of the *Tamarindus indica* (Fam. *Cesalpinaceae*), an evergreen tree found in India and tropical Africa. The fruits are hanging pods, lumpy in relation to the seeds. The seeds are imbedded in a soft, yellowish substance (pulp) with a slightly acid taste and a particular odor. The pulp contains about 20% organic acid in the free form and as potassium salts, mucilaginous substance (20–30%) and sugar. Tamarind laxative is taken in the form of jam or syrup. The dose is 40–60 g for adults and 1–2 g for children, in the case of chronic constipation.

The pulp of **cassia** is obtained from the fruit of the *Cassia fistula* L. (Fam. *Leguminosae*), a tree cultivated in tropical regions. The fruits are cylindrically shaped pods rounded at the extremities. The interior is divided into numerous sections filled with a blackish pulp which has a particular odor and sweetish taste. The pulp contains citric acid, tannic substances, pectin, anthraquinone derivatives (1%) and fructose (70%). It is used in the form of jam or syrup as a mild laxative for children. The dose is 40–60 g (3–5 g for every year of age).

Plums (*Prunus domestica* L., Fam. *Rosaceae*) have an excellent laxative action at doses of 50–100 g. Their laxative effect is due to organic acids (2%), invert sugar (50%) and oxyphenisatin (small amounts). Many other fruits, expecially if not very ripe, act as a laxative probably through a combined action of their fiber and osmotic effects of their natural sugars (12% in figs, 25% in fresh grapes, 70% in raisins and 50% in plums).

Diarrhea

Clinical Picture

- Normally there is only one defecation of 120 g in 24 hours, of which the water content is between 55–70%. Diarrhea is present when stool weight exceeds 200 g and a water content of 70–90%, repeated 2–6 times in 24 hours. Thus diarrhea can be defined as frequent liquid or semi-liquid fecal emission.

- The principal factors responsible for these alterations are intestinal infections. It is known that various pathogenic bacteria release toxins into the intestinal lumen which are able to increase intraluminal secretion or penetrate the intestinal epithelium, reducing absorption. Diarrhea can also arise after swallowing toxic substances or foods which are not well tolerated (milk, eggs, strawberries, shellfish) which stimulate the release of secretagogues by mast cells located along the intestinal lining. There are various medicines which can induce an excessive motor reaction or reduce water and ion absorption if taken regularly and over a long period of time.

Antidiarrheal Drugs

In most cases it is the removal of the cause rather than the use of an antidiarrheal drug which restores intestinal transit and electrolyte disturbances to normal. Antidiarrheal drugs have little effect on iatrogenic or toxic diarrhea. In these cases antidiarrheal therapy actually delays diagnosis of a more serious pathology. Various preparations of opium are potent and effective natural remedies for diarrhea. Their downside, however, is their additional liability and potential life-threatening respiratory depression in instances of overdose. Herbal medicines with antidiarrheal activity are listed in Table 21.5. Most of them are characterized by a high tannin content.

Antidiarrheal Activity of Tannin-containing Herbs

One of the most prominent actions of tannins is their effect on diarrhea. They produce a temporary protective layer of coagulated protein on the mucosal membrane of the gut, possibly desensitizing sensory nerve endings and reducing provocative peristaltic stimuli. Tannins may also have antibacterial activity against enteric pathogens, which is of interest in the treatment of infectious diarrhea. Condensed tannins are also able to bind and to inactivate the hypersecretory activity of some toxins.

Since tannins are polar molecules, they are poorly absorbed through the gastrointestinal tract. Hence the effect is mostly local, within the gastrointestinal lumen. However, decomposition products of tannins are absorbed and do exert quite toxic effects. The poor availability of tannins limits their systemic effects. However, high doses of tannins cause an irritating effect: for these reasons an overdose must be avoided in highly inflamed or ulcerated conditions of the gastrointestinal tract.

Chronic intake of tannins (or drugs containing tannins) is dangerous because (i) they inhibit digestive enzymes which bind to the small intestinal mucosa, (ii) they complex metal ions thus inhibiting their absorption and (iii) they react

Table 21.5
Herbal medicines with antidiarrhoeal activity

Common name	Latin name	Part(s) of plant used	Key constituents	Daily dose
Acacia	*Acacia arabica*	Bark	Tannins	6–10 g
Agrimony*	*Agrimonia eupatoria*	Flowering plant	Tannins, flavonoids	3–6 g
Apple	*Malus domestica*	False fruit	Pectins, tannins, caffeic acid derivatives, fruit acids	a
Banana	*Musa paradisiaca*	Unripe fruit	Pectins	b
Bilberry*	*Vaccinium myrtillus*	Fruits	Tannins, flavonoids	20–50 g
Blackberry*	*Rubus fruticosus*	Leaves	Tannins, flavonoids	3–6 g
Carob	*Ceratonia siliqua*	Seeds	Mucilages, proteic substances, flavonoids	c
Cinquefoil*	*Potentilla erecta*	Rhizome	Tannins, flavonoids, triterpenes,	4–6 g
Coffee charcoal*	*Coffea arabica*	Seeds	Purine alkaloids, hemicellulose derivatives	9 g
Jambolan*	*Syzygium cumini*	Bark	Tannins, triterpenes, flavonoids, steroids	3.6 g
Lady's mantle*	*Alchemilla vulgaris*	Aerial parts	Flavonoids, tannins	5–10 g
Marshmallow*	*Althaea officinalis*	Roots	Mucilages, pectins, starch	6 g
Oak*	*Quercus robur*	Bark	Tannins, coumarins	3 g
Potentilla*	*Potentilla anserina*	Aerial parts	Tannins, flavonoids, coumarins	4–6 g
Psyllium*	*Plantago psyllium*	Seeds	Mucilages, fatty oil, iroidoids, proteic substances	12–40 g
Rhatany	*Krameria triandra*	Roots	Tannins, neolignans	1 g
Tea (green and black tea)	*Camellia sinensis*	Leaves	Purine alkaloids, tannins, volatile oil	8 g
Uzara*	*Xysmalobium undulatum*	Roots	Cardioactive steroid glycosides, pregnane derivates	d
Carrot	*Daucus carota*	Roots	Pectins, carotenoids	e
Witch hazel*	*Hamamelis virginiana*	Bark, roots, branches, dried leaves	Catechins, tannins, volatile oil, flavonoids	f

* supported by German Commission E

a. 1–1.5 kg as a food
b. 1.5–2 fruits per day as a food
c. as a food (a meal made from carob seeds)
d. 45–90 mg of total glycosides
e. 0.5 kg (boiled) as a food
f. tea prepared with 2–3 g in 150 ml water (1 cup, 2–3 times daily)

with thiamin, decreasing their absorption. Pure tannins also seem implicated in the development of esophageal cancer, but this is not the case of tannin-containing drugs. It is prudent to avoid the long-term oral use or the use of high doses of astringent drugs in patients with damaged or inflamed intestines.

Tannin-containing herbal medicines with antidiarrheal activity include agrimony, oak bark, blackberry leaf, Lady's Mantle and tea.

Agrimony consists of the flowering plant of *Agrimonia eupatoria* L. (Fam. *Rosaceae*). The plant is 50–100 cm high, with a villous, erect stem, and indigenous to Middle and Northern Europe, temperate Asia and North America. The drug contains not less than 5% tannins. It also contains flavonoids like quercetin, kaempferol, luteolin and apigenin. Agrimony has a slightly pleasant fragrance and a tangy, bitter taste. Agrimony is supported by German Commission E for the treatment of diarrhea. No side effects are expected. As for the other tannin-containing drugs, excessive quantities could lead to digestive complaints and constipation. The average daily dose is 3–6 g crude drug.

Oak consists of the dried bark of the young branches and lateral shoots of *Quercus robur* L. (= *Q. pedunculata* Ehrh) (Fam. *Fagaceae*), a 50 m high tree which is widespread in Europe, Asia minor and the Caucasus region. The bark is deeply fissured, thick and grey-brown; it contains tannins in a wide range of concentrations (8–20%). Oak bark is supported by German Commission E for the treatment of acute diarrhea. Oak is available as whole, crude and powdered drug form. It is also available in solid pharmaceutical form for oral intake. The daily dose is 3 g drug. A tea can be prepared starting from 1 g powdered drug. No side effects are known in conjunction with the proper administration of designated therapeutic dosage.

Blackberry consists of the leaves of *Rubus fruticosus* L. (Fam. *Rosaceae*), a plant which is indigenous to Europe and is naturalized in America and Australia. The plant is a fast-growing, thorny bush up to 2 m high. The leaves are usually 5-paired pinnate, glabrous above, and grey to white tomentose beneath. Blackberry leaf contains organic acids (including citric and isocitric acids), flavonoids triterpenes and up to 14% tannins. Blackberry leaf is used for non-specific, acute diarrhea and it is supported by German Commission E for such a condition. No side effects are known when used in appropriate dosage. Blackberry leaf is available as crude drug for decoctions and other preparations for internal use. The daily dosage is 3–6 g drug. Like blackberry leaf, raspberry (*R. idaeus*) leaf is still used to treat diarrhea.

Lady's mantle consists of the fresh or dried above-ground parts of *Alchemilla vulgaris* L. (= *A. glabra* Naygenf) (Fam. *Rosaceae*) gathered at flowering time. *A. vulgaris* is an herbaceous plant which grows in various areas of the Northern hemisphere, but it is produced mostly through cultivation. Lady's Mantle is odorless and has an astringent taste. Key constituents include bitter principles, flavonoids and tannins (6–8%). It is supported by German Commission E for the treatment of diarrhea. The daily dose is 5–10 g crude drug. As for the other tannin-containing drugs, no side effects are expected if used in appropriate dosage. Lady's mantle extracts have also antibacterial activity.

Tea (or **Thea**) is the fermented and dried leaf of *Camellia sinensis* (L.) O. Kuntze (or *Thea sinensis* L.) (Fam. *Theaceae*). If growing wild, the tree is 5–10 m tall, but it is also cultivated as a shrub: both have alternate, evergreen leaves. The tea plant is native to Eastern Asia and is now cultivated in other Asiatic regions, in Africa and South America. The plant is marketed as black tea, green tea and "oolong" tea (Box 21.1). Tea occurs in more or less crumpled masses; its odor is agreeable, aromatic, the taste is pleasantly astringent and bitter. It contains 2.5–4.5% caffeine, 0.02–0.04% theophylline, 0.05% theobromine, 5–20% tannins of the catechin type, oxidized polyphenols and about 1% volatile oils which gives the aroma to the tea. The pharmacological activity of tea depends on its geographical origin (Ceylon tea is more active), the age of the tree (10 years old is better) and the leaves (young shoots are preferred to younger or old leaves). The drug is used mainly as a beverage containing about 0.04–0.16 mg of tannins in a cup to 200 ml. The infusion must last for 15–20 minutes, to increase the presence of tannins. In normal individuals one-two litres of tea daily (8 g drug) prolong the intestinal transit time, reduce the excretion of bile acid and produce constipation.

▶ See Appendix B for the use of green tea in cancer prevention

Box 21.1

Preparation of black, green and oolong tea

Black tea is prepared in Ceylon and India from the top shoot and the two uppermost leaves of each branch of the plant. The picking starts when the plant is 3 years old and continues for 30–40 years. The leaves are first dried (may take 15–36 hours), then crushed or rolled: this process puts the enzymes (polyphenol oxidases) in contact with the cell sap and the oxidation that takes places gives a dark color to the end product. The rolled material is then fermented at 30°C for 0.5–2 hours, and heated at 115–120°C (the water content is reduced to 4–5%) to obtain a stable product.

Green tea is prepared in China and Japan: its preparation is different in that the fresh leaves are immediately heated. This destroys the enzymes and the tea becomes green during the subsequent rolling drying processes.

"**Oolong**" tea; this tea, little known in Europe, is only partially fermented.

Other Antidiarrheal Herbs

Uzara consists of the dried, underground parts of 2- to 3-years old plants of *Xysmalobium undulatum* (Fam. *Asclepiadaceae*), a herb native to South Africa. Uzara contains cardioactive steroid glycosides (cardenolides, a mixture referred to as uzarone or xysmalobin and pregnane derivatives). Uzara inhibits intestinal motility. In high dosage, it has a digitalis-like effect on the heart. Uzara is traditionally used as a treatment for dysentery and it is supported by German Commission E for the treatment of diarrhea. If used adequately, Uzara is a safe herb. However, because of the presence of cardioactive glycosides, there is a potential for interaction with other cardiac glycosides such as digoxin. However, there are no reports of such interaction. The drug is available as ethanol-water extracts in liquid form or as a dry extract. Pharmaceutical forms include coated tablets and drops. The daily dose should be equivalent to 45–90 mg total glycosides, calculated as uzarin.

Coffee charcoal is produced by roasting the outer seed parts of the green, dried fruit of *Coffea arabica* L. (Fam. *Rubiaceae*) (and other *Coffea* species) until almost black, then grinding the carbonized product. *Coffea* species are shrubs or small trees with coriaceous leaves and white flowers. The fruit is a drupe, the size of a cherry, which is red when ripe. Coffee charcoal contains purine alkaloids (mainly caffeine), trigonelline and carbonization products of hemicelluloses. It possesses adsorbent and astringent properties. Coffee charcoal is supported by German Commission E for the treatment of diarrhea. There are no risks or side effects following the proper administration of designated therapeutic dosages. However, because of the absorbent properties, coffee charcoal can hinder the absorption of other medicines. The daily dose is 9 g ground drug. The average single dose is 3 g powder.

Green banana. The unripe fruit of green banana (*Musa paradisiaca sapientum* L.; Fam. *Musaceae*) is used in the treatment of various intestinal disorders including diarrhea. Green banana is rich in pectins [a general term designating amylase-resistant polysaccharides (starch)], which are not digested in the small intestine. On reaching the colon, pectins are fermented by resident bacteria into short-chain fatty acids (butyrate, proprionate and acetate) which stimulate salt and water absorption (Figure 21.5), as well as provide energy and induce a trophic effect on the colonic mucosa. A recent randomized double-blind clinical study including a total of 62 boys with persistent diarrhea, showed that cooked fruit of green banana administered into a rice-based diet reduced the amounts of stool and the number of episodes of vomiting and diarrhea duration after 3 days treatment (each child on average consumed 30 g/kg cooked green banana equivalent to 1.5–2 uncooked fruit per day).

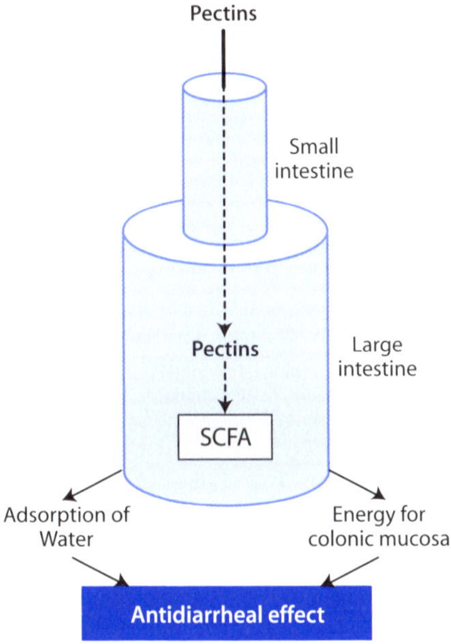

Figure 21.5 ◂ **Antidiarrheal activity of pectins from green banana**
Pectin is a general term designating amylase-resistant polysaccharides (starch) found in the cell wall and intracellular substances in many fruit including green bananas. The pectins present in green bananas are mostly -glucans and dextrin which are hydrolyzed into soluble sugars during the ripening process; however, they are not digested when eaten as unripe fruit. Pectins are not digested in the small intestine. On reaching the colon, they are fermented by resident bacteria into short-chain fatty acids (SCFA, i.e. butyrate, proprionate, and acetate). In the colon SCFA facilitate the absorpion of electrolytes and water and provide an added source of energy, increase protein synthesis, and improve oxygen utilization by the colonic mucosa. Additionally, SCFA could have inhibitory action on colonic motility

Irritable Bowel Syndrome

Clinical Picture

- Irritable bowel syndrome (IBS) is a disturbed state of intestinal motility for which no anatomic cause can be found. It has many manifestations including bloating, constipation, and diarrhea. Usually beginning in the first three decades of life, the disorder occurs in intermittent episodes and may be life-long, but not life-shortening. In some individuals attacks seem to be brought on by stress or emotional difficulties.

Phytotherapy of IBS

Because its etiology is unknown, an evidence-based treatment for IBS is difficult to develop. Treatment is symptomatic: constipation is treated with high fiber diet or bulking agents, diarrhea with antidiarrheal agents or a reduction of fat intake; abdominal pain and spasm are treated with muscle relaxants, and somatoform disorders with antidepressants, but none of these is fully satisfactory. Peppermint oil is the only botanical remedy which has been shown to have a promising efficacy in the treatment of IBS.

Peppermint oil

Botany/Key constituents ▸ Peppermint oil constists of the essential oil of *Mentha piperita* obtained by aqueous steam distillation from freshly harvested, flowering tops and preparations of same. *Mentha piperita* L. (Fam. *Labiatae*) is a perennial, 50–90 cm high herb common in Europe and USA, usually cultivated. Peppermint leaf is harvested several times a year. The maximum leaf harvest and highest oil content is shortly before the flowering season. The harvest is dried mechanically on drying belts at a temperature of 42°C. Chief constituents of peppermint oil include menthol (35–45%), menthone, mentyl acetate, neomenthol, isomenthone, menthofurane.

Mode of action ▸ A primary problem associated with IBS is the hypercontractility of intestinal smooth muscle. The antispasmodic property of peppermint allows these muscles to return to their proper tone, therefore reducing many of the abdominal pains and symptoms. Peppermint oil relaxes isolated gastrointestinal smooth muscle by reducing the influx of Ca^{2+} into muscle cells. In addition to this dihydropyridine-like action, peppermint oil also inhibits the excitability of enteric nerves by reducing calcium uptake into enteric nerves. The active principle of peppermint oil is menthol, a cyclic monoterpene with a Ca^{2+} channel blocking properties.

Clinical efficacy ▸ The efficacy of peppermint oil for irritable bowel syndrome is promising, although not fully conclusive. German Commission E states that peppermint oil can be taken internally for pathologies such as colicky pain in the upper gastrointestinal tract, biliary tract and irritable bowel disease. A meta-analysis retrieved eight randomized placebo-controlled, double-blind randomized controlled trials including a total of 295 patients treated with peppermint oil (approx 0.6–1.2 ml daily) for a period of 2–6 weeks. Collectively they indicate that peppermint oil could be efficacious for symptom relief in irritable bowel syndrome. However, in view of the methodological flaws associated with most studies, no definitive judgment about efficacy can be given.

Adverse reactions/Contraindications ▸ No health hazards are known in conjucnction with the proper administration of designated therapeutic dosages. The intake can lead to gastric complaints in susceptible people. The volatile oil possesses a weak potential for sensitization due to its menthol content. The ingestion of excessive amounts of peppermint oil has been associated with interstitial nephritis and acute renal failure. The minimal lethal dosage of menthol is estimated to be 2 g, although individuals have survived higher dosages (8–9 g).

Susceptible individuals may also experience "heartburn" (gastroesophageal reflux) due to relaxation of the lower esophageal sphincter.

Preparations/Dosage

Enteric-coated capsules (Colpermin®) have been used in most clinical studies. These capsules allow delivery to the intestines and reduce the possibility of heartburn. The dosage is three capsules daily (0.2 ml capsule). Peppermint oil is standardized to contain not less than 44% free menthol.

Further Reading

Afzal M, Al-Hadidi D, Menon M, Pesek J, Dhami MS (2001) Ginger: an ethnomedical, chemical and pharmacological review. Drug Metabol Drug Interact 18:159–190

Borrelli F, Izzo AA (2000) The plant kingdom as a source of anti-ulcer remedies. Phytother Res 14:581–591

Bortolotti M, Coccia G, Grossi G (2002) Red pepper and functional dyspepsia. New Engl J Med 346 (12) :946–948

Bortolotti M, Coccia G, Grossi G (2002) The treatment of functional dyspepsia with red pepper. Aliment Pharmacol Ther 16:1075–1082

Capasso F, Borrelli F, Capasso R, Di Carlo G, Izzo AA, Pinto L, Mascolo N, Castaldo S, Longo R (1998) Aloe and its therapeutic use. Phytoter Res 12:124–127

Eigner D, Scholz D (1999) *Ferula asa-foetida* and *Curcuma longa* in traditional medical treatment and diet in Nepal. J Ethnopharmacol 67:1–6

Ernst E, Pittler MH (2000) Efficacy of ginger for nausea and vomiting: a systematic review of randomized clinical trials. Br J Anaesth 84:367–371

Izzo AA, Gaginella TS, Mascolo N, Capasso F (1998) Recent findings mode of action of laxatives: the role of platelet activating factor and nitric oxide. Trends Pharmacol Sci 19:403–405

Jailwala J, Imperiale TF, Kroenke K. (2000) Pharmacological treatment of the irritable bowel syndrome: a systematic review of randomized, controlled trials. Ann Intern med 18:136–147

Langmead L, Rampton DS (2001) Review article: herbal treatment in gastrointestinal and liver disease – benefits and dangers. Aliment Pharmacol Ther 15:1239–1252

Langner E, Greifenberg S, Gruenwald J (1998) Ginger: history and use. Adv Ther 15:25–44

Mascolo N, Capasso R, Capasso F (1998) Senna. A safe and effective drug. Phytoter Res 12:S143–S145

Pittler MH, Ernst E (1998) Peppermint oil for irritable bowel syndrome: a critical review and meta-analysis. Am J Gastroenterol 93:1131–1135

Saller R, Pfister-Hotz G, Iten F, Melzer J, Reichling J (2002) Iberogast. A Modern Phytotherapeutic Combined Herbal Drug for the Treatment of Functional Disorders of the Gastrointestinal Tract (Dyspepsia, Irritable Bowel Syndrome) - from Phytomedicine to 'Evidence Based Phytotherapy'. A Systematic Review. Forsch Komplementarmed Klass Naturheilkd 9 (Suppl 1):1–20

Rabbani GH, Teka T, Zaman B, Madjid N, Khatun M, Fuchs GJ (2001) Clinical studies in persistent diarrhea: dietary management with green banana or pectin in Bangladeshi children. Gastroenterology 121:554–560

Thomson Coon J, Ernst E (2002) Systematic review: herbal medicinal products for non-ulcer dyspepsia. Aliment Pharmacol Ther 16:1689–1699

Tiran D (2002) Nausea and vomiting in pregnancy: safety and efficacy of self-administered complementary therapies. Complement Ther Nurs Midwifery 8:191–196

Van Gorkom BA, De Vries EG, Karrenbeld A, Kleibueker JH (1999) Review article: anthranoid laxatives and their potential carcinogenic effects. Aliment Pharmacol Ther 13:446–452

Wanitschke R, Goerg KJ, Loew D (2003) Differential therapy of constipation--a review. Int J Clin Pharmacol Ther 41:14–21

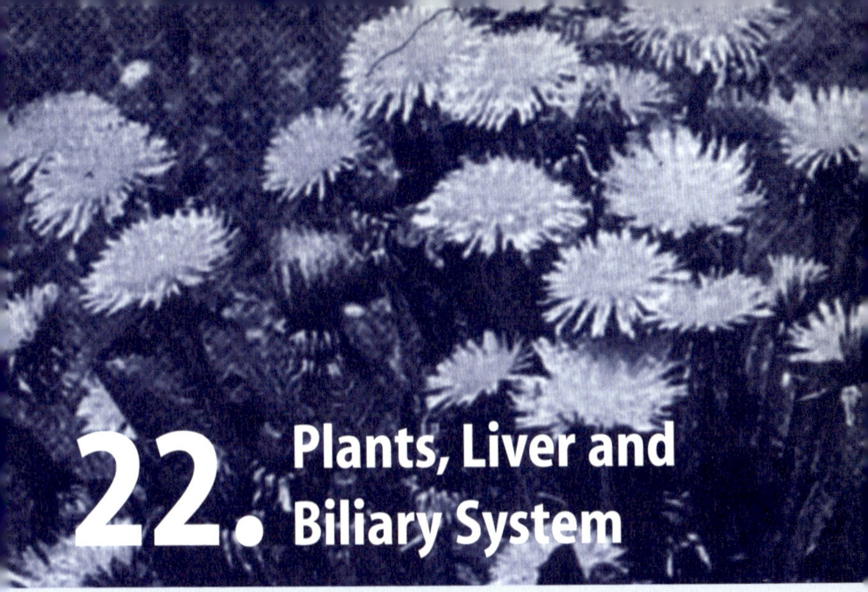

22. Plants, Liver and Biliary System

Introduction

The liver is a gland located in the upper right quadrant of the abdomen immediately beneath the diaphragm. As an exocrine gland it secretes bile. Its other major functions are the synthesis of plasma proteins, heparin, fibrinogen, and prothrombin; destruction of red cells; detoxification; metabolism of proteins, carbohydrates, and fats; and the storage of glycogen and other important substances. The main diseases of the liver include hepatitis and liver cirrhosis.

Diseases of the Liver

Clinical picture

- **Hepatitis** is an inflammation of the liver, involving alteration of hepatocytes, either degenerative or necrotic. Most common is viral hepatitis, which is characterized by inflammation of the liver caused by hepatitis virus A, hepatitis virus B, or by hepatitis virus C. Hepatitis can also be caused by alcohol (alcoholic hepatitis) or drugs (drug-induced hepatitis).
- **Cirrhosis** is a chronic disease of the liver characterized by nodular regeneration of hepatoxytes and diffuse fibrosis. It is caused by parenchymal necrosis followed by nodular proliferation of the surviving hepatocytes. The regenerating nodules and accompanying fibrosis interfere with blood flow through the liver and result in portal hypertension, hepatic insufficiency, jaundice, and ascites.

Hepato-protective Drugs

Hepato-protective drugs are listed in Table 22.1. They are remedies which help to reduce the damage caused to the liver from hepatic stressors and diseases. With the exception of milk thistle (*Silybum marianum*) there is a lack of randomized, placebo-controlled clinical studies.

Table 22.1
Hepato-protective herbal medicines

Common name	Latin name	Part(s) of plant used	Key constituents	Daily dose
Black catnip	*Phyllanthus amarus*	Aerial parts	Tannins, flavonoids, lignans	a
Liquorice	*Glycyrrhiza glabra*	Roots	Triterpene saponins, flavonoids	5–15 g
Milk thistle*	*Silybum marianum*	Seeds	Flavonolignans (silymarin), flavonoids, fatty oil	2–4 g
Picrorhiza	*Picrorhiza kurroa*	Rhizome	Iridoids	0.4–1.5 g
Schizandra	*Schizandra chinensis*	Fruit	Volatile oil, ascorbic acid, lignans	1.5–6 g
Soy	*Glycine max*	Soy lecithin from soy beans	Phospholipids, fatty oil, phytosterols	b
Turmeric	*Curcuma domestica*	Rhizome	Volatile oil, curcuminoids	1.5–3 g

* supported by German Commission E. for dyspeptic and liver complaints
a. no reliable information is available
b. the average dose of phospholipids is 3.5 g

Milk thistle

Botany/Key constituents ▶ Milk thistle is the dried ripe fruit of *Silybum marianum* (L.) Gaertner (Fam. *Asteraceae*), a biennial herb with purple tubulate florets and leaves with white areas. The plant is native to Europe and is cultivated in North Africa and South America (Plate 22.1). *Marianum* refers to the legend that the leaves have a white mottling because a drop of the Virgin Mary's milk landed on them. Milk thistle contains silymarin, which is composed of the flavanolignans silybinin, silydianin, and silychristin, with silybin being the most biologically active and the most abundant (60–70% silymarin). Silymarin is found in highest concentrations in the fruit, but it is also found in the leaves and seeds. Other constituents include taxifolin and other flavonoids.

Mode of action ▶ Milk thistle's hepato-protective effects are accomplished via several mechanisms of action (Figure 22.1). These include increased protein synthesis in hepatocytes and stimulation of liver regeneration, antioxidant effects and anti-inflammatory effects. Regarding the effect on protein synthesis, silymarin stimulates RNA polymerase I activity by activating a promoter site on DNA that the polymerase uses as a template for the synthesis of ribosomal RNA. An increase in the amount of ribosomal RNA results in stimulation of the regenerative capacity of the liver. Silymarin functions as an antioxidant because it is a free-radical scavenger; it increases hepatic contents of glutathione, which detoxifies a variety of substances in the liver, stomach and intestine, and it also increases the enzyme superoxide dismutase (being 10 times more potent as an antioxidant than vitamin E). Finally, silymarin possesses a variety of anti-inflam-

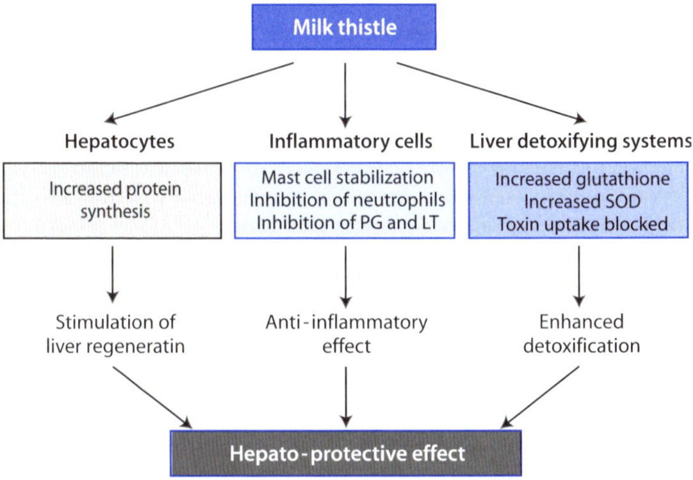

Figure 22.1 ▲ **Hepato-protective effect of milk thistle**
(see text for details) SOD = superoxide dismutase; PG = prostaglandins, LT = leukotrienes

matory effects, including mast cell stabilization, inhibition of neutrophil migration, inhibition of leukotriene and prostaglandin synthesis.

Clinical studies ▸ Milk thistle has been investigated for a number of liver diseases including chronic alcoholic liver disease, viral hepatitis, alcoholic and nonalcoholic cirrhosis and non-specified chronic liver diseases (Box 22.1). In general, the clinical efficacy of milk thistle is not clearly established. Possible benefit has been shown most frequently, but not consistently, for improvement in aminotransferase values, an indicator of abnormal liver function. Survival and other clinical outcome measures have been studied least often, with both positive and negative findings. Available evidence is not sufficient to suggest whether milk thistle may be more effective for some liver diseases than for others or if effectiveness might be related to the duration of therapy or chronicity and severity of liver disease. Nevertheless, silybinin seems to be effective in mushroom poisoning (*Amanita phalloides*) (see note Box 22.1).

Adverse effects/Contraindications ▸ Available evidence suggests that milk thistle is associated with few, and generally minor, adverse effects. In randomized trials reporting adverse effects, the incidence was approximately equal in milk thistle and placebo groups. Adverse effects associated with oral ingestion of milk thistle could include gastrointestinal problems (e.g. nausea, diarrhea, dyspepsia, flatulence, abdominal bloating, abdominal fullness or pain, anorexia, and changes in

Box 22.1

Randomized placebo-controlled, double-blind clinical studies of milk thistle for liver disease[1]

Chronic alcoholic liver disease

Six studies reported the effect of milk thistle on chronic alcoholic liver disease. Four of these reported significant improvement in at least one measurement of liver function (i.e. aminotransferases, albumin, and/or malondialdehyde) or histological findings with milk thistle compared with placebo. However, there were no differences between groups for other outcome measures.

Viral hepatitis

Three studies evaluated milk thistle for viral hepatitis. The one acute viral hepatitis study reported late outcome measures at 28 days and showed significant improvement in aspartate aminotransferase and bilirubin. The two studies of chronic viral hepatitis differed markedly in duration of therapy (7 days and 1 year). The shorter study showed improvement in aminotransferases for milk thistle compared with placebo but not other laboratory measures. In the longer study, milk thistle was associated with a non-significant trend towards histological improvement, the only outcome measure reported.

Alcoholic and nonalcoholic cirrhosis

Two trials included patients with alcoholic and nonalcoholic cirrhosis. Milk thistle showed a trend towards improved survival in one trial and significantly improved survival for subgroups with alcoholic cirrhosis or Child's group A severity. The second study reported no significant improvement in laboratory measures and survival for other clinical subgroups.

Alcoholic cirrhosis

Two trials specifically studied patients with alcoholic cirrhosis. Duration of therapy was unclear in the first study, which reported no improvement in laboratory measures of liver function, hepatomegaly, jaundice, ascites, or survival. However, there were non-significant trends favoring milk thistle in incidences of encephalopathy and gastrointestinal bleeding and in survival for subjects with concomitant hepatitis C. The second study, after treatment for 30 days, reported significant improvements in aminotransferases but not bilirubin for milk thistle compared with placebo.

Hepatotoxic drugs

Three trials evaluated milk thistle in the setting of hepatotoxic drugs: one for therapeutic use and two for prophylaxis with milk thistle. Results were mixed among the three trials.

Chronic liver disease

Available data were insufficient to sort six studies into specific etiological categories; these were grouped as chronic liver disease of mixed etiologies. In three of the six studies that reported multiple outcome measures, at least one outcome measure improved significantly with milk thistle compared with placebo, but there were no differences between milk thistle and placebo for one or more of the other outcome measures in each study. Two studies indicated a possible survival benefit.

[1] A remarkable use of silybinin is the treatment of *Amanita* mushroom poisoning. Clearly, for such condition, placebo-controlled, double-blind clinical studies are prohibited. Case reports have demonstrated a dramatic lower death rate after infusion of silybinin.

bowel habits), headache, skin reactions (pruritus, rash, urticaria, and eczema), neuropsychological events (e.g. asthenia, malaise, and insomnia), arthralgia, rhinoconjunctivitis, impotence and anaphylaxis. The incidence of such events is extremely low. At higher doses (> 1500 mg/day) silymarin may produce a laxative effect due to increased bile flow and secretion. Milk thistle increases liver function and thus may influence drug metabolism.

Preparations/Dosage

The oral daily dose is 12–15 g dried crude drug, corresponding to 200–400 mg silymarin. Silymarin is poorly soluble in water, so it is typically administered as an encapsulated extract and not as a "tea" . Milk thistle extracts are usually standardized to contain 70–80% silymarin (Legalon®). For *Amanita* posoning silymarin is given by infusion. For such use the dose is 20 mg silybinin per kg body-weight over a 24-h period, divided into 4 infusions, each administered over a 2-h period.

Other Hepato-protective Drugs

Picrorhiza. The name is given from the rhizome of *Picrorhiza kurroa* (Fam. *Scrophulariaceae*), a small perennial herb that grows in North-East India on the slopes of the Himalayas. The most important constituents of picrorhiza are the iridoid glycoside picrosides I, II, and kutkoside, known collectively as kutkin. The mechanism by which picrorhiza affords protection to the liver is not completely understood, but several possibilities have come to light. Like milk thistle, picrorhiza possesses antioxidant activity, stimulates liver regeneration and possesses anti-inflammatory activity. Picrorhiza is a more potent choleretic and anticholestatic agent than silymarin. Picrorhiza is a traditional Ayurvedic medicine widespread in India, however, no reliable data for human liver disease exist. Picrorhiza is poorly soluble in water and so it is not usually taken as a tea. It is soluble in ethanol and so can be taken in tincture form (very bitter), but is usually administered as an encapsulated standardized extract (4% kutkin, Picrovir). The usual adult dosage is 400–1500 mg/day. No major adverse effects have been reported in Ayurvedic medicine.

Black catnip. The black catnip herb is the aerial part of *Phyllanthus amarus*, an Indan herb which also grows in Africa, America and other Asiatic regions. Key constituents include tannins, flavonoids, lignans including the extremely bitter compound phyllanthin (0.8%) and hypophyllanthin. Phyllanthin and hypophyllanthin possess antiviral properties. The drug possesses antiviral properties. An acqueous extract of *Phyllanthus amarus* inhibited woodchuch hepatitis virus DNA polymerase and surface antigen expression. A recent systematic review identified 22 randomized clinical trials involving 1947 patients with chronic hepatitis B virus infection. The results of this review showed that *Phyllanthus* species (*P. amarus*, *P. urinaria*, *P. niruri*) had a positive effect on clearance of serum HbsAg compared with placebo or no intervention. There was no significant difference on clearance of serum hepatitis B surface antigen (HbsAg), hepatitis Be antigen (HbeAg) and hepatitis B virus (HBV) DNA between *Phyllanthus* species and the reference drug (interferon). *Phyllanthus* species were better than non-specific treatment or other herbal medicines for the clearance of serum HbsAg, HbeAg, HBV DNA, and liver enzyme normalization. However, the evidence is not strong due to the general low methodological quality of the trials and the variation of the herbal medicine. No health hazards are known in conjunction with the proper administration of designated therapeutic dosages. The drug can be given as decoction (10 plants to 1 liter water); however, no exact doses are known.

Schizandra (Wu-Wei-Zi). *Schizandra chinensis* (Turcz) Baillon (Fam. *Schizandraceae*) is a liana plant indigenous to China and Korea. Key constituents include a volatile oil, vitamin C and lignans (schizandrine A to C, schizandrol A and B). Some studies indicate that the fruits have hepato-protective effects. The lignan components would act by inhibiting lipid peroxidation. Both the ethanolic extract and schizandrines/schizandrols have undergone clinical studies and are used to treat hepatitis. A daily dose of 1.5–6 g crude drug is recommended. The drug is well tolerated. No specific side effects are known.

► *See Chapter 19 for the adaptogenic action of schizandra*

Liquorice is the dried roots and rhizome of *Glycyrrhiza glabra* L. (Fam. *Fabaceae*). A group of saponins related to glycyrrhizin and lectins from liquorice has been used for over 20 years to treat chronic viral hepatitis in Japan. The standardized aqueous extract (Stronger Neo-Minophagen C), administered parenterally for 2 weeks at a daily dose of 80 mg can normalize aspartate transaminase and alanine transaminase in over 60% of patients with chronic hepatitis. In a retrospective analysis of 84 patients with chronic hepatitis C virus infection who were treated with intravenous glycyrrhizin 2 to 7 times weekly for a median of 10.1 years, comparison with a matched group of 109 patients who remained untreated over 9.2 years revealed a 2.5-fold reduction of the relative risk of hepatocellular carcinoma. According to German Commission E, the maximum recommended dose of glycyrrhizin is 100 mg/day. Because of its aldosterone-like activities, use of the drugs requires caution and monitoring for hypertension, hyperkalemia, and worsening ascites.

► *See Chapter 21 for the antiulcer properties of liquorice*

Biliary Tract

Clinical Picture

- Bile is secreted by the liver and is stored in the gallbladder. It reaches the duodenum through the cholecystic duct. Bile consists of approximately 65–90% bile salts, 5–25% cholesterol and 2–25% phospholipids, bilirubin, fatty acids, electrolytes and water. The bile, in virtue of its surfactant activity emulsifies fatty foods, rendering them more sensitive to pancreatic enzyme lipase, thus facilitating the digestion and absorption. When bile produced from the liver is scarce or bile has difficulty in reaching the intestinal lumen (presence of gallbladder stones, inflammation of cholecystitis, atonia of biliary ducts), this may cause pain in the upper portion of the stomach and dyspeptic complaints.

Table 22.2
Therapeutic use of cholagogues[1]

Dyspepsia	Post-prandial epigastric weight, slowness digestion, eructations, swelling
Small hepatic insufficiencies	Poor digestion, bad taste in the mouth, nausea, somnolence, asthenia
Biliary dyskinesia	Altered motility of choleystitis and bile-ducts
Headache	Of digestive nature
Intestinal ailments	Constipation, poor intestinal motility, irritable colon
Gallbladder complaints	Moderate cholecystitis*

1 Cholagogues are not recommended in cases of diarrhea, obstruction of bile ducts, inflammation or degeneration of hepatic disease

* Inflammation of the gallbladder. It may be acute or chronic and is most commonly associated with cholelithiasis (biliary stones)

Cholagogue/Choleretic Drugs

Stimulating the bile flow can have some therapeutic application (Table 22.2). There is a traditional differentiation between cholagogues and choleretics. **Cholagogues** are agents that stimulate the flow of bile that has already been formed, particularly by contracting the gallbladder. **Choleretics** are agents that promotes bile secretion by hepatocytes. Most of the choleretics have cholagogue properties. Choleretic/cholagogue herbal drugs are listed in Table 22.3. There is very little interest in choleretics and cholagogues in modern medicine. Nevertheless, randomized clinical trials have shown a promising evidence of efficacy in treating dyspepsia for some herbal choleretic/cholagogues including celandine (*Chelidonium majus*) and turmeric (*Curcuma longa*).

Artichoke consists of the fresh or dried leaves of *Cynara scolymus* L. (Fam. *Asteraceae*), one of the world's oldest cultivated vegetables, grown by the Greeks and the Romans in the hayday of their power. The drug contains caffeic acid derivatives, flavonoids and sesquiterpene lactones. Clinical studies have demonstrated that artichoke leaf extract causes an increase of bile secretion into the duodenum of healthy volunteers. This action is most likely due to increased production of bile acid. In a surveillance study carried out in 553 patients with dyspeptic syndrome, treatment with artichoke extract significantly reduced the considered symptoms (vomiting, nausea, abdominal pain, constipation, flatulence, meteorism, fat intolerance). German Commission E cites dyspeptic complaints as indication for artichoke leaf preparations (tincture, fluid extracts and other forms) and recommends a daily dose of 6 g crude drug. It is well tolerated and has few side effects (flatulence, feeling of weakness and hunger). Artichoke also possesses hepato-protective properties. According to the German Commission E, artichoke is contraindicated in patients with cholelithiasis and bile duct occlusion. Colic may occur when the patient suffers from gallstones. Patients allergic to *Asteraceae* are potentially at risk of an allergic reaction to artichoke.

▶ *See Chapter 15 for the antilipidemic properties of artichoke*

Boldo consists of the dried leaves of *Peumus boldus* Mol. (Fam. *Monimiaceae*), a small tree (an evergreen shrup) native to Chile. The drug contains about 2% volatile oil composed of monoterpenoids flavonoids and alkaloids (0.2–0.5%) including boldine. Boldine is the component responsible of the choleretic activity of boldo: it increases the biliary secretion in anesthetized rats. Boldo extract also inhibits lipid peroxidation in rat hepatocyte culture and protects hepatocytes against damage by different xenobiotics. Boldo extract is an ingredient of proprietary drugs used in the treatment of dyspepsia, combretum, abdominal cramps, constipation and hepatic ailments. Boldo is generally combined with cholagogues and laxatives. A recent systematic review identified one randomized placebo-controlled clinical trial (n = 359 subjects with mild to moderate func-

Table 22.3
Choleretic/Cholagogue herbal medicines

Common name	Latin name	Part(s) of plant used	Key constituents	Daily dose
Artichoke**	*Cynara scolymus*	Leaves	Caffeic acid derivatives, flavonoids, sesquiterpene lactones	6 g
Boldo *	*Peumus boldus*	Leaves	Boldine, flavonoids, volatile oil	2–3 g
Celandine**	*Chelidonium majus*	Aerial parts	Coptisine, berberine, chelidonine, protopin	2–4 g
Curcuma**	*Curcuma xanthorrhizia*	Rhizome	Volatile oil, curcuminoids	2 g
Dandelion*/**	*Taraxacum officinale*	Roots, leaves	Sesquiterpene lactones, triterpenes and sterols, flavonoids	3–5 g
Devil's claw*	*Harpagophytum procumbens*	Secondary roots	Iridoids, triterpenes, phenols	4.5 g
Fumitory**	*Fumaria officinalis*	Aerial parts	Flavonoids, isoquinoline alkaloids, fumaric acid	6 g
Horehound*	*Marrubium vulgare*	Aerial parts	Marrubin, caffeic acid derivatives, flavonoids	4.5 g
Immortelle*	*Helichrysum arenarium*	Flowers	Flavonoids, phthalides, pyrones, caffeic acid derivatives	3 g
Japanese Mint**	*Mentha arvensis* var. *piperascens*	Oil from aerial parts	menthol, menthone, limonene, α- and β-pinene	3–6 drops oil
Peppermint */**	*Mentha piperita*	Leaves, oil from leaves	Volatile oil (menthol, menthone, limonene, α- and β-pinene) flavonoids, caffeic acid	3–6 g (0.6 ml oil)
Milk thistle*/**	*Silybum marianum*	Fruits	Flavonolignans (silymarin), flavonoids, fatty oil	12–15 g
Turmeric*	*Curcuma domestica*	Rhizome	Volatile oil, curcuminoids	1.5–3 g
Wormwood*/**	*Artemisia absinthium*	Aerial parts	Volatile oil, sesquiterpene bitter principles (absinthine)	3–5 g
Yarrow*/**	*Achillea millefolium*	Aerial parts	Volatile oil, sesquiterpene lactones, polyynes, flavonoids	3–4.5 g

* supported by German Commission E for dyspeptic complaints
** supported by German Commission E for liver and gallbladder complaints

tional disorders of the gastrointestinal tract) in which a combination of four herbal medicines (boldo, cascara, gentian and rhubarb) produced significant improvements in the loss of appetite, dyspepsia and constipation, whereas boldo alone improved symptoms of constipation only. Boldo is taken as a tea prepared with 2–3 g drug in 150 ml water. The drug is contraindicated in cases of obstruction of the biliary tract and lithiasis. The administration of boldo is contraindicated in patients who have gallstones. Neither boldo oil nor boldo distillates must be used because ascaridole, which is present in these preparations to the extent of about 40%, is believed to be toxic.

Turmeric is the dried rhizome of *Curcuma longa* L. = *Curcuma domestica* Val.) (Fam. *Zingiberaceae*), a perennial herb cultivated in India, Pakistan, China and Malaya. The primary and secondary rhizomes are dug up, steamed (or boiled) and dried. Turmeric has an aromatic odor and a warm bitterish taste; it is the main ingredient in curry powder. Turmeric contains about 5% curcuminoids (curcumin is the most significant); 4.2–14% volatile oil consisting of sesquiterpenes (zingiberine), ketones and monoterpenes; sugars (fructose 12%, glucose 2%, etc.). Turmeric is an old remedy used for a variety of liver conditions. Several experimental studies show that the drug increases bile secretion and flow. Such effect is attributed to its volatile oil, while the cholekinetic effect is due to curcumin. Curcumin is a potent anti-inflammatory agent; its mechanism of action includes: (i) an indirect action via the adrenal cortex, (ii) an inhibition of cortisone metabolism in the liver and consequently an increase of circulating cortisone and (iii) an inhibition of production of interleukins and tumor necrosis factor (TNF). Curcumin is active at relatively low concentration, but it is not well absorbed when given orally. The poor absorption of curcumin and other curcuminoids emphasizes the main role of the volatile oil constituents in the activity of turmeric. The drug is used as a digestive aid. A recent systematic review identified one randomized placebo-controlled clinical trial, in which 116 patients (diagnosed with acid dyspepsia, flatulent dyspepsia or atonic dyspepsia) received capsules of turmeric (2 g/day) or placebo for 7 days. Significantly more patients reported an overall favorable resolution or improvement of symptoms following treatment with turmeric than placebo. Because both volatile oil and curcuminoids are relatively water-insoluble turmeric teas are seldom used. The drug is employed in the form of tinctures, hydroalcoholic fluid extract, or encapsulated powders. The dose is 1.5–3.0 g turmeric daily. Turmeric appears to have no adverse effects. Prolonged use may occasionally result in gastric disturbance. Individuals with gallstones or blockage of the bile duct should avoid consuming turmeric (or curry powder which contains 28% turmeric).

Dandelion is the dried root (and leaves) of *Taraxacum officinale* G.H. Weber (Fam. *Asteraceae*), a perennial herb native to Europe (Plate 22.2). Dandelion contains triterpenoids (e.g. taraxacin and taraxerol), chlorogenic and caffeic acids, inulin, vitamins, minerals, phytosterols, flavonoid glycosides. The roots are best collected between June and August when they are most bitter. Dandelion root has been used in the management of liver and digestive disorders and to stimulate appetite and dandelion leaves as a diuretic in cases of edema. Dandelion is both choleretic and a cholagogue. Experimental studies tend to support these properties. A product including dandelion among other ingredients has been used to treat hepatitis. The drug is employed in the form of infusion or decoction (3–5 g dried root in 150 ml water) three times daily and of tincture (3–4 mg of crude drug) three times daily. Dandelion should be used with caution in cases of occlusion of the bile ducts, gallbladder, empyema and paralytic ileus. The drug can lead to gastric complaints and possess a weak potential for sensitization reactions.

Celandine (Greater celandine) consists of the aerial parts of *Chelidonium majus* L. (Fam. *Papaveraceae*), a 30–120 cm high plant found throughout Europe and the temperate and subarctic regions of Asia. The roots and the fresh rhizome are traditionally used to alleviate toothache. Key constituents of the aerial parts include isoquinoline alkaloids [coptisine (main alkaloid), berberine, chelidonine, sanguinarine, chelerythrine] and caffeic acid derivatives (coffeoyl-malic acid). Animal experiments suggest a direct anti-spasmolytic action on smooth muscle and a stimulation of bile flow that can contribute to celandine efficacy in the treatment of dyspepsia. A recent systematic review identified one randomized placebo-controlled, double-blind clinical trial in which a standardized celandine extract was used. The participants were 60 patients with functional epigastric complaints and cramp-like pains in the region of the biliary and gastrointestinal tract. After 6 weeks of treatment, patients treated with the celandine extract reported fewer gastrointestinal symptoms compared with the placebo group. The symptoms that showed most improvement were stomach pains, bilious complaints, flatulence, nausea and sensation of fullness. Celandine is approved by the German Commission E for the treatment of liver and gallbladder complaints. Nevertheless, case reports have highlighted the possibility of acute hepatitis following treatment with celandine. The daily dose of celandine is 2–4 g crude drug in liquid or solid extracts, equivalent to 12–30 total alkaloids calculated as chelidonine.

Further Reading

Bean P (2002) The use of alternative medicine in the treatment of hepatitis C. Am Clin Lab 21:19–21

Brent J (1999) Three new herbal hepatotoxic syndromes. J Toxicol 37:715–719

Flora K, Hahn M, Rosen H, Benner K (1998) Milk thistle (silybum marianum) for the therapy of liver disease. Am J Gastroenterol 93:139–143

Langmead L, Rampton DS (2001) Review article: herbal treatment in gastrointestinal and liver disease-benefits and dangers. Aliment Pharmacol Ther 15:1239–1252

Liu J, Lin H, McInthosh H (2001) Genus Phyllanthus for chronic hepatitis B virus infection: a systematic review. J Viral Hepat 8:358–366

Liu J, McInthosh H, Lin H (2001) Chinese medicinal herbs for chronic hepatitis B: a systematic review. Liver 21:280–286

Luper Scott (1998) A review of plants used in the treatment of liver disease: part I. Altern Med Rev 3:410–421

Luper Scott (1999) A review of plants used in the treatment of liver disease: part II. Altern Med Rev 4:178–188

Rao AV, Gurfinkel DM (2000) The bioactivity of saponins: triterpenoid and steroidal glycosides. Drug Metabol Drug Interact 17:211–235

Roeder E (2000) Medicinal plants in China containing pyrrolizidine alkaloids. Pharmazie 55:711–726

Saller R, Meier R, Brignoli R (2001) The use of silymarin in the treatment of liver diseases. Drugs 61:2035–2063

Schuppan D, Jia Ji-D, Brinkhaus B, Hahn EG (1999) Herbal products for liver diseases: a therapeutic challenge for the new millennium. Hepatology 30:1099–1104

Shibata S (2000) A drug over the millenia: pharmacognosy, chemistry and pharmacology of licorice. Yakugaku Zasshi 120:849–862

Stickel F, Egerer G, Seitz HK (2000) Hepatotoxicity of botanicals. Public Helath Nutr 3:111–113

Thomson Coon J, Ernst E (2002) Systematic review: herbal medicinal products for non-ulcer dyspepsia. Aliment Pharmacol Ther 16: 1689–1699

Thyagarajan S, Jayaram S, Gopalakrishnan V, Hari R, Jeyakumar P, Sripathi M (2002) Herbal medicines for liver diseases in India. J Gastroenterol Hepatol 17:S370–S376

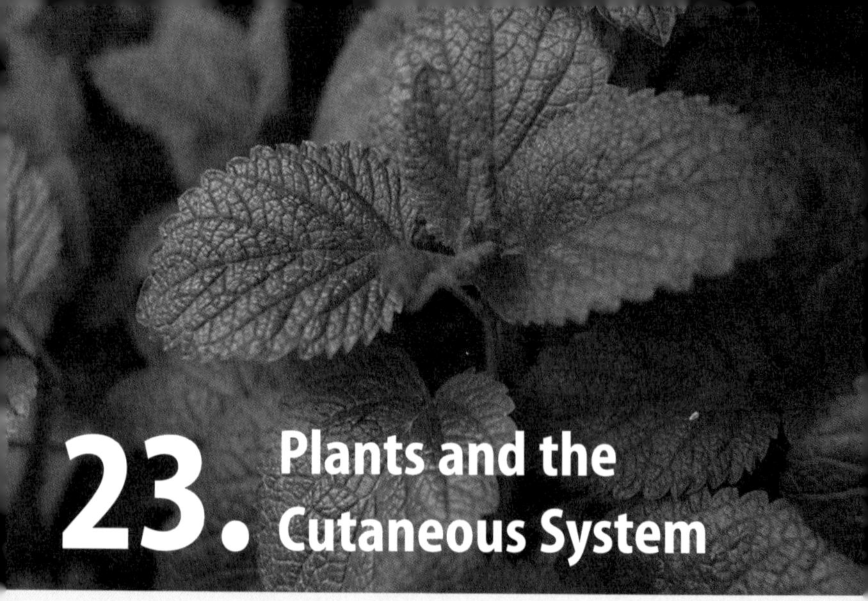

23. Plants and the Cutaneous System

Introduction

The tegumental apparatus is composed of skin and cutaneous attachments (nails, hair and various glands) which are distributed over it with different organizations and functions. The skin in turn is composed of two layers, one superficial (epidermis) and the other deep (dermis). The epidermis consists of 5 layers, from the outside to the inside: horny, shiny, thorny, granulous and germinative. The germinative layer is the only one to reproduce itself and form new cells which are gradually transformed into horny cells. The horny layer in turn flakes off, a necessary process to maintain constant thickness of the epidermis. In some cases the horny layer of the skin can thicken due to irritative phenomena, thus causing the formation of 'callosity'.

The dermis consists of connective tissue in which there is a dense network of vessels, nerves, glands (sudoriferous and sebaceous) and piliferous follicles. Inflammations, infections, rashes, lesions, ulcers, excrescences, burns and other traumas can temporarily alter the cutaneous strata causing more or less serious trouble according to their gravity and length. Cutaneous disturbances can also arise due to organic causes and excessive perspiration of the cutaneous layer.

Cutaneous lesions are visible and easily accessible. Topical treatment is therefore preferred as it does not usually cause systemic effects and is sufficient to improve or heal the 'disturbance'. Medicines to treat skin disorders are applied in the form of a paste, ointment, emulsion, lotion and glycerolate, etc. (Table 23.1). The vehicle used for the preparation of these pharmaceutical forms must be devoid of pharmacological action. Figure 23.1 shows some herbal remedies used in specific conditions.

To obtain a good local action the medicine should be retained within the epidermis and dermis. This avoids systemic effects. However, significant absorption of active drugs can occur when the surface of application is large, when the skin is not intact and when the product is applied in such a way that facilitates absorption (friction, massage).

Table 23.1

Pharmaceutical preparations for topical use

Pharmaceutical form	Preparation	Indication (condition)
Paste	Liquids/fats mixed with inert powders in percentages of 20–30%	Edema
Ointment	Fats are mixed with inert powders in percentages not over 10%	Dry and flaky skin
Emulsion	Two non-miscible liquid phases are mixed : water and oil	Exudative forms
Lotion	Inert powders are suspended (10–30%) in water or water and alcohol and adding glycerine or starch	Exudative forms
Powder	As described in paragraph 9.2.3	Rash

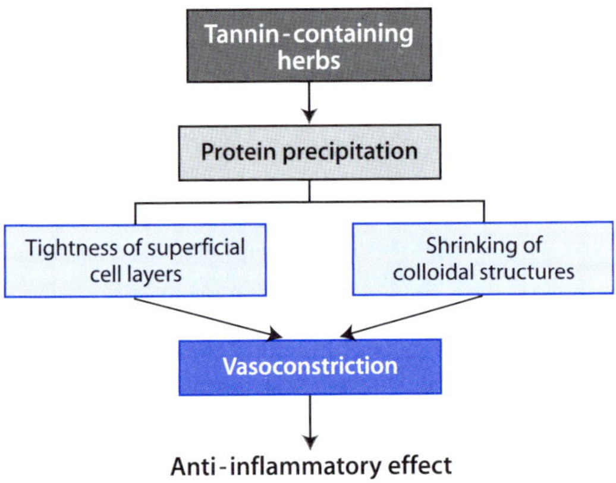

Figure 23.1 ▲ **Anti-inflammatory activity of tannin-containing herbs**
Applied topically to broken skin or mucous membranes, tannins induce a protein precipitation that tightens up superficial cell layers and shrinks colloidal structure, causing capillary vasoconstriction. The decrease in vascular permeability leads to a local anti-inflammatory action. The astringent action on the tissues deprives bacteria of a favorable growth medium, producing an indirect antibacterial

Inflammatory Skin Diseases

Clinical Picture

- **Eczema** and **dermatitis** are interchangeable terms and describe an inflammatory skin reaction characterized clinically by a variety of features, including pruritus, erythema, clustered papules or vesicles, hyperkeratosis, exudation of serum, and crusting. Eczema is characterized histologically by epidermal spongiosis, permeated by an inflammatory infiltrate. Treatment includes the use of emollients (to reduce transepidermal water loss, which is increased as a result of spongiosis) and anti-inflammatory and vasoconstricting drugs (to reduce inflammation). Herbal medicines used to treat dermatitis are listed in Table 23.2.
- **Acne** is a term used to describe any chronic inflammatory disease of the pilosebaceous follicles, characterized by keratinous obstruction of the upper part of the pilosebaceous gland. Acne is characterized by comedones (keratin plugs in the sebaceous duct opening), inflammatory papules, pustules, nodules, cysts, and scars. Acne occurring in adolescence is the result of androgenic stimulation of the pilosebaceous follicles in genetically predisposed subjects and the active pilosebaceous follicles are heavily colonized by *Propionilbacterium acnes*. Treatment of acne includes keratolytics (to eliminate the keratin plug which blocks the sebaceous follicle), antibiotics, antiseptics/anti-inflammatories. Herbal medicines used to treat acne are listed in Table 23.3.

Table 23.2
Herbal medicines used to treat eczema/dermatitis

Common name	Latin name	Part(s) of plant used	Key constituents
Aloe gel	*Aloe spp.*	Leaves	Mucillages, aloins
Bittersweet nightshade*	*Solanum dulcamara*	Stems	Alkaloids, steroid saponins
German chamomile	*Matricaria recutita*	Flower heads	Volatile oil, flavonoids, mucillages, coumarins
Evening primose	*Oenothera biennis*	Oil from the seeds	Linoleic acid, palmitic acid, oleic acid, γ-linoleic acid
Marigold	*Calendula officinalis*	Flowers	Triterpene saponins, flavonoids, volatile oil, triterpene alcohols
Tea tree	*Melaleuca alternifolia*	Oil from the leaves	Terpin-1-en-4-ol
Witch hazel	*Hamamelis virginiana*	Leaves, bark	Tannins, volatile oil, flavonoids, procyanidins

* supported by German Commission E for the treatment of eczema, foruncles, acne and warts

Table 23.3
Herbal medicines used to treat acne

Common name	Latin name	Part(s) of plant used	Key constituents
Bittersweet nightshade*	*Solanum dulcamara*	Stems	Alkaloids, steroid saponins
Eucalyptus	*Eucalyptus globulus*	Oil from leaves	1-8 cineol, α-pinenes, limonene, geraniol, camphene
Heartsease	*Viola tricolor*	Aerial parts	Flavonoids, phenol carboxylic acid, mucilage, tannins
Tea tree	*Melaleuca alternifolia*	Oil from stems	Terpin-1-en-4-ol

* supported by German Commission E

Psoriasis is an inflammatory-hyperproliferative skin disease which is characterized by (i) lesion in the form of a well-demarcated plaque, usually dull red or dark salmon pink in color and covered with silvery scales, (ii) capillary dilatation in the papillary dermis, (iii) an inflammatory infiltrate. Any part and any proportion of the skin surface may be affected. Treatment include the use of keratolytics (to reduce the hyperkeratosis), anti-inflammatory/immunosuppressants to reduce inflammatory cell infiltration and antiproliferative agents.

Anti-inflammatory Drugs

Several herbal medicines have been used to treat inflammatory conditions of the skin. Some of those supported by the German Commission E are listed in Table 23.4. Anti-inflammatory preparations represent a logical choice for topical treatment of most skin diseases.

Aloe gel

Botany/Key constituents ▸ This is obtained from the parenchymal layer of the leaves of *Aloe barbadensis* (*vera* or *vulgaris*) (Fam. *Liliaceae*), a plant originating in North Africa and introduced into the Antilles (Plate 23.1). The parenchymal layer of the leaves contains above all mucilages (about 30%) which once extracted produce a gel. This is not to be confused with latex which is also obtained from the leaves of aloe (from the pericyclic tubers which are found exactly under the epidermis of the leaves), and which has catarthic properties due to the presence of anthrachinones. The gel is obtained after eliminating the outermost tissues of the leaf. Aloe gel also contains 25% polysaccharides, 22% aloins, resinous substances, vitamins, enzymes and fiber.

Table 23.4

Antinflammatory herbal medicines and their use in dermatology accordi Commission E

Common name	Latin name	Part(s) of plant used	Key constituents	Use
Agrimony	*Agrimonia eupatoria*	Flowering plant	Catechin tannins	Inflammation of the skin
Arnica	*Arnica montana*	Flowers	Sesquiterpene lactones	Inflammation of the skin, blunt injuries
English plantain	*Plantago lanceolata*	Aerial parts	Iridoide monoterpenes, tannins, mucilages, flavonoids	Inflammation of the skin
Fenugreek	*Trigonella foenum-graecum*	Seeds	Mucilages, flavonoids, saponins, trigonelline	Inflammation of the skin
Flax	*Linum usitatissimum*	Seeds	Fatty oil, mucilages, lignans	Inflammation of the skin
German chamomille	*Matricaria recutita*	Flower heads	Volatile oil, flavonoids, mucilages, coumarins	Inflammation of the skin, wounds and burns
Heartsease	*Viola tricolor*	Aerial parts	Flavonoids, mucilages, tannins	Inflammation of the skin
Jambolan	*Syzygium cumini*	Bark	Steroids, tannins, triterpenes, flavonoids	Inflammation of the skin
Oak	*Quercus robur*	Bark	Tannins	Inflammation of the skin
Oats	*Avena sativa*	Straw from aerial parts	Polysaccharides, silicic acid, steroid saponins, flavonoids	Inflammation of the skin, warts
St. John's wort	*Hypericum perforatum*	Aerial parts (fatty oil)	Anthracene derivatives, flavonoids, phloro-glucinol derivatives	Blunt injuries, wounds and burns, inflammation of skin
Walnut	*Juglans regia*	Leaves	Tannins , naphthalene derivatives, flavonoids	Inflammation of the skin
Witch hazel	*Hamamelis virginiana*	Leaves	Tannins, flavonoids, procyanidins	Inflammation of the skin, wounds and burns

Mode of action ▶ Substances in aloe gel are able to penetrate cutaneous tissue, perhaps inhibiting the production of kinins and prostanoids. Aloe gel also has antibacterial, antifungal and antiviral properties; it also dilates capillaries thus improving blood flow and it has local anaesthetic action. It is used externally to combat sunrashes, sores, ulcers and other cutaneous complaints. Moreover, it facilitates the healing of wounds by stimulating cell proliferation and/or by its protective/hydrating properties due to its high water content.

Clinical efficacy ▶ A recent systematic review reports positive (although preliminary) results for wound healing management of full-face dermabrasion patients

Box 23.1

Randomized clinical studies of aloe gel in dermatological conditions (topical use)[1]

Wound healing

Two studies reported the wound-healing properties of aloe gel. In the first study, the faces of full-faced 17 dermabrased patients with acne vulgaris were divided in half. One side was treated with a standard polyethylene oxide gel wound dressing, while the other side was treated with a polyethylene oxide saturated with aloe vera. After 48 hours with the aloe vera dressing, intense vasoconstrition and a reduction in edema was noted; less exudate and crusting was evident by the fourth day. By the fifth day, re-epithelialization was complete at 90% on the aloe side, compared with 40–50% on the control side. Overall, wound healing was approximately 72 hours faster at the aloe side. In another study 40 women with complications of wound healing after gynecological surgery used a standard wound management protocol with and without aloe vera. The mean healing time in the conventional care group (53 days) was significantly shorter than in the aloe gel group.

Psoriasis

One study was performed. 60 patients with mild to moderate chronic psoriasis received either an aloe vera or placebo cream. The cream was self-applied three times per day for four weeks. Patients were subsequently followed up for 12 months. The cure rate in the aloe group was 83% and only 7% in the placebo group.

Radiation-induced skin injury

Two studies by the same authors were performed. In the first study 194 women receiving radiation therapy were treated with aloe gel or placebo, self-administered to the radiation-exposed skin twice daily. After 10 weeks treatment there were no differences between the two groups. The second study, performed on 108 women, was similar to the first, except that the control group received no topical therapy at all. The trial was therefore not blind. Again, the results were negative.

Genital herpes

Two studies were performed of the effect of aloe vera in the treatment of first genital herpes episodes. In the first study 120 men were divided into three parallel groups. Each patient applied either aloe vera cream (aloe vera extract 0.5% in hydrophilic cream), aloe gel, or placebo three times daily for two weeks. Aloe vera cream showed shorter mean duration of healing than aloe gel and placebo (4.8 days versus 7.0 and 14.0 days, respectively). The numbers of cured patients were 70%, 45%, and 7.5% respectively. Of the 49 patients healed at the end of this trial period, six had a relapse after 21 months of follow-up. The second study included 60 men who were randomized into two groups. The trial compared aloe vera extract 0.5% in a hydrophilic cream versus placebo. The aloe vera cream group had both significantly shorter healing time (4.9 days versus 12 days) and a higher number of cured patients (66.7% versus 6.7%) compared with the placebo group. Of the 22 healed patients, three showed recurrence after 158 months.

[1] Data from Vogler and Ernst (1999)

(reduction in edema, less crusting, rapid re-epithelialization) for the treatment of mild and moderate psoriasis and for the treatment of genital herpes episodes. However, aloe gel was not able to prevent radiation-induced skin injury (Box 23.1).

Adverse events/Contraindications ▸ Adverse effects have very rarely been reported. Some patients experienced burning contact dermatitis and mild itching, after topical application. All adverse effects were reversible. However, individuals predisposed to allergic reactions should avoid topical application of aloe gel. One case of cathartic effect after local application of aloe gel has been described.

Preparations/Dosage

The gel is widely used in ointments and creams: a minimum of 70% concentration of aloe gel is necessary for wound healing and anti-inflammatory effects. The gel is also used in cosmetic products (sun lotions, shaving creams, lip balm, etc.). It is sold commercially in powder or concentrated liquid form.

▸ *See Chapter 15 for the use of aloe in diabetes mellitus*
▸ *See Chapter 21 for the use of aloe in mouth inflammation*

Chamomile

Botany/Key constituents ▸ Chamomile consists of the flower-heads of *Matricaria recutita* (German chamomile) (Fam. *Compositae*) (Plate 23.2). The plants originate from Southern Europe and is cultivated in many parts of the world. Argentina, Egypt, and Hungary are big producers of German chamomile. The drug contains flavonoids (e.g. apigenin) and a volatile oil, the main constituents of which is bisabolol and its oxides. The oil also contains proazulenes (e.g. matricin).

Mode of action ▸ *In vitro* studies have determined that at least part of the anti-inflammatory activity of chamomile extracts is due to constituents which block the formation of prostaglandins and leukotrienes and have antioxidant activity.

Bisabolol and apigenin appear to be responsible, in part, for this activity. Chamazulene also displays anti-inflammatory activity. Moreover, several polysaccharides of chamomile have demonstrated anti-inflammatory activity when applied topically. Chamomile also possesses antimicrobial activity, the effect being due to the synergistic effect of bisabolol, bisabolol oxides, chamazulene and dicycloethers.

Clinical efficacy ▶ Chamomile preparations are used to treat bacterial and non-bacterial inflammations of the skin, poorly healing wounds and inflammations of the oral cavity. Chamomile may also be used in the case of eye irritation. German Commission E suggests the use of chamomile for inflammations of the skin and mucous membranes and bacterial diseases involving the skin and oral cavity, irritation of the respiratory tract (administration by inhalation) and diseases of the anogenital region (administration by bathing or douching). Clinical studies have shown positive results in the treatment of eczema, skin ulceration and healing of wounds.

Adverse events/Contraindications ▶ Despite reports of skin reactions and dermatitis from topical use of chamomile, the likelihood of chamomile preparation causing a contact allergy is low. However, persons with known sensitivity to other members of the *Compositae* family (such as feverfew, marigold) should avoid topical application of chamomile. Chamomile preparations must not be used in cases of sharp pain in the eye, direct blow to the eye or when the irritation is accompained by pus.

Preparations/Dosage

In a supplement to its 1990 monograph, the German Commission E gives these dosage recommendations: use of 3–10% infusion for douches; 5 g/l as a bath additive; semisolid preparations should have a 3–10% content crude drug.

▶ *See Chapter 13 for the anxiolytic/seditive properties of chamomile*
▶ *See Chapter 21 for the gastric antacid properties of chamomile*

Evening primrose oil

Botany/Key constituents ▶ Evening primrose oil is the fixed oil obtained from the seeds of *Oenothera* species including *O. biennis* (Fam. *Onagraceae*), which grows to a height of about 1 m (Plate 23.3). The seeds, small (1–2 x 0.5–1 mm) and angular, contain up to 25% of an oil, rich in unsaturated fatty acids [linoleic acid (65–75%) and gamma-linolenic acid (8–10%), oleic acid (6–11%)].

Mode of action ▸ Gamma-linolenic acid (GLA) may suppress inflammation at least through two distint mechanisms: (i) competitive inhibition of the activity of cyclooxygenase and lipoxygenase enzyme, resulting in a decreased production of the pro-inflammatory substances prostaglandins and leukotrienes, (ii) production of prostaglandin E_1, which, although possessing an acute pro-inflammatory effect, can have inhibitory effects on pro-inflammatory cells.

Clinical efficacy ▸ The efficacy of evening primrose oil in the treatment of atopic eczema is well documented: a meta-analysis involving ten placebo-controlled studies, five parallel and five crossover (total of about 200 patients) showed that evening primrose oil was superior to placebo. A number of signs of inflammation, including dryness, scaliness and particularly itching were reduced by treatment with evening primrose oil.

Adverse events/Contraindications ▸ Evening primrose oil appears to be well tolerated with very few side effects reported. Mild gastro-intestinal effects, indigestion, nausea, softening of stools, and headache have occasionally occurred.

Preparations/Dosage

The doses are based on a standardized GLA content of 8%. Low to medium dosage should be used for conditions such as atopic eczema: 2–3 g/daily of evening primrose oil (corresponding approximately to 160–240 mg GLA). Higher doses should be used for other conditions such as arthritis. In Germany, capsules containing 500 mg evening primrose oil (40 mg GLA) have been approved for the treatment and symptomatic relief of atopic eczema.

▸ *See Chapter 17 for the use of evening primrose oil in rheumatoid arthritis*
▸ *See Chapter 20 for the use of evening primrose oil in menopausal symptoms*

Anti-inflammatories with "Astringent" Mechanism (Tannin-containing Drugs)

Astringents are substances which applied to skin and mucous membranes excercise a local anti-inflammatory action. Astringents must not be absorbed in order to retain their local action and not cause harm to the organism (systemic effects). They bring about coarctation and drying of the affected tissue; the mucous membranes become dry (due to precipitation of proteins), with a reduction in exudation and secretions. In practice they coagulate the superficial tissue layer creating a protective layer; they coagulate the exudate, if present, forming a further protective layer; they slow up cell exchange by reducing cellular permeability; they reduce capillary permeability and constrict the arteries, reducing hyperemia, edema and hemorrhages (Figure 23.1).

Astringents lower the sensitivity of sensory nerve fibers, attenuating pain. They also have a disinfectant action. All these actions attenuate local phagocytosis until it ceases altogether, while the dried tissue forms an extremely unfavorable sub-layer for the development of microbes. These effects are caused by the precipitation of proteinaceous substances with which the astringents come into contact, modifying the colloidal state of the live material. In high concentrations, however, astringents may coagulate live cells, causing necrosis limited to the zone of application. The astringents, therefore, behave as caustics if used in high doses.

Tannin-containing drugs include witch hazel (leaves or bark of *Hamamelis virginiana*), oak bark (bark of *Quercus* species), walnut leaves (leaves of *Juglans regia*), krameria (rhatany) (root of *Krameria trianda*) and tormentil (root of *Potentilla tormentilla*). These are used as a local therapy for dermatitis and phlogosis of the skin and accessible mucous membrane and for slight hemorrhages of the epithelium and tissues.

Witch hazel

Botany/Key constituents ▶ Witch hazel consists of the leaves (or bark) of *Hamamelis virginiana* (Fam. *Hamamelidaceae*), a shrub or small tree (up to 7 m high) occurring in eastern North America. Key constituents include a mixture of tannins (3–10%) including gallotannins, hamamelitannins and procyanidins. The drug also contains an essential oil (0.05%) and flavonoids (astragalin, myricitrin).

Mode of action ▶ Witch hazel is known to possess astringent (vasoconstrictive) and hemostatic properties, which have been attributed to the tannin constituents. The anti-inflammatory activity could be due, in part, to a vasoconstrictor activity. Moreover, hamamelitannins and procyanidins possess anti-inflammatory activity through inhibition of 5-lipoxygenase and PAF biosynthesis, respectively.

Clinical efficacy ▶ Witch hazel is supported by the German Commission E for the treatment of hemorrhoids, inflammation of the skin, venous disturbance, wounds and burns. The leaves, but not the bark, are recommended for the treatment of inflammation of the mouth and pharynx. The clinical efficacy of witch hazel has been demonstrated in several non-randomized clinical studies. Application of witch hazel leaf cream has been shown to be effective in forms of eczema or atopic neurodermatitis, with clear improvement in the symptoms investigated (redness, scaling, lichenification, pruritus, infiltration).

Adverse events/Contraindications ▶ Contact dermatitis caused by the topical use of witch hazel has been reported in rare cases. In a study of 1032 consecutively tested patients, four were found to react to an ointment containing a 25% extract of witch hazel. Two of these patients reacted positively to the wool fat in the ointment base.

Preparations/Dosage

Dried bark and leaves are available as a decoction, extract and distilled extract for topical use. The recommended dosage is 2 g leaf or bark by infusion three times daily; 2–4 ml three times daily of *Hamamelis* liquid extract (1:1 in 45% alcohol). The drug is also used in cosmetics as Hamamelis Water or Distilled Witch hazel extract and promoted (BPC 1973) for local application as an astringent.

► *See Chapter 14 for the use of witchhazel in the treatment of hemorrhoids*

Wound Healing and Post-traumatic Drugs

Table 23.5 and Table 23.6 list some medicinal herbs supported by the Commission E for treating wounds and burns or which are useful for post-traumatic and postoperative conditions. Among these is hydrocotyle (*Centella asiatica*). Clinical trials or a robust traditional use have given particular value to hydrocotyle for the treatment of wounds and burns, and arnica (*Arnica montana*) and bromelain (from the pineapple tree *Ananas comosus*) in post-traumatic conditions.

Table 23.5

Some herbal medicines supported by German Commission E for the treatment of wounds and burns

Common name	Latin name	Part(s) of plant used	Key constituents
Cajeput	*Maleleuca leucadendra*	Oil from the leaves and twigs	Eucalyptol, terpineol, terpineol valerate
Echinacea	*Echinacea purpurea*	Aerial parts	Polisaccharides, flavonoids, caffeic acid derivatives
German chamomile	*Matricaria recutita*	Flower heads	Volatile oil, flavonoids, mucilages, coumarins
Horsetail	*Equisetum arvense*	Aerial parts	Flavonoids, caffeic acid ester, silicic acid, pyridine alkaloids
Marigold	*Calendula officinalis*	Flowers	Saponins, flavonoids, volatile, triterpene alcohols
Peruvian balsam	*Myroxylon balsamum*	Balsam from trunk	Cinnamein (an ester mixture), resins, volatile oil
Pineapple	*Ananas comosus*	Fruits	Proteases (bromelain)
St. John's wort	*Hypericum perforatum*	Aerial parts (olive oil solution)	Anthracene derivatives, flavonoids, phloroglucinol derivatives
Witch hazel	*Hamamelis virginiana*	Leaves, bark	Tannins, flavonoids, procyanidins

Table 23.6

Some herbal medicines approved by German Commission E for the treatment of blunt injuries

Common name	Latin name	Part(s) of plant used	Key constituents
Arnica	*Arnica montana*	Flowers	Sesquiterpene lactones (henelanin), flavonoids, volatile oil
Comfrey	*Symphytum officinale*	Aerial parts	Allantoin, mucilages, tannins, triterpene saponins, pyrrolizidine alkaloids
Pineapple	*Ananas comosus*	Fruit	Proteases (bromelain)
St. John's wort	*Hypericum perforatum*	Aerial parts (fatty oil)	Anthracene derivatives, flavonoids, phloroglucinol derivatives
Sweet clover	*Melilotus officinalis*	Aerial parts	Coumarins, flavonoids, triterpene saponins

Gotu kola (Hydrocotyle)

Botany/Key constituents ▸ This is obtained from the leaves and caulis of *Centella asiatica*, a perennial creeping plant that flowers between August and September; its flowers are of a light violet color. The grey to brownish-green plant has a smell that is reminiscent of tobacco leaves. The plant is distributed in India, Madagascar and Indonesia. It contains triterpenic compounds (asiacoside, madecassoside), amino acids, flavonoids and a trace of volatile oil.

Mode of action ▸ Experimental studies have shown that topical application of gotu kola is associated with accelerated wound healing in abnormal conditions of the skin associated with a reduction in granuloma weight, and increase in the force needed to produce rupture. In addition, other studies have revealed an increase in the synthesis of collagen (a substance which permits the epithelium to interact with the connecting layer, favoring epithelization and therefore the correct repairing of the wounds), intracellular fibronectin content and an increase in mitotic activity of the germ layer (resulting in an increased re-epithelization). Triterpenic compunds (i.e. asiacosides, medacassoids) are believed to be responsible of these activities.

Clinical efficacy ▸ The clinical efficacy of gotu kola is very promising. The wound-healing properties of hydrocotyle have been documented in clinical trials, although a definitive conclusion cannot be drawn. In some studies, in addition to local treatment (ointment or powder), the patients received i.m. injections of asiacoside.

Adverse events/Contraindications ▸ Side effects in the form of a burning sensation at the time of the application were noted. Allergic reactions are also observed, but in rare cases.

Preparations/Dosage

The usual dose of gotu kola is 0.6 g dried leaf by infusion three times daily. Centellase® is an extract prepared from *Centella asiatica* (total triterpene fraction), comprising madecassic acid (30%), asiatic acid (30%), and asiaticosides (40%). Centellase® is marketed in the form of an ointment (1%) or powder (2%).

▶ *See Chapter 14 for the use of gotu kola in chronic venous insufficiency*

Arnica

Botany/Key constituents ▶ Arnica consists of the flower of *Arnica montana* L. (Fam. *Asteraceae*), a perennial 30–60 cm high herbaceous plant that is native to the mountainous regions of Europe. The plant is rare and protected in several European countries. Key constituents include sesquiterpenoid lactones (helenalin and dihydrohelenalin), flavonoids and a volatile oil.

Mode of action ▶ Arnica possesses anti-inflammatory and antimicrobial activity. The anti-inflammatory activity is due to an inhibitory action on neutrophil cells and to inhibition of lysosomal enzymatic activity in neutrophils. At high concentration, inhibition of cyclooxygenase may occur. A series of sesquiterpene lactone, including helenalin and dihydrohelenalin are believed to be responsible of the anti-inflammatory action. Helenalin could be responsible, at least in part, for the antimicrobical activity of arnica.

Clinical efficacy ▶ Despite the widespread use of arnica in post-traumatic conditions (treatment of injuries), there is a paucity of reports dealing with the clinical efficacy of arnica. In twelve male volunteers externally applied arnica was superior to placebo for muscle ache. German Commission E states that arnica flower preparations are indicated for external use in the treatment of post-traumatic and postoperative conditions such as hematomas, sprains, bruises, contusions, fracture-related, and rheumatic ailments of the muscle and joints. Arnica is also recommended by German Commission E for the treatment of inflammation of the mouth and pharynx and inflammation of the skin.

Adverse events/Contraindications ▶ Topical application of arnica has been known to cause allergic or irritant contact dermatitis. The sesquiterpene lactones are the proven sensitizing agents. There are also reports of cross-sensitivity to other *Asteraceae* plants (i.e. calendula, feverfew, chamomile). Prolonged treatment of damaged skin can cause edematous dermatitis. At high concentration, formation of vesicles or even necrosis may occur. It should only be applied to unbroken skin and as a tincture. Arnica and its preparations are poisonous if taken internally; they cause headaches, abdominal pains, palpitations and breathing difficulties.

Preparations/Dosage

Arnica has traditionally been used in the form of tincture (1:5, 45%, application of 2–4 ml). Arnica oil is obtained by macerating one part of arnica flowers in five parts of vegetable oil. To prepare a poultice 2–3 g arnica is covered with 150 ml hot water and strained after 10 minutes. Bandages, gauze or cotton are soaked in the infusion and then placed on the affected area of the body (bruises, echymoses, petechiease, sprains and sunburns). Arnica preparations must not be applied near the eyes and mouth or on open wounds.

Bromelain

Botany/Key constituents ▶ Bromelain is a preparation containing a number of sulfhydryl proteolytic enzymes. It is prepared from the juice of the pineapple, *Ananas comosus* (L.) Merr. (Fam. *Bromeliaceae*). This set of enzymes occurs in the stem of ripe and unripe fruit. Bromelain is a mixture of glycoproteins in which the protein moiety is not very different from that of papain. The main component of stem bromelain is a glycoprotein also named bromelain.

Mode of action ▶ Bromelain is an effective anti-inflammatory and fibrinolytic agent. Bromelain's fibrinolytic activity has been attributed to the enhanced conversion of plasminogen to plasmin, which limits the spread of the coagulation process by degrading fibrin. This minimizes venous stasis, facilitates drainage, increases permeability and restores the tissues' biological continuity (Figure 23.2). In addtion to the fibrinolytic/anti-inflammatory effect, topical bromelain separates eschar at the interface with living tissue. It is hypothesized that bromelain activates colagenase in living tissue which then attacks the denatured collagen in the eschar. This produces a demarcation between living and dead tissue (Figure 23.3). A non-proteolytic component of bromelain, referred as to escharase, is responsible for this effect. Moreover, bromelain stimulates cytokine production and this may assist in generating an acute-stage healing response.

Clinical efficacy ▶ The therapeutic benefits of bromelain in treating musculoskeletal injuries, burns, inflammation and surgical traumas are well documented. The German Commission E states that the therapeutic efficacy has been established for "acute postoperative and post-traumatic swelling, especially of the nose and paranasal sinuses".

Adverse events/Contraindications ▶ Bromelain is considered extremely safe. Side effects consist of gastric upset, diarrhea, and occasional allergic reactions. However, the allergenic potential of proteolytic enzymes should not be underestimated, for they cause, in particular, IgE-mediated respiratory allergies. Inhalation (but not ingestion) of bromelain could cause asthma in workers involved in bromelain production.

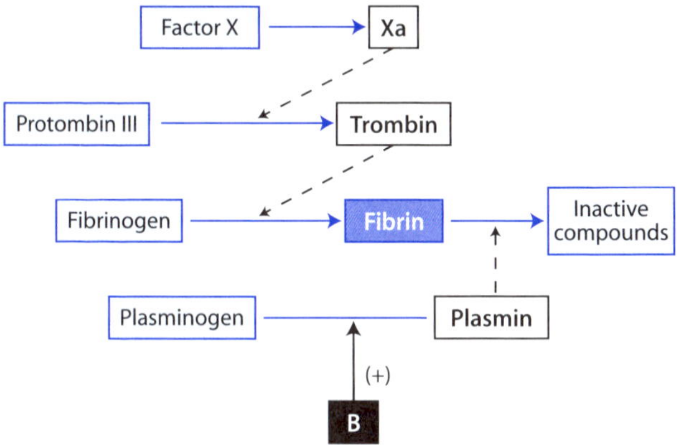

Figure 23.2 ▲ **Fibrinolytic action of bromelain**
Fibrin forms a protective matrix around the injured area. This matrix inhibits tissue drainage, promotes edema and blocks circulation of blood flow. Bromelain's fibrinolytic activity has been attributed to the enhanced conversion of plaminogen to plasmin, which degrades fibrin

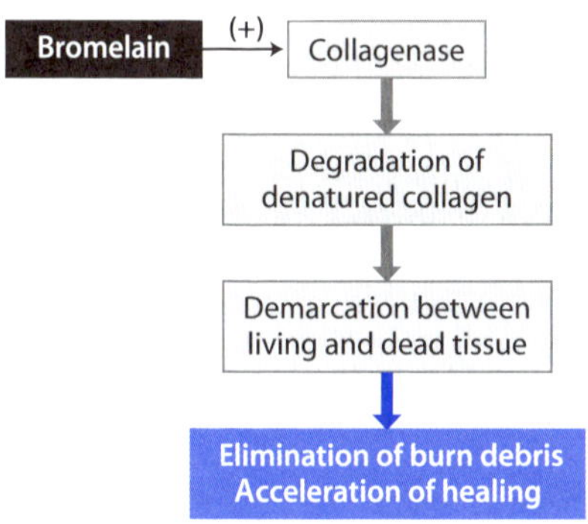

Figure 23.3 ◀ **Debridement action of bromelain**
Topical bromelain separates eschar at the interface with living tissue. It is hypothesized that bromelain activates collagenase in living tissue which then attack the denatured collagen in the eschar. This produces a demarcation between living and dead tissue

Preparations/Dosage

The usual dosage of bromelain is 100–250 mg/day (or 500,000 U/day), divided in three oral doses per day. The drug is used in form of enteric-coated tablets (sometimes combined with antibiotics). It is generally recommended that bromelain be taken without food because it may act as a digestive enzyme and its therapeutic benefit might be diminished.

Other Anti-inflammatory and/or Wound-healing Herbs

Hypericum oil (red oil) is made by macerating the fresh flowering tops of the plant (*Hypericum perforatum*) in olive oil (25:100 ratio) and then placing them in the sun until the oil acquires a reddish color. The red color is caused not only by hypericins, but by various naphtodianthrone derivatives. However, the exact composition of the oil is not known. Hypericum oil has long been used for the healing of wounds and burns, due in part to its antimicrobial activity. This preparation was even used by the surgeons to clean foul wounds, and was official in the first *London Pharmacopoeia*. Hypericum oil is supported by the German Commission E for the treatment of inflammation of the skin, blunt injuries, wounds and burns.

► *See Chapter 13 for the antidepressant use of St John's wort*

Marigold is obtained from the flowers of the 30–50 cm high herb *Calendula officinalis* L. (Fam. *Asteraceae*). The original habitation is obscure but it is found as a garden escape on waste, cultivated and arable land and along roadsides. It contains triterpenes (the principal group of compounds), a volatile oil and flavonoids, which may contribute to the anti-inflammatory effect. However, the active principle that promotes wound healing has not been identified. Despite its long history of use to facilitate wound healing and to solve local skin inflammatory problems, there are almost no studies regarding the efficacy of calendula in humans. Marigold is supported by the German Commission E for the treatment of inflammation of the mouth and pharynx and wounds and burns. Marigold is also reported to be useful in the treatment of fungal vaginal infections. The recommended dosage for internal use is 1–2 g dried herb (in three doses) or application of 2–5% cream. There have been no reports in Western literature describing serious reactions to the use of calendula. In Russia, there was one report of anaphylaxis in a patient who gargled with calendula. Theoretically, it could produce allergic cross-reaction with other members of the *Asteraceae/Compositae* family (e.g. feverfew, chamomile).

Lemon balm (melissa) is obtained from the leaves of *Melissa officinalis* L. (Fam. *Lamiaceae*), a 40–50 cm high herb native into Southern Europe and commonly seen growing in many European or American gardens (Plate 23.4). It displays white and yellow flowers and bright, green leaves that emit a lemon smell. The main active component in lemon balm is caffeic acid. Other components include flavonoids and rosmarinic acid. There are many uses of lemon balm. It is most often used as a mild sedative to relieve insomnia and anxiety or as antispasmodic to treat intestinal colic. Externally, it is applied to wounds as an antimicrobical agent. It is also used as an antiviral agent against herpes simplex virus Type 1 and 2 and the varicella zoster virus. The antiviral action is due to caffeic acid. In Germany lemon balm is available as a 70:1 extract cream for herpes sim-

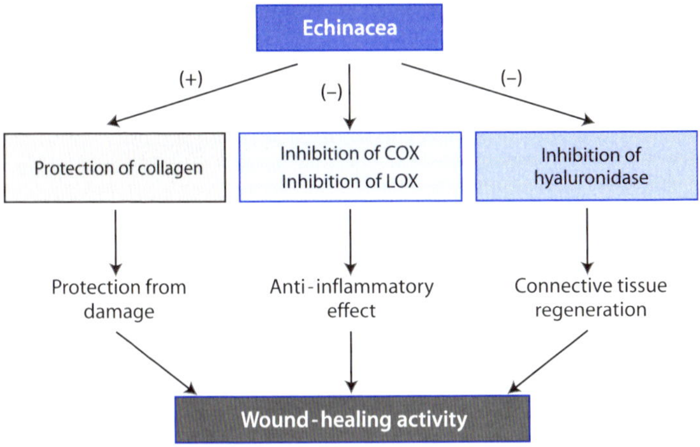

Figure 23.4 ▲ **Wound-healing properties of Echinacea**
(see text for details)

plex infection. Lemon balm is also available as 2% solution for the treatment of the varicella zoster viral infection. No adverse effects are expected.

Echinacea preparations derive from the aerial parts of *Echinacea purpurea*, *pallida*, or *angustifolia*. Echinacea possesses more than one action which may explain the wound-healing properties (Figure 23.4). Echinacea possesses anti-inflammatory activity via inhibition of cyclooxygenase and lipoxygenase enzymes and this effect is in part due to the presence of polyunsaturated alkylamides. Moreover, caffeic acid esters and *E. purpurea* extracts possess antihyaluronidase activity and protect collagen from damage caused by superoxide and free radicals. According to the German Commission E, semisolid preparations containing at least 15% juice expressed from the aerial parts are applied locally for the treatment of superficial, poorly healing wounds.

► *See Chapter 18 for the use of echinacea in the treatment of cold and flu*

Antiseptic Herbal Drugs

All volatile oils containing phenolic and terpenic compounds have antiseptic disinfectant properties; they also possess a revulsive and anaesthetic action. Essential oils are oily substances, insoluble in water, volatile and of a particular odor. They are obtained by pressure, extraction with solvents and by steam distillation.

Their most widespread use is as an antiseptic, not only for the urinary and bronchial tracts but also for the oral cavity; they are also used for the treatment of scalds, insect bites, athletes foot and wounds. They are used as such or in galenic preparations of the plants which contain them. Table 23.7 reports some herbal antiseptics used in the treatment of infections of the skin and skin structure. Among these, tea tree oil should be mentioned in particular.

Table 23.7
Herbal antiseptics used in the treatment of infections of the skin and skin structures

Common name	Latin name	Part(s) of plant used	Key constituents
Coconut palm	*Cocos nucifera*	Fixed oil from the seeds	Myristic acid, lauric acid, palmitic acid
Goa powder	*Andira araroba*	Latex from the trunk	Anthrone derivatives
Jack-in-the-pulpit	*Arisaema atrorubens*	Rhizome	Poysaccharides, pungent substances
Oak gall	*Quercus infectoria*	Galls	Tannins, phenol carboxylic acids
Pasque flower	*Pulsatilla pratensis*	Aerial parts	Protoanemonine-forming agents, triterpene saponins
Tea tree	*Melaleuca alternifolia*	Oil from steam	Terpin-1-en-4-ol
Thuja	*Thuja occidentalis*	Oil from leaves	Tujone, fenchone
Virola	*Virola theiodora*	Bark	Tryptamine derivatives

Tea tree oil (TTO)

Botany/Key constituents ► Tea tree (*Melaleuca alternifolia* Cheel; Fam. *Myrtaceae*) is a small tree native to the North-east of New South Wales (Australia). The name "tea tree" may cause confusion because in Australia such term is used for other species of the genus *Melaleuca* as well as for species of a related genus (*Leptospermum*). The leaves contain 1.8% essential oil (tea tree oil, TTO) which can be obtained by steam distillation. The oil contains more than 48 compounds, the main constituent including terpin-1-en-4-olo (not less than 30%, 1,8-cineole, gamma-terpinene, p-cymene and cineole (not more than 15%).

Pharmacological activity ► The oil possesses both antiseptic and antifungal activity. It is effective against a number of pathogens including *Candida albicans*, *Propionibacterium acnes*, *Pseudomonas aeruginosa*, *Staphylococcus aureus*, *Streptococcus pyrogens* and *Trichomonas vaginalis*.

Clinical efficacy ► Four randomized clinical trials (including a total of 421 patiens) were retrived and analyzed in a systematic review. The results suggest that TTO may be effective as a treatment of acne and fungal infections (Box 23.2). The evidence is promising but by no means compelling.

Box 23.2

Randomized clinical trials of tea tree oil (TTO) in dermatological conditions (topical use)[1]

Acne

A single-blind randomized trial of TTO (5% water-based TTO gel for three months) versus the reference drug benzoyl peroxide lotion was performed in 124 patients with mild to moderate acne. The results of this trial suggest that both treatments were equally effective. The number of inflamed and non-inflamed lesions dropped sharply during treatment. The effect of TTO tended to take longer to become clinically apparent. The percentage of patients experiencing adverse effects with TTO was lower than in the control group (44% vs 79%).

Tinea pedis

Tinea is a fungal infection of the skin, hair, or nails in humans that is caused by a fungus of one of the dermatophytes: *Microsporum*, *Trichophyton* or *Epidermophyton*. The fungal infection is confined to the keratinized tissues, but the clinical appearance is produced by a variable degree of inflammation in the living epidermis and dermis. Tinea pedis is tinea of the foot, in particular the lateral clefts between the toes and the soles. A double-blind trial with three parallel treatment groups was performed. Patients with tinea pedis applied either a 10% TTO cream, a 1% tolnaftate or a placebo cream twice daily for 4 weeks. Clinical improvement was experienced by 65% of the TTO group, 58% of the tolnaftate group and 41% of the placebo group. There was statistical significance between the TTO group and placebo. Skin tolerance was excellent in all three groups, and no adverse effects were reported.

Subungual onychomycosis

Onychomycosis is defined as any fungal infection of the nails. Usually, invasion of the nail plate rather than just the nail fold is involved. In a study, 117 patients with subungual onychomycosis received either topical 100% TTO or 1% clotrimazole twice daily for 6 months. At the end of the trial period, 18% of patients treated with TTO and 11% of control patients had negative culture (no fungal infection). Full or partial resolution of symptoms was experienced by 60% (treated with TTO) and 61% (treated with clotrimazole). At 3-months follow-up these figures had declined to 56% and 55% respecively.

Toenail onychomycosis

In one study, 60 patients with at least 25% fungal infection of a toenail received either 5% TTO cream or placebo for 8 weeks. Toenails were examined weekly up to week 16, thereafter patients were examined monthly up to 9 months. The main outcome measure was defined as "overall cure" consisting of resolution of clinical symptoms, negative fungal culture and progressive growth of normal nail. The overall cure rates after 9 months were 80% in the TTO group and 0% in the placebo group. 93.3% of patients did not experience any side effects. Four patients in the TTO group experienced mild inflammation.

[1] Data from Ernst and Huntley (2000)

Adverse events/Contraindications ▶ The adverse effects of TTO are usually mild and transient. There are numerous reports of contact dermatitis after exposure to tea tree oil. In a series of 28 healthy volunteers, 3 tested strongly positive to tea tree oil. Serious anaphylactic reactions have so far not been documented. Oral (accidental) application of TTO leads to toxicity with symptoms such as ataxia and drowsiness, confusion and inability to walk. TTO posioning requires less than 10 ml oral ingestion of 100% pure tea tree oil.

Preparations/Dosage

TTO is available in various preparations: 5% water-based TTO gel to be applied daily (for acne and skin infections), 100% TTO twice daily or 10% TTO cream twice daily for fungal nail infections, 40% tea tree oil solution emulsified with isopropyl alcohol and water for vaginal infections.

Protective Herbal Drugs

These are substances which due to their physical properties have only a local action when applied to cutaneous tissue, forming a protective skin which reinforces the defensive capacity and reduces skin sensibility.

Protective medicines are chemically inert substances, insoluble in water and not absorbable. In addition they have absorbent properties and can increase the softness and elasticity of the tissue to which they are applied (emollient properties); they can also reduce swelling (demulcent properties) and sensibility of the treated tissue.

The protectives are of particular therapeutic interest in cases of desquamation, inflammation and ulcerization and are used for skin and mucous membrane infections, scalds and sores. Both scalds and sores require treatment which facilitates the regeneration of tissue, relieves pain and prevents infection.

Some powders (starch) and the mucilages (aloe gel, holly hock, mallow, Iceland moss, salep, etc.) behave as protectives. The powders absorb toxins and exudates; they are sometimes used internally to absorb, for example, intestinal gas. Mucilages absorb water and form absorbent colloids which have an adhesive capacity and high viscosity.

Further Reading

Amenta R, Camarda L, Di Stefano V, Lentini F, Venza F (2000) Traditional medicine as a source of new therapeutic agents against psoriasis. Fitoterapia 71:S13–S20

Barre DE (2001) Potential of evening primrose, borage, blackcurrant, and fungal oils in human health. Ann Nutr Metab 45:47–57

Bedi MK, Shenefelt PD (2002) Herbal therapy in dermatology. Arch Dermatol 138:232–242

Capasso F, Borrelli F, Capasso R, Di Carlo G, Izzo AA, Pinto L, Mascolo N, Castaldo S, Longo R (1998) Aloe and its therapeutic use. Phytoter Res 12:S124–S127

Ernst E (2000) Adverse effect of herbal drugs in dermatology. Br J Dermatol 143:923–929

Ernst E, Huntley A (2000) Tea tree oil: a systematic review of randomized clinical trials. Forsch Komplementärmed 7:17–20

Ernst E, Pittler MH, Stevinson C (2002) Complementary/alternative medicine in dermatology: evidence-assessed efficacy of two diseases and two treatments. Am J Clin Dermatol 3:341–348

Levin C, Maibach H (2002) Exploration of "alternative" and "natural" drugs in dermatology. Arch Dermatol 138:207–211

Lovell CR (1998) Some biblical plants of dermatological importance. Clin Dermatol 16:33–40

Mantle D, Gok MA, Lennard TW (2001) Adverse and beneficial effects of plant extracts on skin and skin disorders. Adverse Drug React Toxicol Rev 20:89–103

Maurer HR (2001) Bromelain: biochemistry, pharmacology and medical use. Cell Mol Life Sci 58:1234–1245

Millikan LE (2002) Complementary medicine in dermatology. Clin Dermatol 20:602–605

Pribitkin ED, Boger G (2001) Herbal therapy: what every facial plastic surgeon must know. Arch Facial Plast Surg 3:127–132

Reynolds T, Dweck AC (1999) *Aloe vera* leaf gel: a review update. J Ethnopharmacol 68:3–37

Thomson KF, Wilkinson SM (2000) Allergic contact dermatitis to plant extracts in patients with cosmetic dermatitis. Br J Dermatol 142:84–88

Vogler BK, Ernst E (1999) *Aloe vera*: a systematic review of its clinical effectiveness. Bri J Gen Prat 49:823–828

Vonau B, Chard S, Mandalia S, Wilkinson D, Barton SE (2001) Does the extract of the plant *Echinacea purpurea* influence the clinical course of recurrent genital herpes? Int J STD AIDS 12:154–158

Young GL, Jewell D (2000) Creams for preventing stretch marks in pregnancy. Cochrane database Syst Rev 2:CD00066

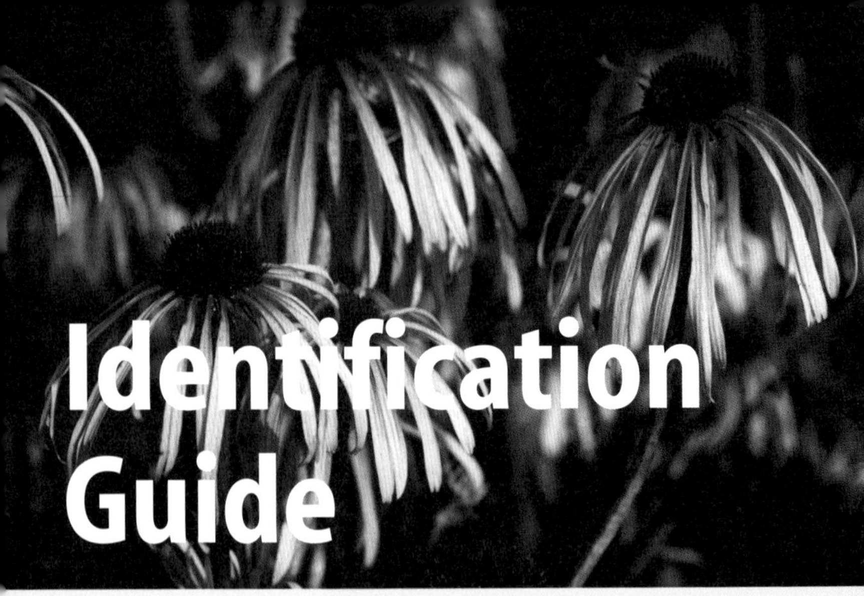

Identification Guide

Plants

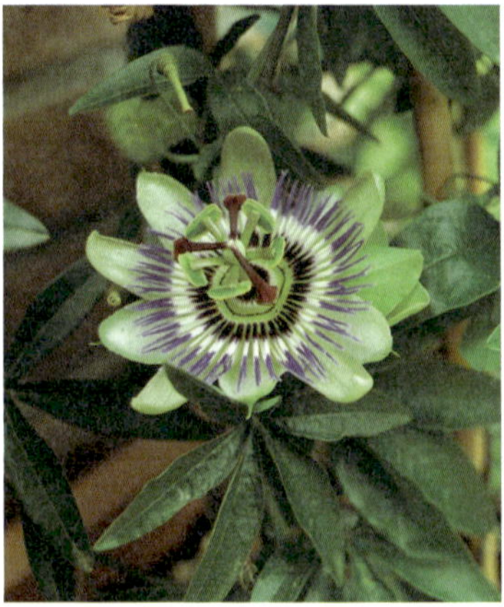

13.1 Passion flower
(Passiflora incarnata)

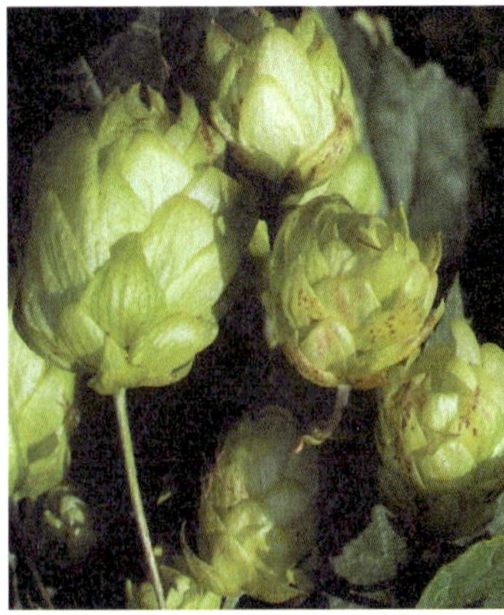

13.2 Hops
(Humulus lupulus)

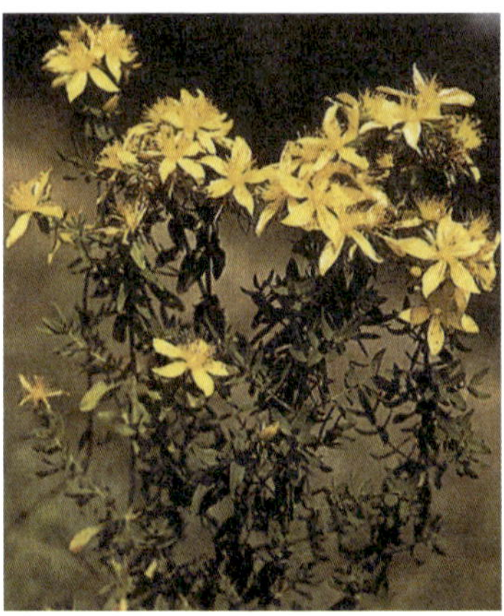

13.3 St John's wort
(Hypericum perforatum)

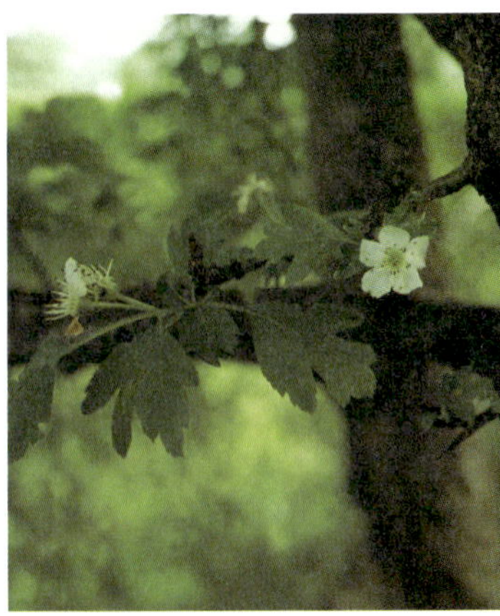

14.1 Hawthorn
(Crataegus laevigata)

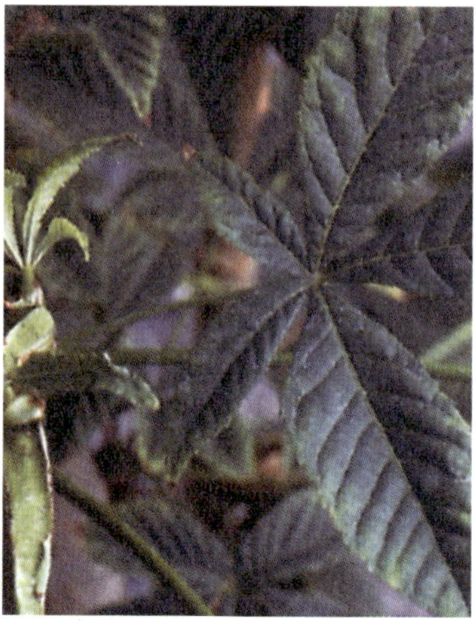

14.2 Horse chestnut
(Aesculus hippocastanum)

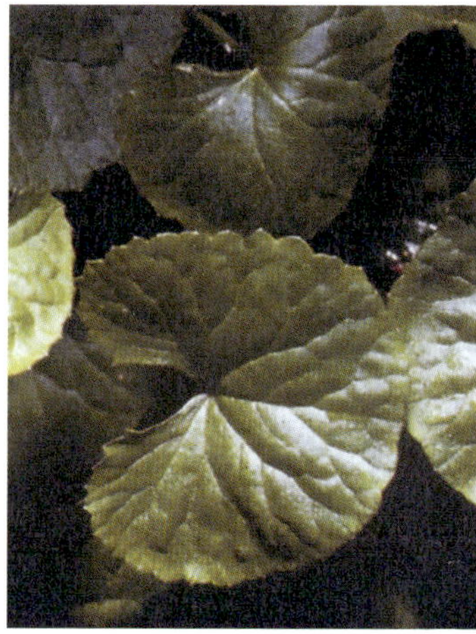

14.3 Gotu kola
(Centella asiatica)

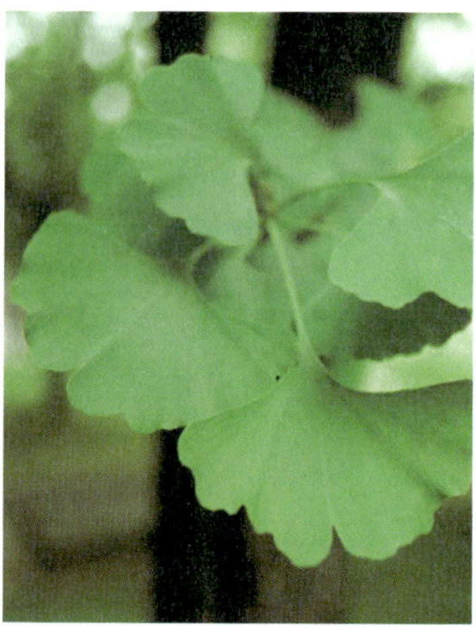

14.4 Ginkgo
(Ginkgo biloba)

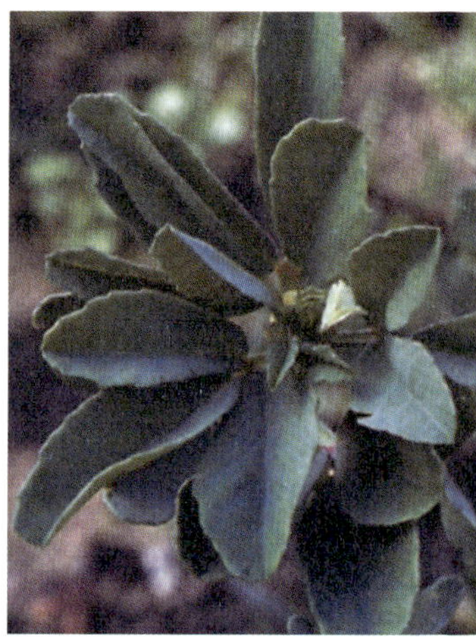

15.1 Fenugreek
(Trigonella foenum-graecum)

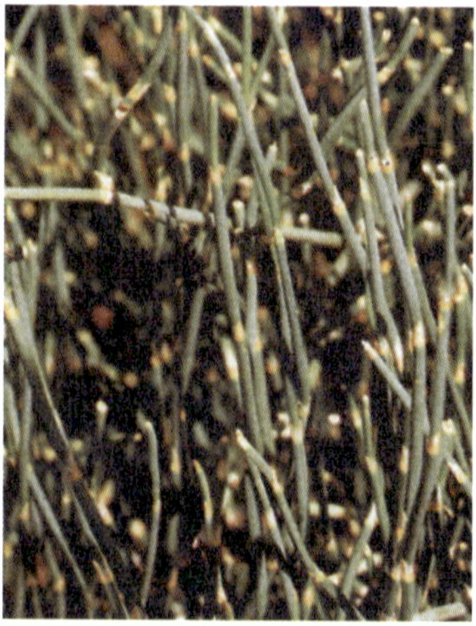

15.2 Ephedra
(Ephedra sinica)

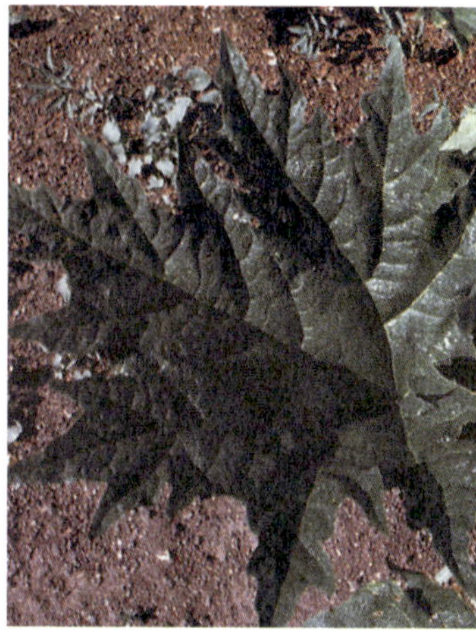

15.3 Rhubarb
(Rheum palmatum)

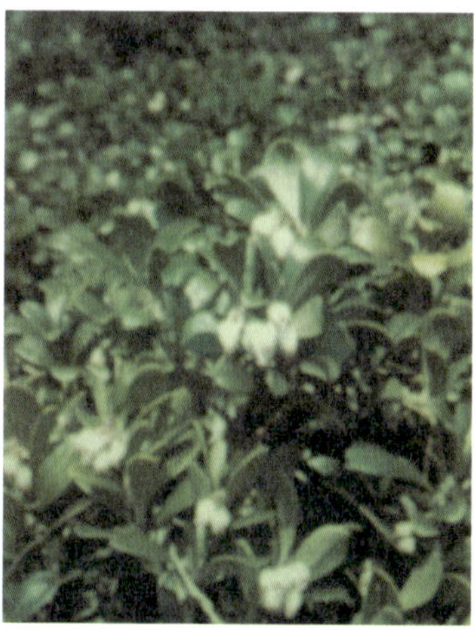

16.1 Bearberry
(Arctostaphylos uva-ursi)

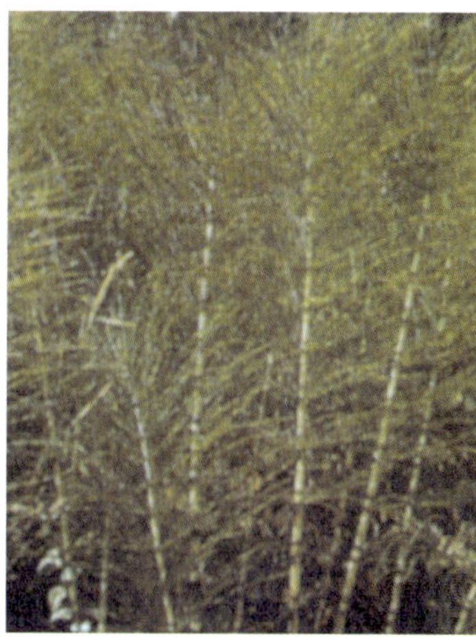

16.2 Horsetail
(Equisetum arvense)

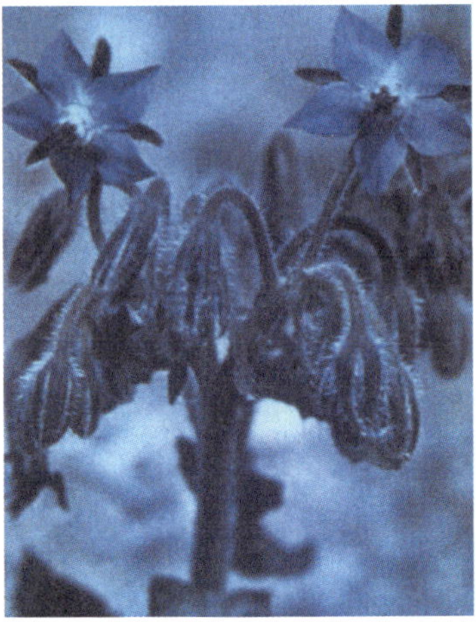

17.1 Borage
(Borago offinicalis)

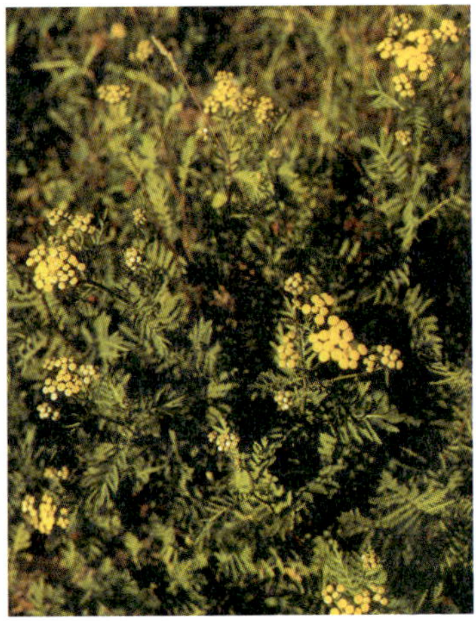

17.2 Feverfew
(Tanacetum parthenium)

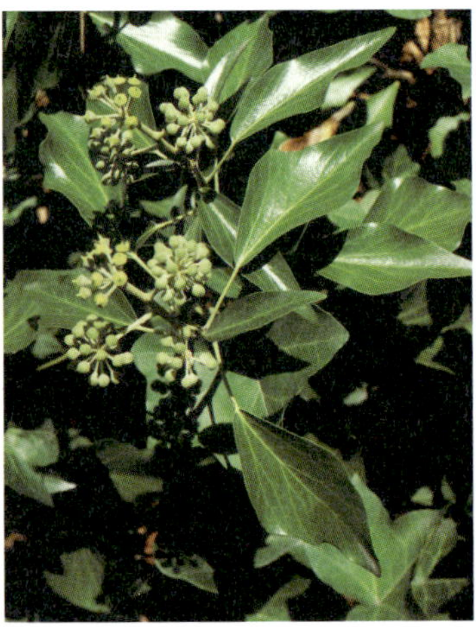

18.1 Common ivy
(Hedera helix)

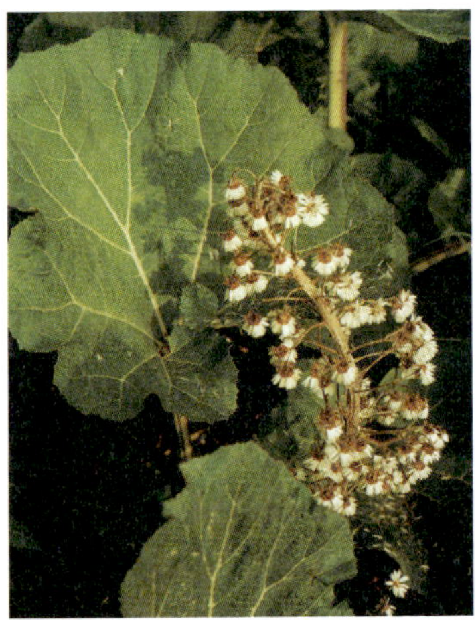

18.2 Butterbur
(Petasites hybridus)

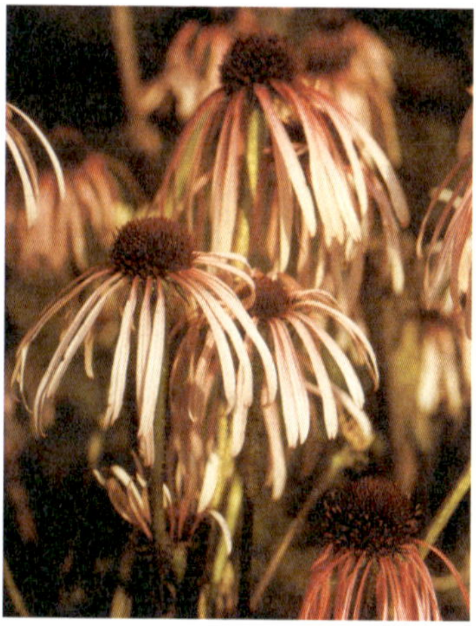

18.3 Echinacea
(Echinacea angustifolia)

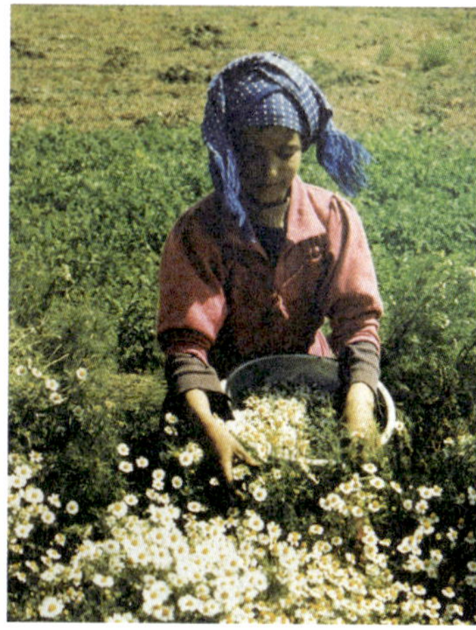

19.1 Ginseng
(Panax ginseng)

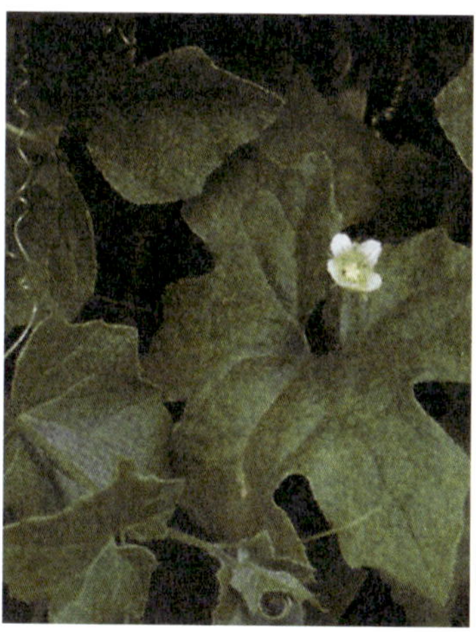

19.2 White bryony
(Bryonia alba)

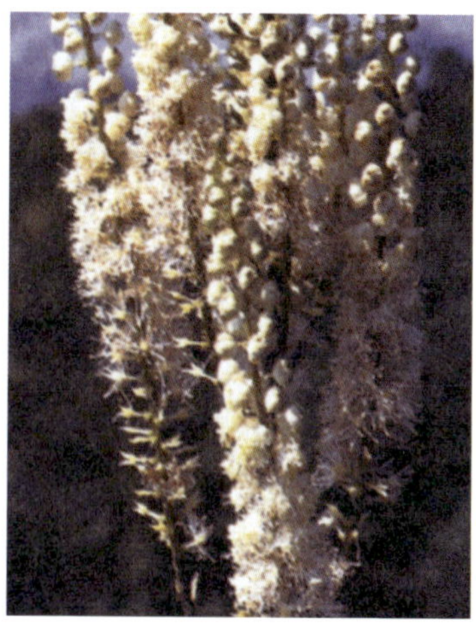

20.1 Black cohosh
(Cimicifuga racemosa)

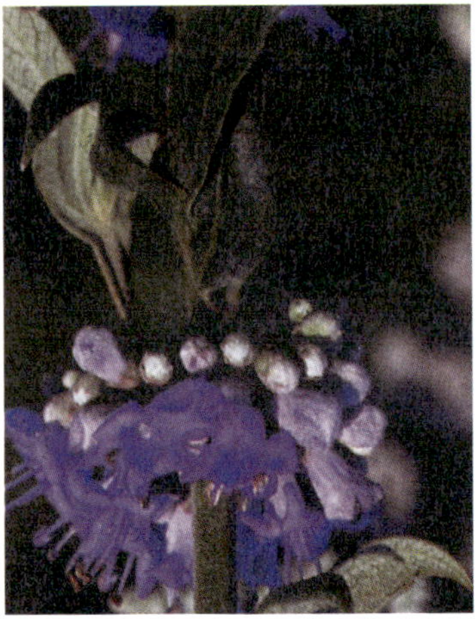

20.2 Chasteberry
(Vitex agnus-castus)

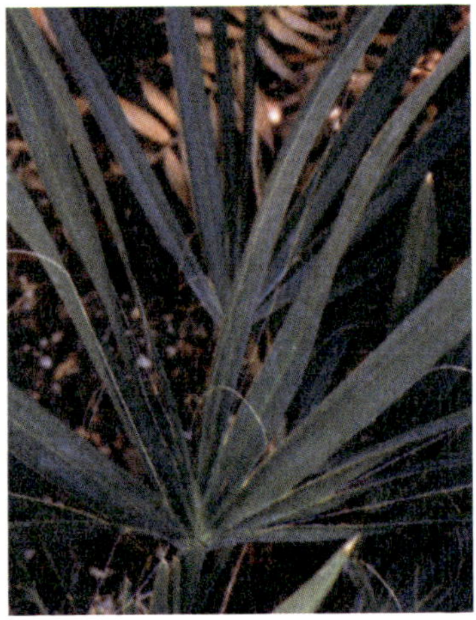

20.3 Saw palmetto
(Serenoa repens)

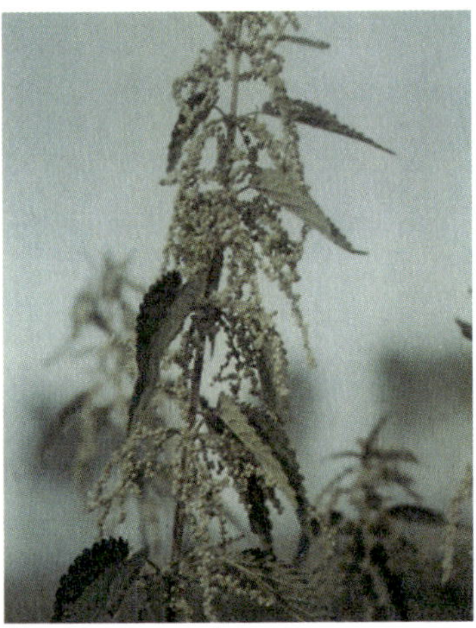

20.4 Stinging Nettle
(Urtica dioica)

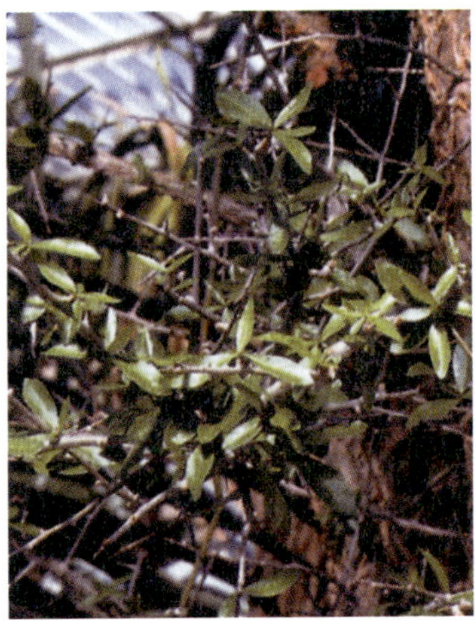

21.1 Mirrh
(Commiphora myrrha)

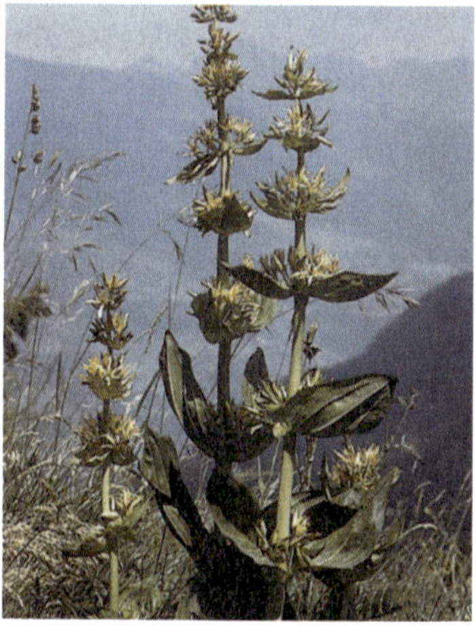

21.2 Gentian
(Gentiana lutea)

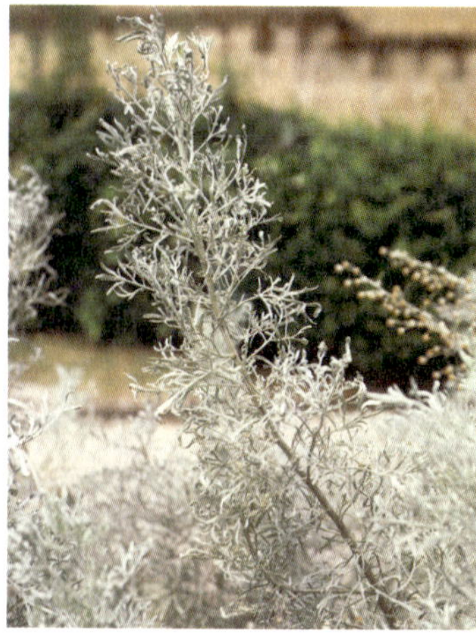

21.3 Wormwood
(Artemisia absinthium)

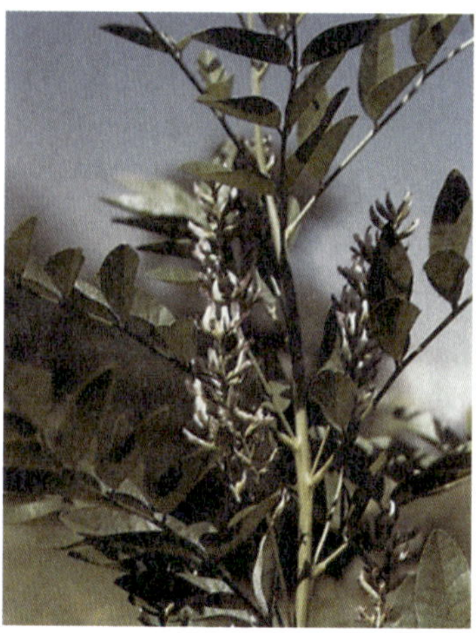

21.4 Liquorice
(Glycyrrhiza glabra)

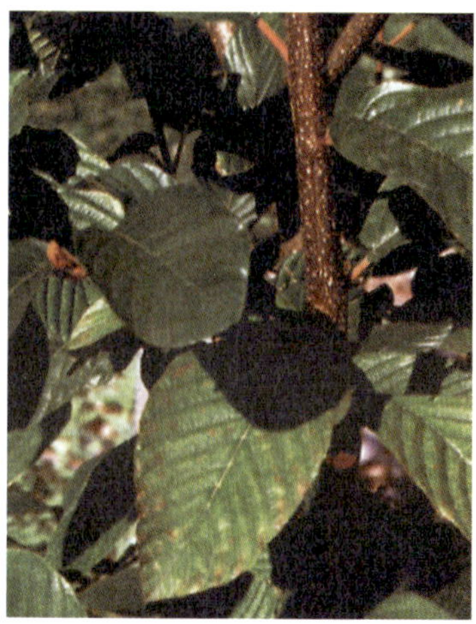

21.5 Cascara
(Rhamnus purshiana)

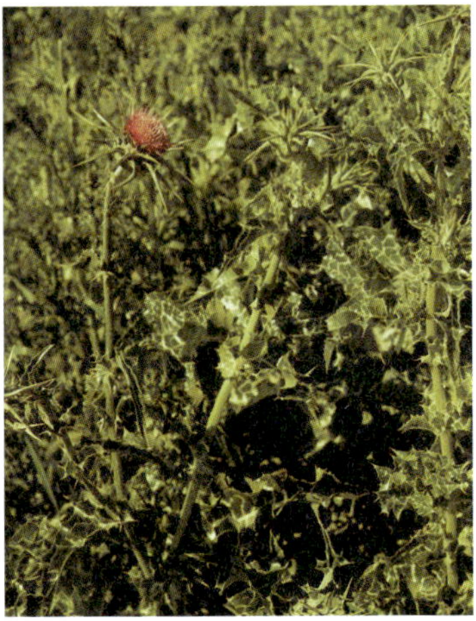

22.1 Milk thistle
(Silybum marianum)

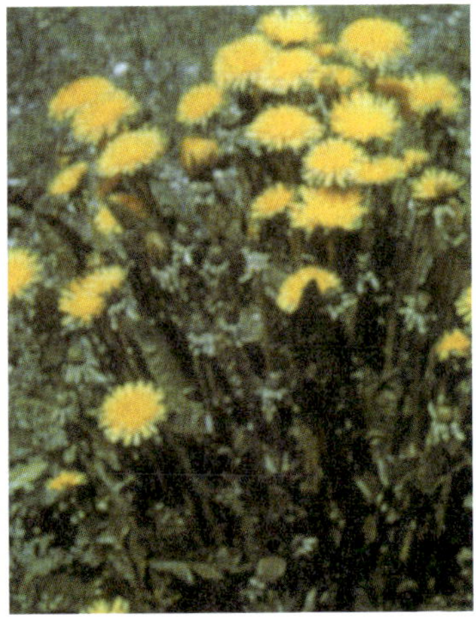

22.2 Dandelion
(Taraxacum officinale)

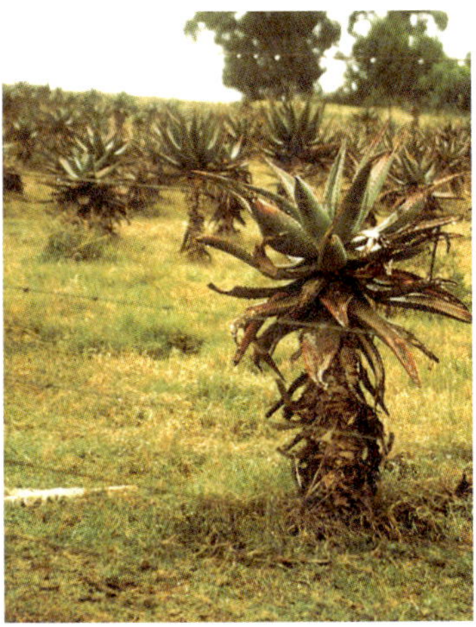

23.1 Aloe vera
(Aloe barbadensis)

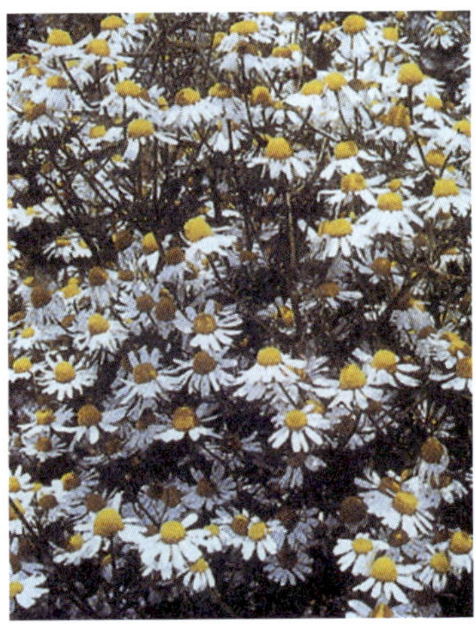

23.2 Chamomile
(Matricaria recutita)

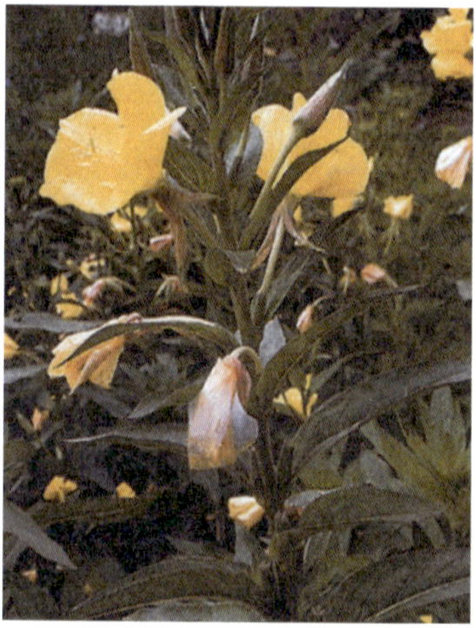

23.3 Evening primrose
(Oenothera biennis)

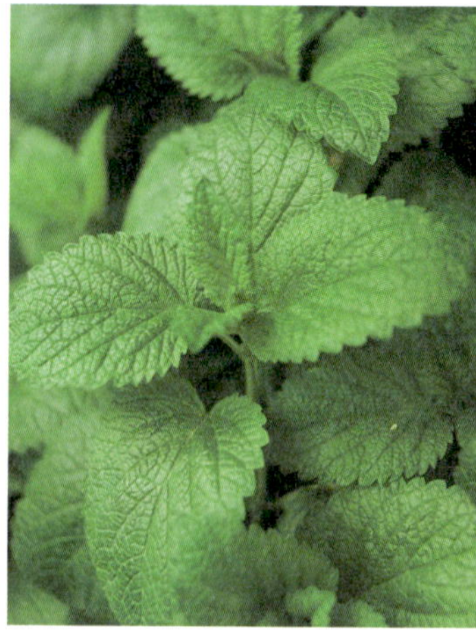

23.4 Lemon balm
(Melissa officinalis)

Crude Drugs

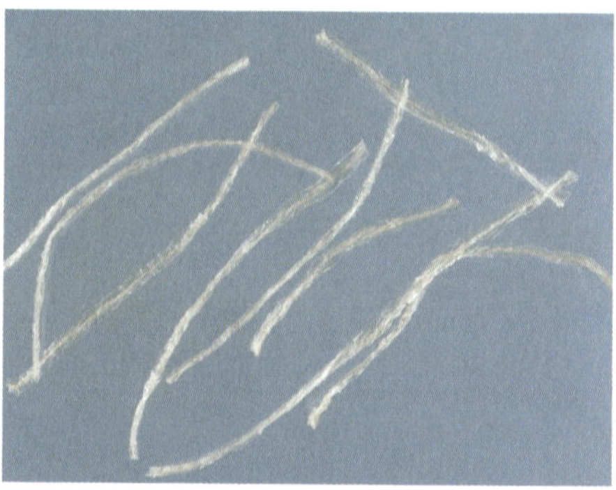

Agar
(Gelidium amansii)

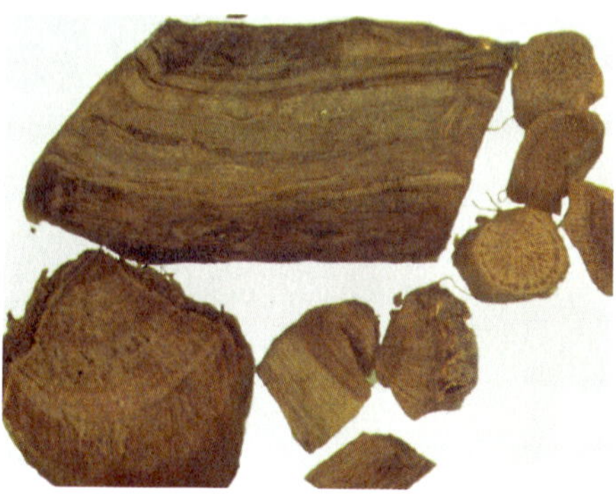

Althea
(Althea officinalis radix)

Ashvagandha
(Withania somnifera radix)

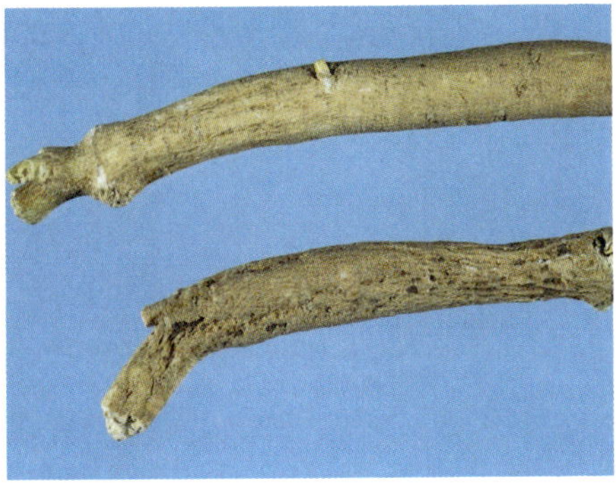

Bearberry
(Arctostaphylos uva-ursi folium)

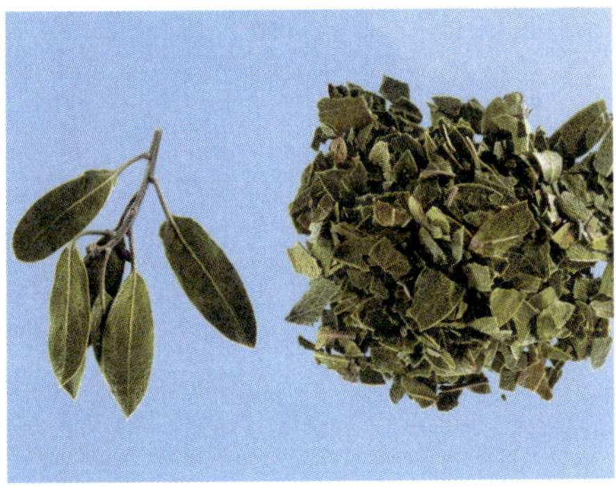

Boldo
(Peumus boldus folium)

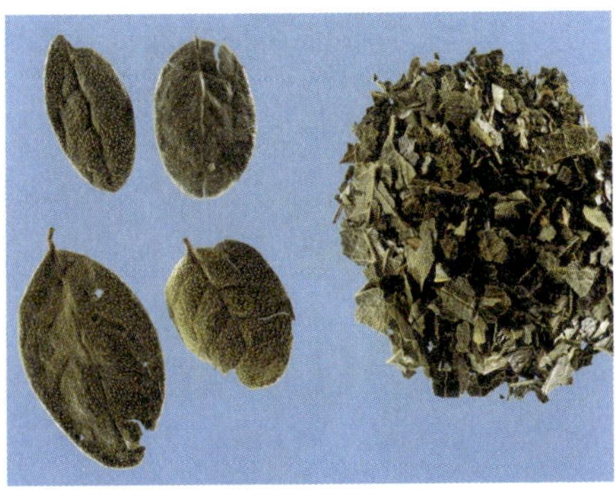

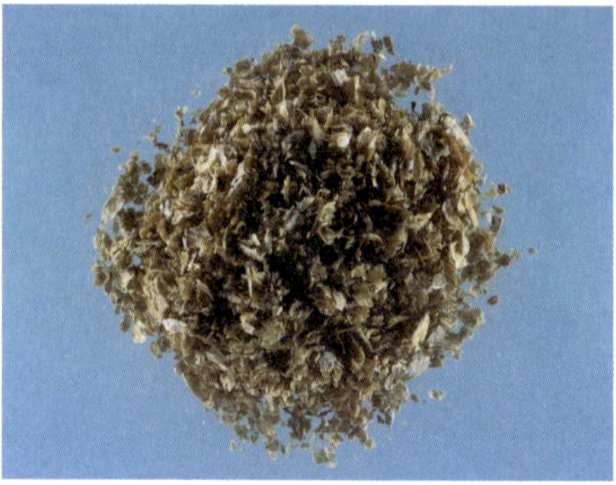

Bran
(Triticum aestivum seminin pericarpum)

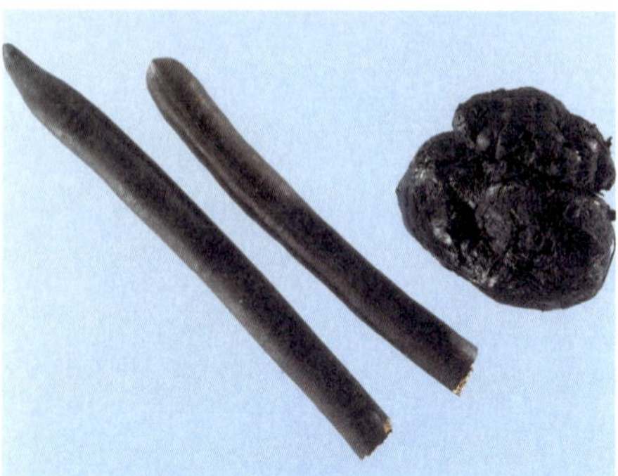

Cassia
(Cassia fistula fructus)

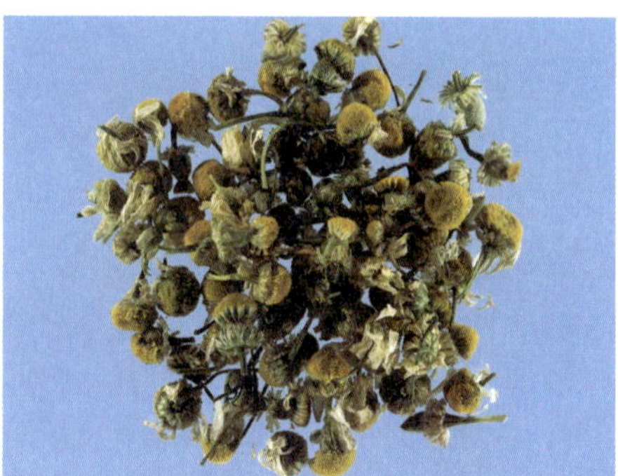

Chamomile
(Matricaria chamomilla flos)

Common ivy
(Hedera helix folium)

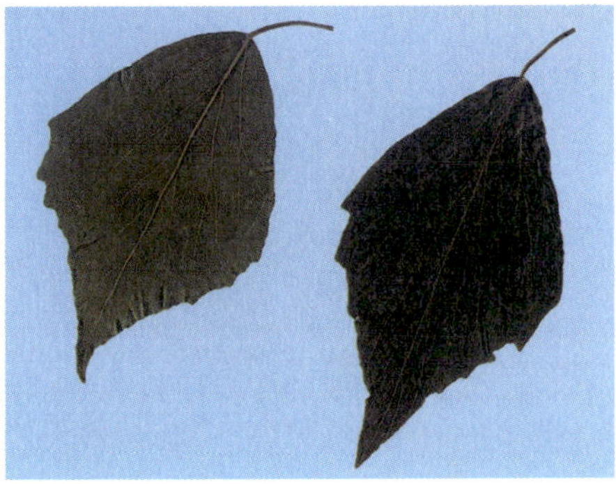

Dandelion
(Taraxacum officinale radix)

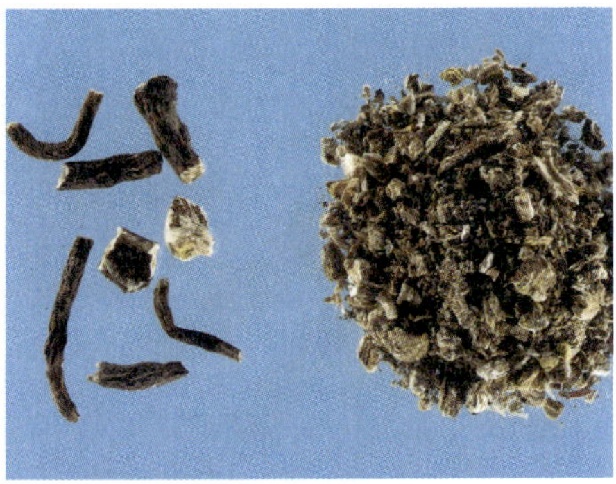

Devil's claw
(Harpagophytum procumbens fructus)

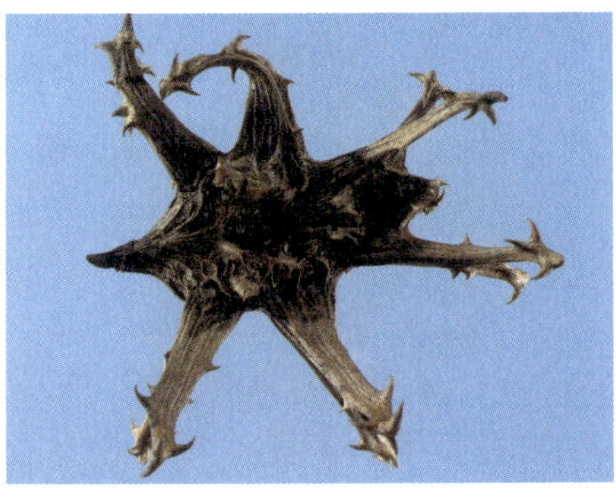

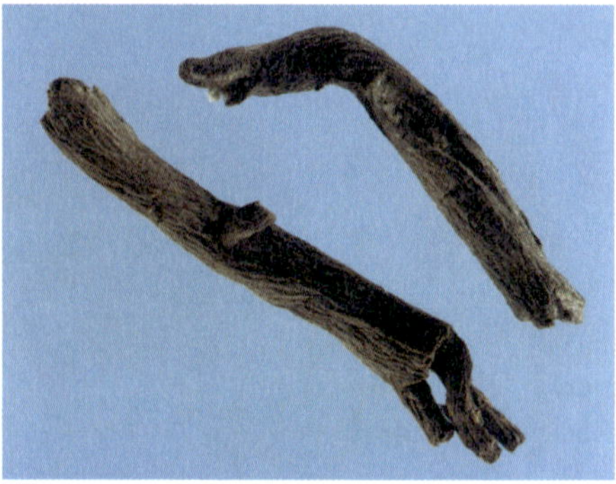

Echinacea
(Echinacea angustifolia radix)

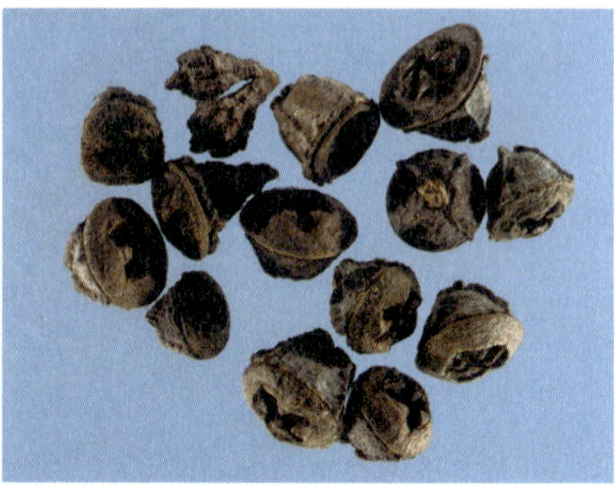

Eucalyptus
(Eucalyptus globulus folium)

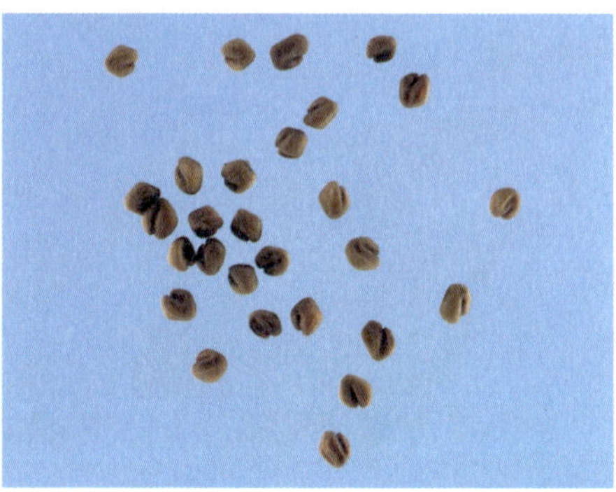

Fenugreek
(Trigonella foenum-graecum semen)

Frangula
(Rhamnus frangula cortex)

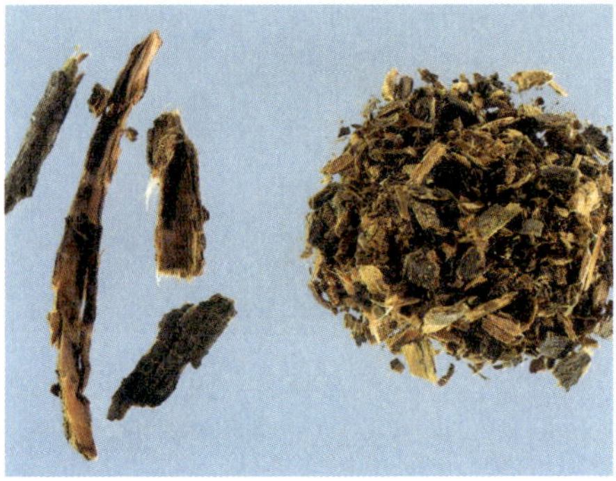

Gentian
(Gentiana lutea radix)

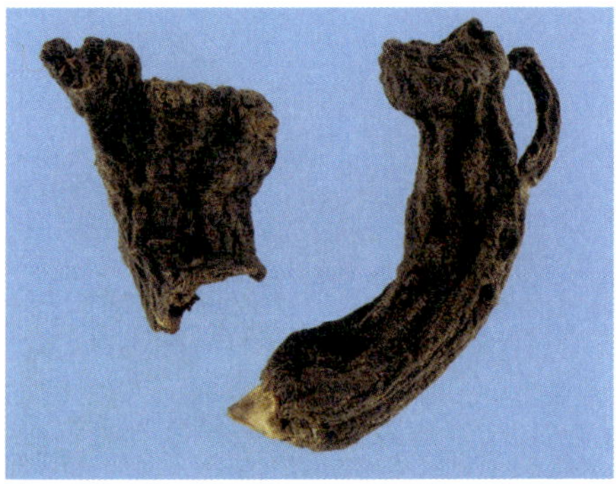

Ginger
(Zingiber officinale rhizoma)

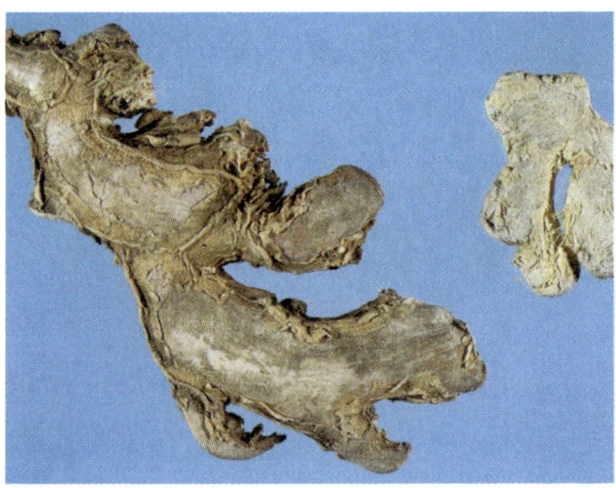

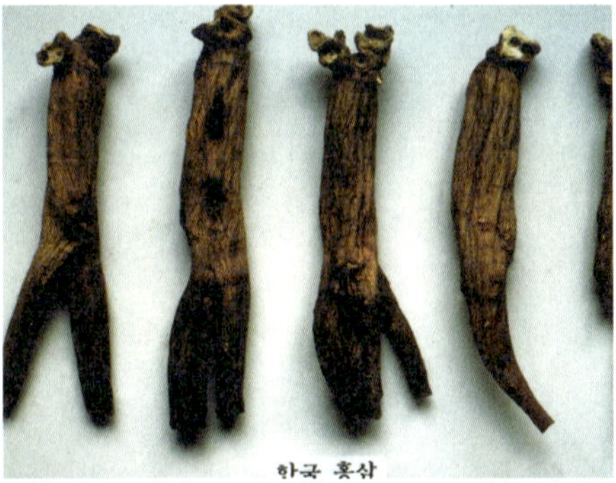

Ginseng (red ginseng)
(Panax ginseng radix)

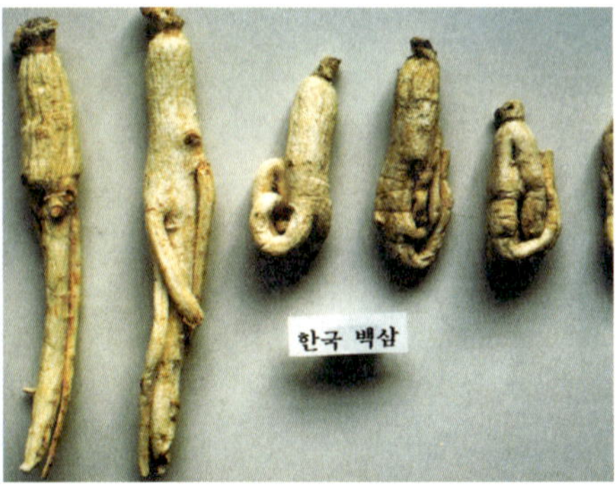

Ginseng (white ginseng)
(Panax ginseng radix)

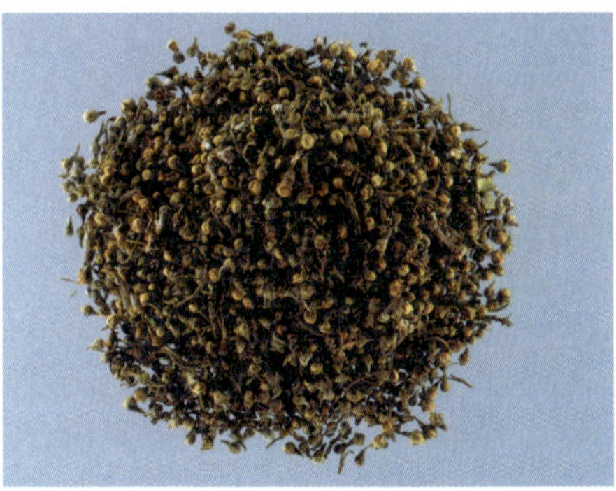

Hawthorn
(Crataegus monogyna flos)

Hops
(Humulus lupulus inflorescentia)

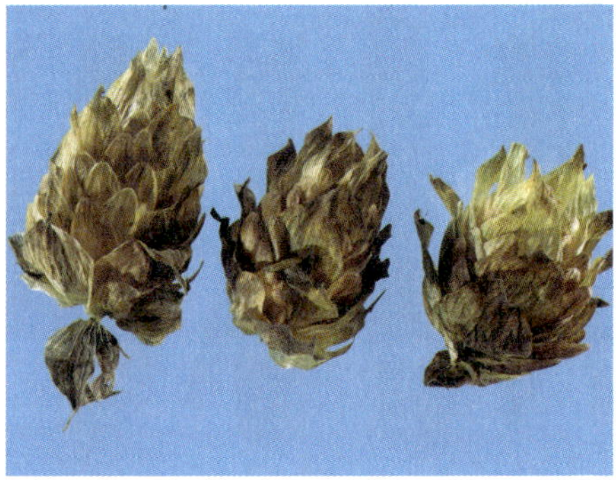

Horse chestnut
(Aesculus hippocastanum semen)

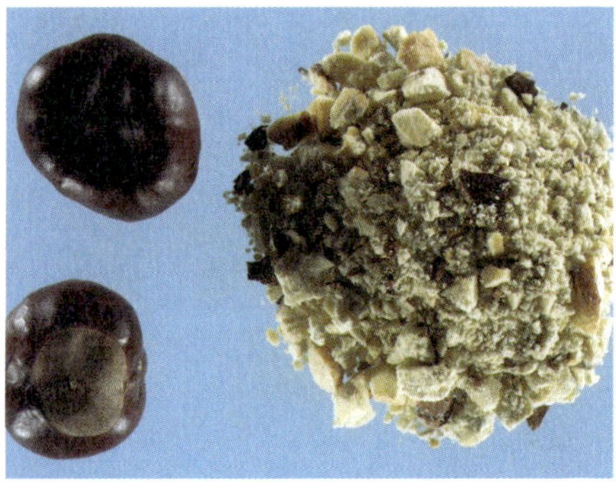

Horsetail
(Equisetum harvense herba)

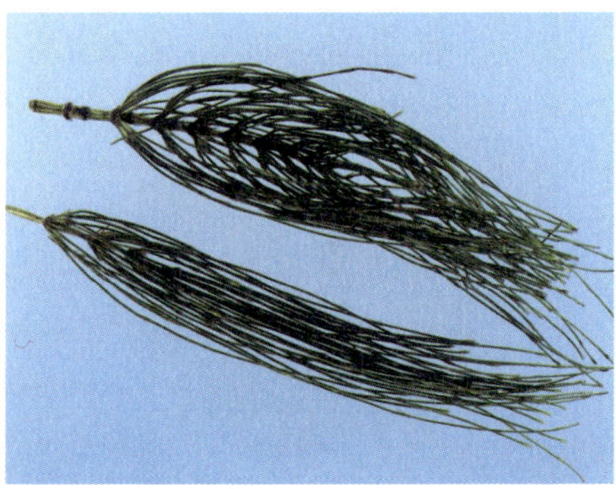

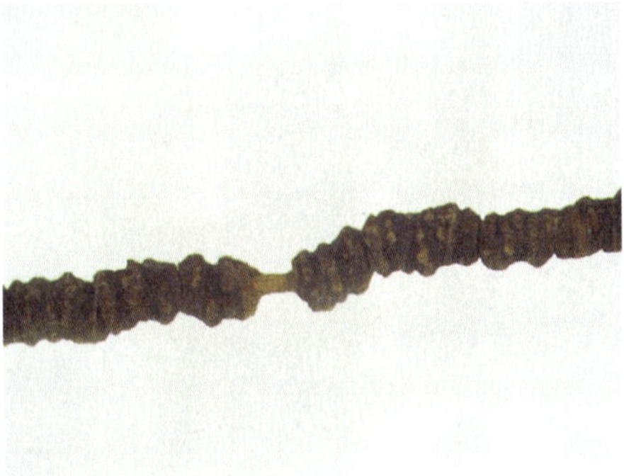

Ipecac
(Caephalis ipecacuana radix)

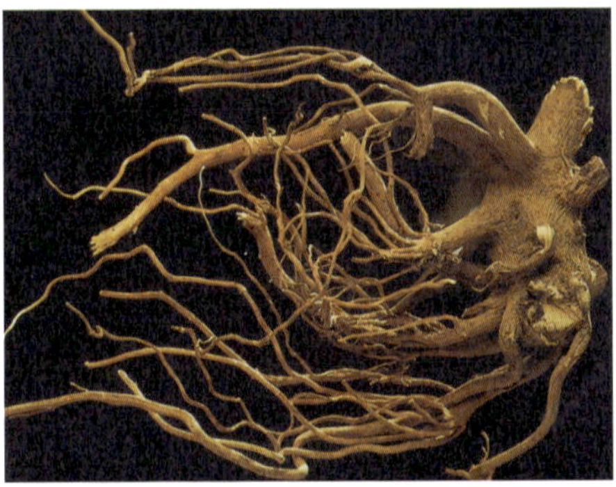

Kava
(Piper methysticum rhizoma)

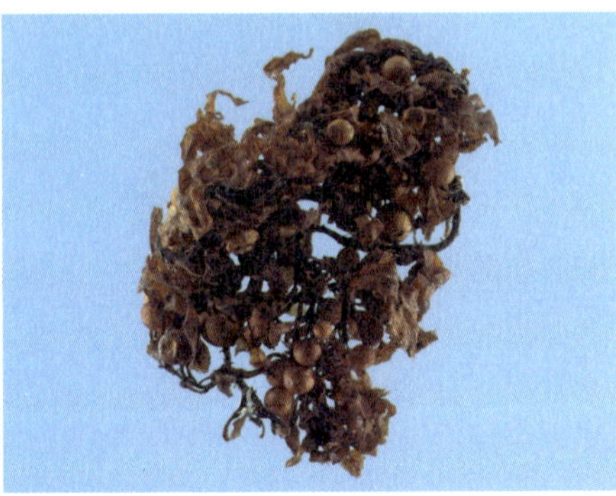

Kelp
(Fucus vesiculosus thallus)

Lavender
(Lavandula officinalis inflorescentia)

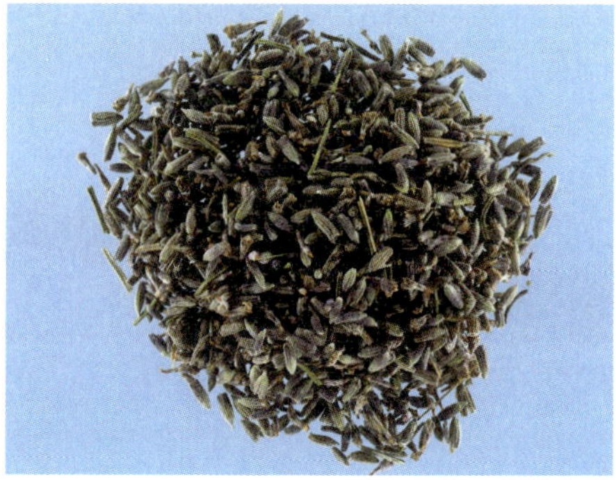

Lemon balm
(Melissa officinalis folium)

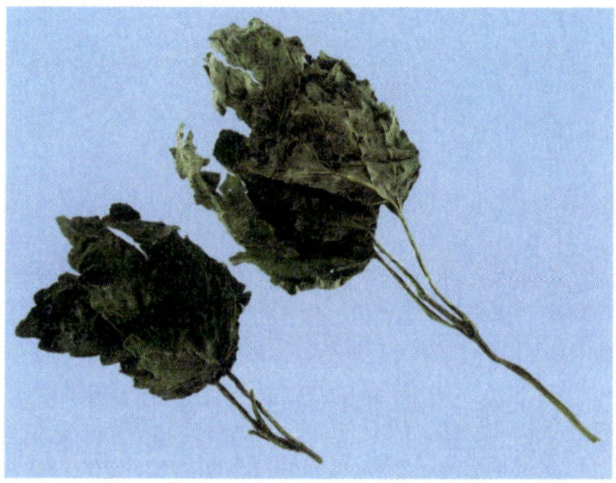

Liquorice
(Glycyrrhiza glabra radix)

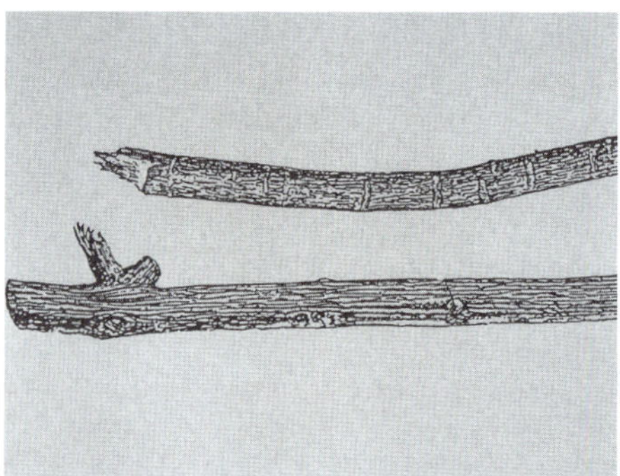

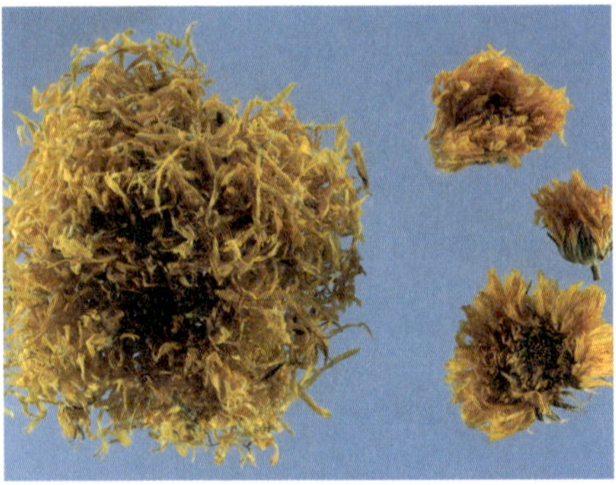

Marigold
(Calendula officinalis flos)

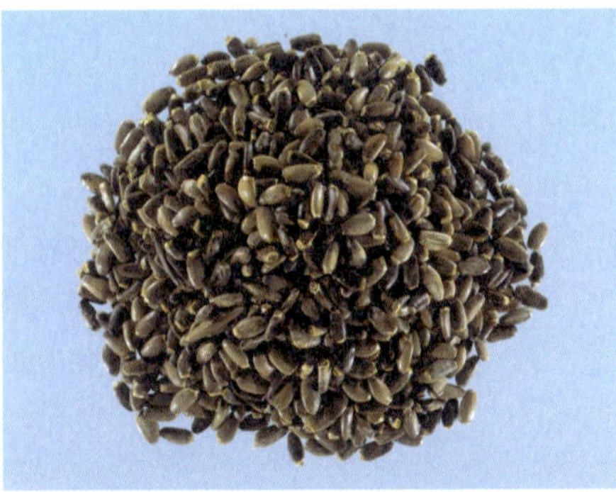

Milk thistle
(Silybum marianum achaenium)

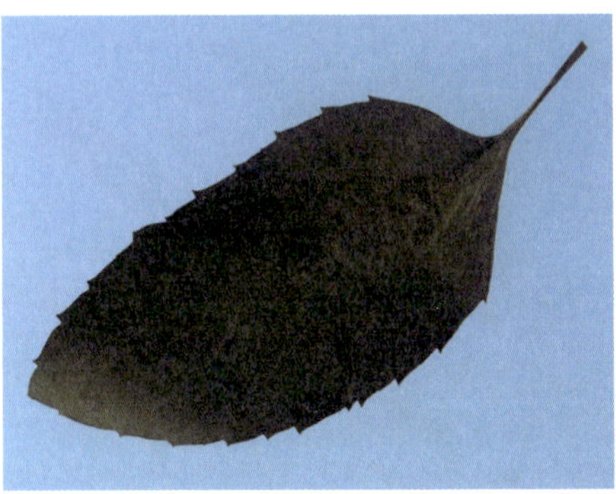

Peppermint
(Mentha piperita folium)

Picrorhiza
(Picrorhiza kurroa radix)

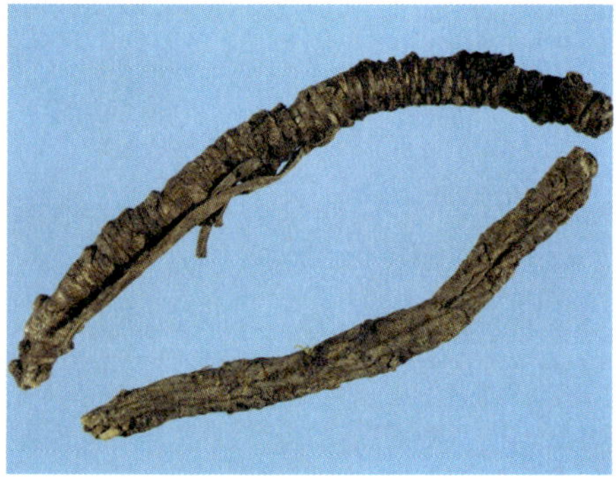

Psyllium
(Plantago psyllium semen)

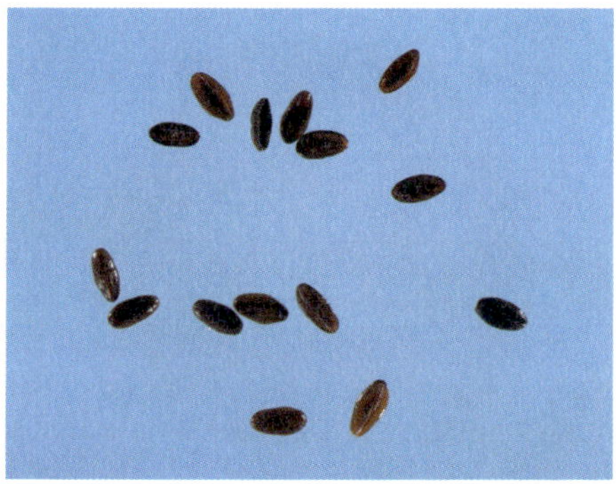

Quassia
(Quassia amara lignum)

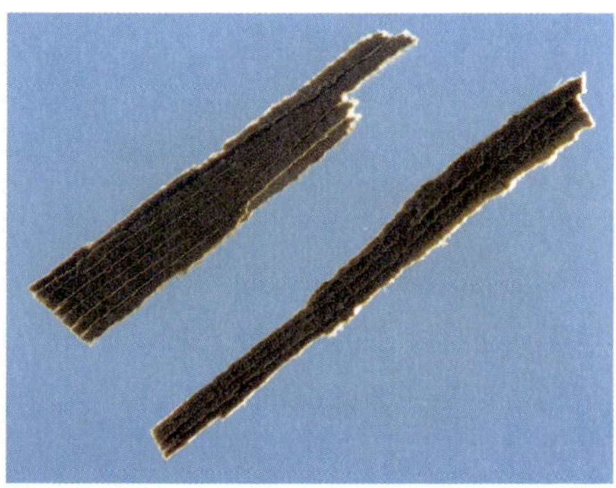

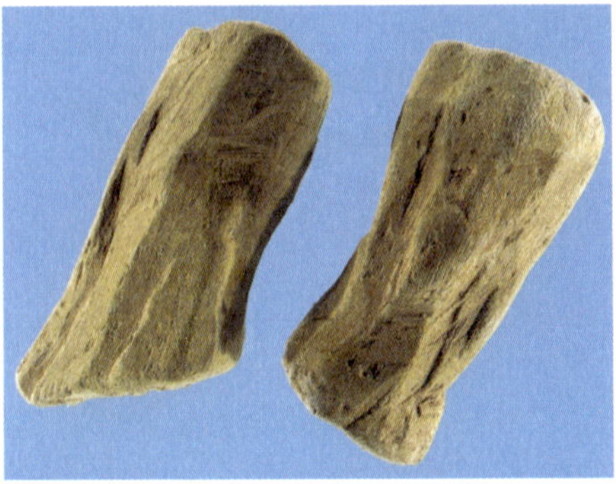

Rhubarb
(Rheum palmatum rhizoma)

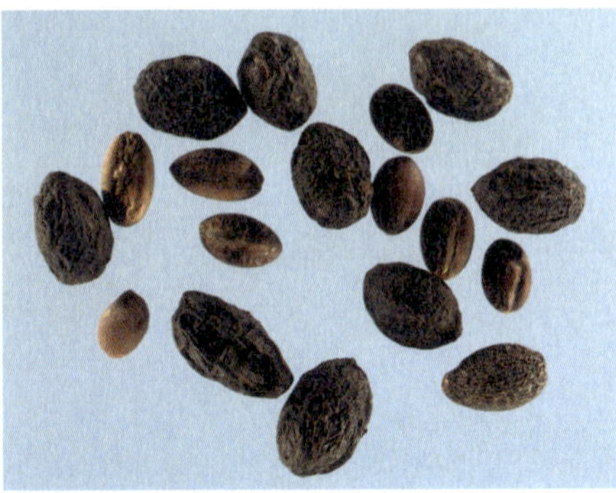

Saw palmetto
(Serenoa repens fructus)

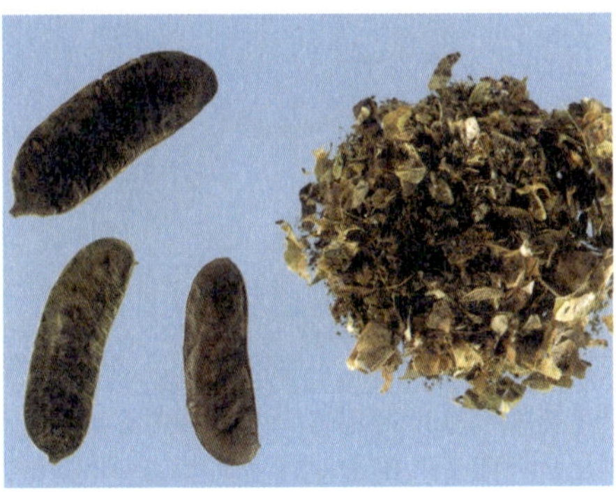

Senna
(Cassia angustifolia fructus)

Snakeroot
(Polygala senega radix)

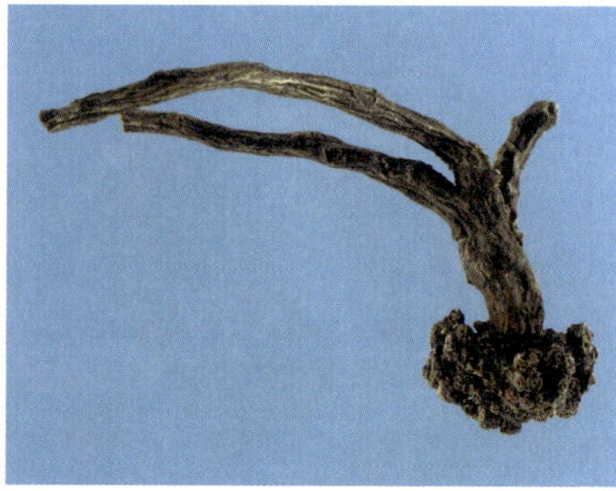

St John's wort
(Hypericum perforatum flos)

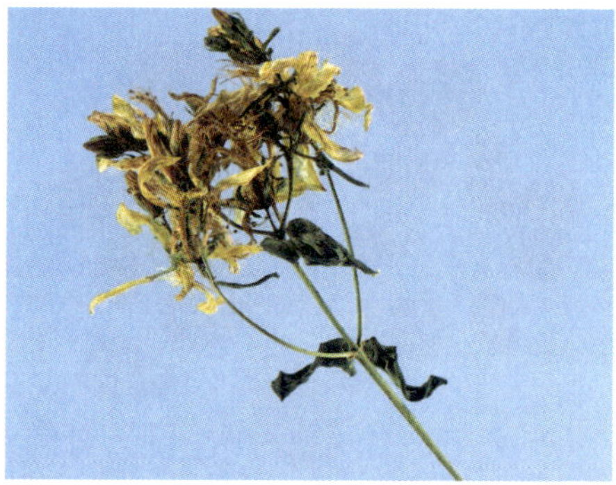

Tamarind
(Tamarindus indica fructus)

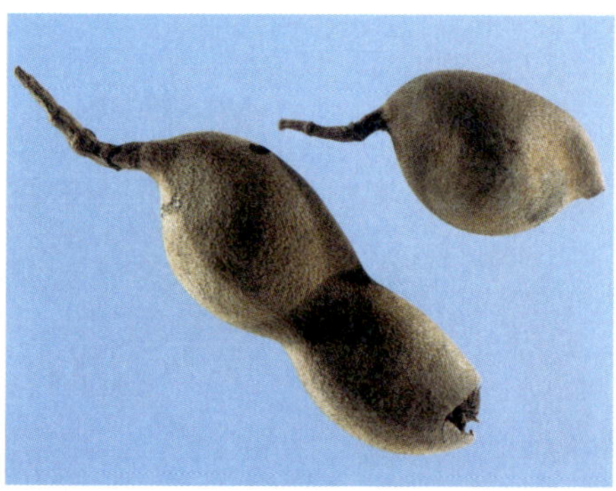

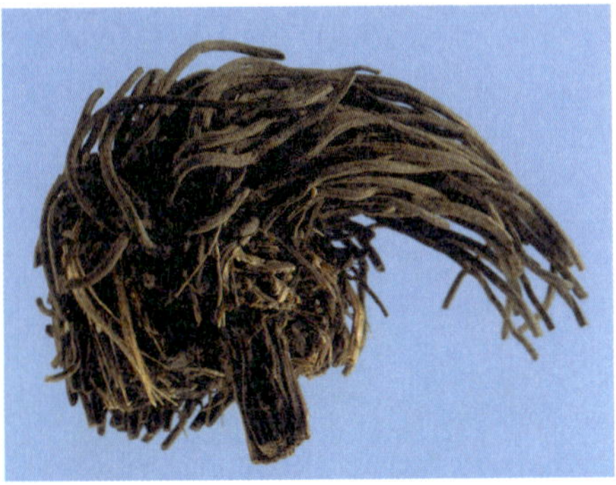

Valerian
(Valeriana officinalis radix)

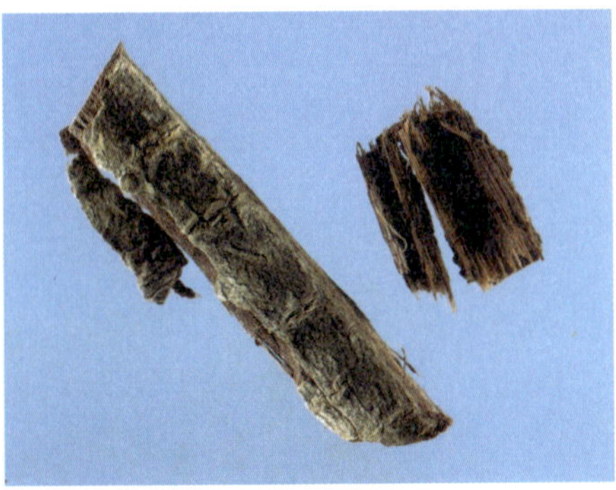

Witch hazel
(Hamamelis virginінana cortex)

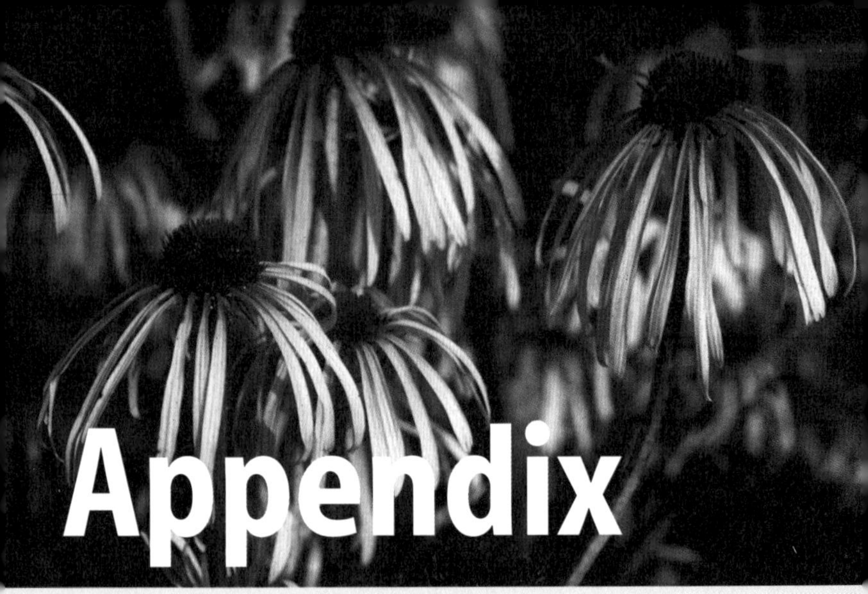

Appendix

Appendix A

Nutraceuticals and Herbal Supplements

People have always believed that certain foods and their components may have prophylactic and/or healing properties. However, only in the last 50 years foods are being scientifically investigated for their ability to prevent or reduce the risk of "life style-related diseases" such as cardiovascular diseases, diabetes and cancer. Actually there is great interest and much scientific activity on the possible health benefits of food and their substances.

The term nutraceuticals was coined by the Foundation for Innovation in Medicine in 1989 to indicate this area of biomedical research and means "any substance that may be considered a food or part of a food which provides medical or health benefits, including the prevention and treatment of disease". Nutraceuticals cover a broad list of terms including:

- functional foods (or medicinal foods), i.e. foods that encompass potentially healthy products including any modified food or food ingredient that may provide health benefits beyond the traditional nutrients it contains. Medical food also includes food as a delivery system for pharmaceutical agents and vaccines.
- medical foods, i.e. special dietary foods intended for use solely under medical supervision to meet nutritional requirements in specific medical conditions.
- dietary supplements, i.e. products that are intended to supplement the diet that bear or contain one of the following dietary ingredients: (i) a vitamin, (ii) a mineral, (iii) an herb, (iv) a dietary substance (flavonoid, carotenoid, terpenoid, cathechin, vanilloid, isothiocyanade, polyphenol, phytoestrogen, protease inhibitor) for use by man to supplement the diet by increasing the total dietary intake, (v) a concentrate, metabolite, constituent, extract, or combination of any ingredient described.

Nutraceuticals are viewed as the center of the continuum between food and medicine and their use are moving towards the pharmaceutical sector and competing with medicines on a global basis. This is why there is an urgent need to rationalize the standardization of these products and give correct information on them to both physicians and consumers. Two types of products exist: potential and established nutraceuticals. The former may become established nutraceuticals only after clinical data have demonstrated a benefit. Obviously the usefulness of nutraceuticals depends on their ability to have a precise impact on the prevention and treatment of disease as well as other health benefits (e.g. increased energy). Actually nutraceuticals are not closely regulated or standardized; therefore these products may be defined and formulated differently by manufacturers. Nutraceuticals must be standardized, i.e. contain the same amount of active compounds per dose. Some Pharmacopoeias also refer to standards of identity and quality which include microbial limit test, disintegration and dissolution of nutritional substances, weight variation of nutritional substances and manufacturing practices.

Nutraceuticals are used not only to prevent or reduce the risks of some diseases, but also to help individuals who have general weakness (with no specific disease), children (particularly infants who need more of certain specific nutrients, including vitamins and minerals, than do adults), the elderly (illness, multiple medicines, and the ageing process itself may require consumption of more nutrients than that recommended for their age), women during pregnancy and breast-feeding [women may need to take adequate amounts of vitamin (especially folic acid), minerals and amino acids] or people who use specific medicines (Table 1).

Table 1

Medicines that may induce a deficit in nutrients

Medicine	Nutrients
Antibiotics	Vitamin K, vitamin H
Anticonvulsants	Folic acid, calcium phosphate, vitamin B, vitamin D_3, vitamin K
Corticosteroids	Calcium, potassium, vitamin C, vitamin B_6, vitamin D_3, zinc
Diuretics	Calcium, magnesium, potassium, zinc
Oral contraceptives and estrogens	Folic acids, vitamin B_6, vitamin B_{12}, vitamin C

Alcohol and smoking may induce a deficit in folic acid and vitamin B_6

From a scientific point of view, many nutraceuticals have proved to be effective, although little is known about their mechanism of action. However, some people may also need to take certain herbs to maintain good health and well-being. The DSHEA (Dietary Supplement and Health Education Act) of 1994 has provided for herbs and botanical preparations to be available for sale as dietary supplements and as such they do not have to be subject to FDA regulation before marketing. Herb supplements are currently being used by more than 80% of the global population. The most popular herbal supplements currently used in the world are presented in Table 2.

Table 2
Examples of herbal supplements

Common name	Latin name	Part of plant	Main constituent(s)	Promoted use	Administration
Ginseng	*Panax ginseng*	Roots	Ginsenosides	Cancer prevention	Fresh consumption once a month or more
Garlic	*Allium sativum*	Bulb	Alliins	Cancer prevention	Regular consumption
Grape seeds	*Vitis vinifera*	Seeds	Polyphenols (proanthocyanidins)	Prevention of arteriosclerotic disease	40–80 mg/daily proanthocyanidins
Green tea	*Camellia sinensis*	Leaves	Polyphenols	Cancer prevention	6–10 cups daily
Liquorice	*Glycyrrhiza glabra*	Roots	Glycyrrhizin	Antiulcer (supportive treatment), expectorant	Beverage prepared using 2 g roots in 150 ml water
Onion	*Allium cepa*	Bulb	Alliins	Cancer prevention	Regular consumption
Psyllium	*Plantago psyllium*	Seeds	Mucilage	Constipation, Hypercholesterolemia	Juice or milk beverage from the stirred seeds
Red clover	*Trifolium pratense*	Flower heads	Phytoestrogens	Menopausal symptoms	40 mg isoflavones daily (500 mg/extract or infusion or 3 cups infusion starting from 4 g crude drug)
Soy	*Glycine max*	Seeds	Phytoestrogens	Menopausal symptoms, Hypercholesterolemia, Cancer prevention	40–100 mg isoflavones daily (60 g/day soy protein)

Top-selling herbal supplements include grape seeds (*Vitis vinifera*), plants containing **phytoestrogens** such as soy (*Glycine max.*), red clover (*Trifolium pratense*), and green tea (*Camellia sinensis*).

▸ *See Appendix B for the use of herbal supplements in cancer prevention*

Grape Seeds are the seeds of *Vitis vinifera* L. (Fam. *Vitaceae*). Epidemiological studies suggest that red wine has a protective effect on arteriosclerotic disease. This evidence has been revealed mostly from the evaluation that the low incidence of cardiovascular disease in France is paralleled by a very high dietary intake of lipids, but concomitantly by an elevated consumption of red wine. This is commonly referred to as "the French Paradox" and is thought to be due to polyphenols (proanthocyanidins) which are highly concentrated in grape seeds. Grape seeds and proanthocyanidins have been reported to posses a broad spectrum of pharmacological properties against oxidative stress in both *in vitro* and *in vivo* experimental models. Proanthocyanidins are better free radical scavengers than vitamins C, E and beta-carotene and have demonstrated cytotoxicity towards human breast, lung and gastric adenocarcinoma and protection against ischemia/reperfusion injury. There is some clinical evidence that the antioxidant activity in blood samples from healthy volunteers can be increased by supplementation of grape seed extracts. There are no safety concerns associated to grape seed extract consumption. However, grape seed extracts are contraindicated during pregnancy and lactation. Extract of grape seeds concentrated 100-fold and standardized to contain 80—85% proanthocyanidins are commercially available and are usually taken at a daily dose of 40—80 mg.

Soy beans are obtained from *Glycine max.* (L.) Merr. (Fam. *Fabaceae*), a herb native to East Asia and nowadays cultivated in the United States as well as in South America and India. Soy beans are very rich in **phytoestrogens** (non-steroidal plant-derived compounds with diverse chemical structures possessing a weak estrogenic activity), mainly the isoflavones genistein and diadzein. Asian people consume 10—100 times more isoflavones than Western people, and osteoporosis-related fractures are less frequent in Asian than Western communities, possibly because of the large amounts of phytoestrogen-rich soy beans and vegetables in the Asian diet. The major source of isoflavones in Asian soy products are soybean curd, fermented soybeans, and soybean paste. Indirect evidence for studies of ipriflavone, an isoflavone derivative, suggests a potential benefit of isoflavones in preventing osteoporosis.

Clinical evidence suggests the potential beneficial effect of soy isoflavone in the treatment of menopausal symptoms, to prevent heart disease and cancer. A number of case-control studies suggest a link between soy phytoestrogen consumption and reduced risk of breast and other cancers. A meta-analysis of 38 controlled trials reported that consumption of soy is associated to decreased serum concentrations of total cholesterol, LDL cholesterol and triglycerides.

Several randomized clinical trials reported a reduction of menopausal symptoms, particularly hot flushes, with dietary soy product, although these results need confirmation. A study performed on 478 postmenopausal Japanese women who reported soy consumption (mean isoflavones intake: 54.3 mg/day) reported that high consumption of soy products is associated with increased bone mass in postmenopausal women and might be useful for preventing hypoestrogenic effects.

There are no contraindications for phytoestrogens consumed as part of the diet, but their use can cause flatulence. Concentrated isoflavone supplements should be avoided during pregnancy or lactation. Theoretically, large quantities of phytoestrogens may affect the reproductive system. The recommended daily intake of isoflavone is 40—100 mg. Soyselect® is a special patented extract containing 13—17% isoflavones (genistein:daidzein, 3:2).

Further Reading

Adleurcreutz H (2002) Phyto-oestrogens and cancer. Lancet Oncol 3:364–373

Bagchi D, Bagchi M, Stohs S, Ray SD, Sen CK, Preuss HG (2002) Cellular protection with proanthocyanidins derived from grape seeds. Ann N Y Acad Sci 957:260–270

Ewies AA (2002) Phytoestrogens in the management of the menopause: up-to-date. Obstet Gynecol Surv 57:306–313

Renaud SC, Gueguen R, Siest G, Salamon R (1999) Wine, beer and mortality in middle-aged men from Eastern France. Arch Intern Med 159:1865–1870

Scalbert A, Deprez S, Mila I, Albrecht AM, Huneau JF, Rabot S (2000) Proanthocyanidins and human health: systemic effects and local effects in the gut. Biofactors 13:115–120

Somekawa Y, Chiguchi M, Ishibashi T, Takeshi A (2001) Soy intake related to menopausal symptoms. Obstet Gynecol 97:109–115

Appendix B

HERBAL MEDICINES AND CANCER PREVENTION

Cancer is a general term to define any disease characterized by malignant tumor formation or proliferation of anaplastic cells. It is estimated that 25% of the population of the United States will face a cancer diagnosis during their lifetime; a 5-year survival of cancer patients is about 40%, ranking cancer second only to cardiovascular disease as a cause of mortality.

For the past 50 years, the main weapons in the war against cancer have been early detection and surgical removal, radiotherapy, chemotherapy, and attempts to develop gene therapy. However, the results so far are less than ideal; in most cases, these therapies produce only a regression of the disease, and relapse may eventually lead to death.

Cancer patients are very often desperate and may try any treatment that offers hope; therefore, many cancer patients use herbal medicines. Table 1 lists some herbal remedies promoted as "cancer cures", but none of these treatments are backed up by convincing clinical evidence. A different strategy is to switch from therapeutic approaches to prevention of cancer by identifying effective natural products as chemopreventive agents.

HERBAL CHEMOPREVENTIVE AGENTS

Green tea is obtained by the dried leaf of *Camellia sinensis* (L.) Kuntze (also named *Thea sinensis* L.) (Fam. *Theaceae*). When growing wild, the plant is a 5–10 m tall tree, but in cultivation it is maintained as a shrub, through constant picking of the top shoots and young leaves. Green tea is the main type of tea used in Eastern Asia. Its preparation differ from that of black tea in that the fresh leaves are immediately heated. This destroys the enzymes responsible for breaking down the colour pigments in the leaves and allows the tea to maintain its green colour during the subsequent rolling and drying processes. Green tea exhibits anticancer effects in animal experiments. This effect is due to its polyphenol constituents, such as epigallocatechin-3-gallate (the major polyphenolic constituent of green tea). Mechanisms proposed to underlie the inhibition of carcinogenesis by green tea include: (1) the modulation of signal transduction pathways that lead to the inhibition of cell proliferation and transformation;

Table 1
Herbal medicines used in cancer treatment. None of these herbal medicines has shown convincing clinical evidence

Herbal medicine	Description	Main constituent(s)	Pharmacological studies	Clinical evidence	Safety concern
Essiac	This is a formula which consists of four herbal medicines: burdock root (*Arctium lappa*), rhubarb root (*Rheum palmatum*), sheep sorrel (*Rumex acetosella*) and slippery elm bark (*Ulmus fulva*)	Phytoestrogens, anthraquinones, flavonoids, polysaccharides	Experimental studies with individual herbs and isolated compounds (e.g. phytoestrogens, anthraquinones, flavonoids) have detected antioxidant, immunostimulant and antitumor actions	There are no published clinical studies. Evidence of anticancer activity is limited to anecdotal reports recorded for some 40 years in Canada. Individual case reports suggest that essiac improves the quality of life and alleviates pain among cancer patients	Essiac is unlikely to cause serious side-effects
Mistletoe	Mistletoe is obtained from the leaves, branches and berries of *Viscum album*, a semiparasitic evergreen shrub	Mistletoe lectins (viscumin), viscotoxins	Viscumin and viscotoxins stimulate the production of immunostimulant cytokines and inhibit tumor colonisation	Two systematic reviews have found only a few clinical trials (bronchial, colorectal, gastric, breast and genital carcinoma), none of which was conclusive due to significant methodological flaws. Overall, the use of mistletoe extract in the treatment of cancer patients is not recommended	Bradycardia, dehydration, delirium, diarrhea, gastroenteritis, hallucinations, hepatitis, hypo- and hypertension, fever, leukocytosis, mydriasis, myosis, nausea, seizures, vomiting. The injectable preparations are burdened with potentially dramatic allergic reactions

continued on page next page

Table 1

Herbal medicines used in cancer treatment. None of these herbal medicines has shown convincing clinical evidence (*continued*)

Herbal medicine	Description	Main constituent(s)	Pharmacological studies	Clinical evidence	Safety concern
PC-SPES	The herbal formula PC-SPES contains eight herbal medicine: *Dendrathema morifolium* (Chrysanthemum), *Isatis indigotica* (Dyer's woad), *Glycyrrhiza glabra* (Liquorice), *Ganoderma lucidum* (Reishi), *Panax pseudoginseng* (San-Qi ginseng), *Rabdosia rubescens* (Rubescens), *Serenoa repens* (saw palmetto), *Scutellaria baicalensis* (Baikal skullcap)	Polysaccharides, phytosterols, fatty acids, flavonoids	Isolated substances from PC-SPES possess immunostimulant and antitumoral activity. PC-SPES lowers prostate-specific antigen in patients with prostate cancer and inhibits the growth of prostate cancer cells *in vitro*	The encouraging pre-clinical studies require confirmation in clinical trials in patients with prostate cancer	Reduced libido, hot flashes, diarrhea, dyspepsia, leg cramps, gynecomastia, nipple tenderness, pulmonary emboli, vein thrombosis
Shosaiko-to (Chinese name:Xiao-Chai-Hu-Tang)	Shosaiko-to is a Kampo (Japanese herbal) mixture of seven different medicinal plants: *Buplerum falcatum* root (thorowax), *Glycyrrhiza baicalensis* root (liquorice, gan cao), *Panax ginseng* root (ginseng), *Pinellia ternata* rhizome (ban xia), *Scutellaria baicalensis* root (Chinese skullcap), *Zingiber officinale* rhizome (ginger) *Zizyphus jujuba* fruit (jujube)	Polysaccharides, ginsenosides, flavonoids, essential oils, saponins	Shosaiko-to has direct cytostatic and cytotoxic effects on hepatocellular carcinoma cell lines. It stimulates the synthesis of immunostimulant cytokines	A study on 260 patients with hepatocellular carcinoma and cirrhosis has been performed. The 5-year survival rate showed a non-significant trend to be higher in patients treated with Shosaiko-to (compared to patients treated with conventional drugs)	Although Shosaiko-to has long been considered to have very few, and only minor, side effects, in recent years a number of cases of acute pneumonitis have been reported

(2) the induction of apoptosis of pre-neoplastic and neoplastic cells and (3) the inhibition of tumour invasion and angiogenesis. Epidemiological studies suggest that the regular consumption of green tea conveys a moderate reduction of cancer risk, particularly oesophageal cancer. Epidemiological studies also suggest an inverse association between green tea consumption and some pre-neoplastic conditions, such as chronic gastritis and intestinal adenomatous polyps. The bulk of such evidence stems from data on drinking tea (6–10 cups daily) rather than consuming tea leaf supplements. By contrast, there is currently no clear epidemiological evidence to support the suggestion that green tea plays a role in the prevention of stomach and colon cancer. It is important to emphasize that there is no good clinical evidence for the ability of green tea to change the course of the existing disease. There are no serious safety concerns associated to green tea consumption; however, due to its caffeine content, insomnia may occur.

► *See Chapter 21 for the antidiarrheal activity of tea*

Ginseng is the root of *Panax ginseng* C.A. Meyer (Fam. *Araliaceae*), an ancient Chinese medicine, employed as a kind of panacea. On the basis of the hypothesis that the life-prolonging effect of ginseng reported by Shennong's Ancient Chinese medical book could be due to its efficacy in preventing the development of cancer, Korean researchers have, since 1978, carried out extensive long-term anticarcinogenicity experiments in animals and confirmed the antitumoral action of ginseng. Ginseng extract and ginsenosides exert a tumor-protective effect through stimulation of the immune system. A study carried out in a Ginseng-growing region in Korea, where 4634 inhabitants were assessed by questionnaire on ginseng intake, showed a reduced risk of cancer in individuals who regularly consumed fresh ginseng. These studies, however, are not ultimately convincing. Ginseng is not entirely free of risk. Adverse effects of ginseng can include insomnia, diarrhea, vaginal bleeding, mastalgia, swollen tender breasts, manic episodes, and Stevens-Johnson syndrome. Overdose of ginseng is defined as "ginseng abuse syndrome" with symptoms including hypertension, sleeplessness, skin eruptions, morning diarrhea and agitation.

► *See Chapter 14 for the use of ginseng in the treatment of angina*
► *See Chapter 19 for the adaptogenic properties of ginseng*

Garlic and onion are well known perennial herbs used as food. There are several lines of evidence to suggest that the regular consumption of *Allium* vegetables (Fam. *Alliaceae*) is tumor-protective. *Allium* derivatives regulate immune function and inflammation, in addition to cellular proliferation. Experimental studies have shown that alliins, abundant in garlic (*Allium sativum* L.) and onion (*Allium cepa* L.), inhibits chemically-induced stomach cancer in animals. Site-

specific case-control studies and cohort studies suggest a preventive effect of *Allium* vegetables consumption against stomach, colorectal and prostate cancer, although evidence for a protective effect against cancer at other sites, including the breast, is still lacking.
It is noteworthy that a population-based, case-control study (n = 238 subjects with prostate cancer) showed that men in the category of highest intake of total *Allium* vegetables (> 10 g/day) had a statistically significant lower risk of contracting prostate cancer than did those in the category of lowest intake (< 2.2 g/day).

► *See Chapter 14 for the use of garlic in hypertension*
► *See Chapter 15 for the use of garlic in the treatment of hypercholesterolemia*

Further Reading

Borchers AT, Sakai S, Henderson GL, Harkey MR, Keen CL, Stern JS, Teresawa K, Gerhwin ME (2000) Shosaiko-to and other Kampo (Japanese herbal) medicines: a review of their immunomodulatory activities. J Ethnopharmacol 73:1–13

Bushman JL (1998) Green tea and cancer in humans: a review of the literature. Nutr Cancer 31:151–159

Ernst E, Cassileth BR (1999) How useful are unconventional cancer treatments? Eur J Cancer 35:1608–1613

Ernst E (2000) The role of complementary and alternative medicine in cancer. Lancet Oncol 1:176–180

Fleischauer AT, Arab L (2001) Garlic and cancer: a critical review of the epidemiologic literature. J. Nutr 131:1032S–1040S

Fujiki H, Suganuma M, Imai K, Nakachi K (2002) Green tea: cancer preventive beverage and/or drug. Cancer Lett 188:9–13

Hsing AW, Chokkalingam AP, Gao YT, Madigan MP, Deng J, Gridley G, Fraumeni JF Jr (2002) Allium vegetables and risk of prostate cancer: a population-based study. J Natl Cancer Inst 94:1648–1651

Izzo AA, Capasso F (2003) Herbal medicine, cancer prevention and cyclooxygenase 2. Trends Pharmacol Sci 24:218–219.

Pandha HS, Kirby RS (2002) PC-SPES: phytotherapy for prostate cancer. Lancet 259:2213–2215

Tamayo C, Richardson MA, Diamond S, Skoda I (2000) The chemistry and biological activity of herbs used in flor-essence herbal tonic and essiac. Phytother Res 14:1–14

Yang CS, Maliakal P, Meng X (2002) Inhibition of carcinogenesis by tea. Annu Rev Pharmacol Toxicol 42:25–54

Yun T-K (2001) Panax ginseng. A non organ specific cancer preventive. Lancet Oncol 2:49–55

Appendix C

Herbs in Traditional Chinese and Indian Medicine

Plants have long been the principal tools of traditional medical systems. Although ancient in origin, many traditional medical systems have evolved into quite sophisticated healing systems and in Western countries chemical drugs have generally replaced traditional herbal medicine.

In many parts of the world, such as China and India, traditional medicine is still used to provide a major part of primary health care. The World Health Organisation has estimated that the majority of the world's population depends on botanical medicines for basic health care needs. Reasons for this include cultural compliance, cheaper price as compared to chemical drugs, and belief in efficacy.

The paucity of studies to support the efficacy and safety of individual plants or plant mixtures constitutes a major criticism of non-Western botanical healing systems. Rigorous studies include randomized clinical data on efficacy as well as information on toxicity, dosage, method of use, and adverse reactions.

Herbs in Traditional Chinese Medicine (TCM)

Traditional Chinese Medicine is based on the rationalization of certain philosophical concepts of the universe and all known facts are related and incorporated into these theories. TCM represents one aspect of the Chinese medical philosophy that is characterized by its emphasis on maintaining and restoring body balance. Without an understanding of the philosophical basis of TCM it is very difficult for Western culture to evaluate the value of TCM as a system of medicine.

Medicinal plants play an key role in TCM. In recent years, following the expansion of the market for Chinese herbal medications, a great deal of research has been carried out on traditional Chinese herbs. Table 1 lists some traditional Chinese herbal medicines. Most Chinese formulations contain a mixture of herbs.

Most Westerners do not take TCM seriously, considering it unscientific in its understanding of the human body and the nature of disease and its treatment. The adoption of TCM in industrialized countries is impeded by a lack of quality

Table 1
Examples of traditional Chinese herbal medicines

Latin name	Chinese name	English name	Main constituent(s)	Conditions frequently treated
Acanthopanax gracilistylus	Pi Wu Jia	Acanthopanax	Pregnanes	Rheumatic arthritis, scrotal oedema
Acanthopanax senticosus (*Eleutherococcus senticosus*)	Ci Wu Jia	Siberian ginseng	Eleutherosides	Immunodeficiency, cancer, obesity, stress states
Aconitum charmichaelii	Chuan Wu Tou	Aconite (monkshood)	Aconitine	Cardiac disease, pain, diarrhea
Adenophora tetraphylla	Sha Seng	Ladybell	Stigmasterol	Cough
Adonis chrysocyathus	Fu Shou Cao	Adonis	Cymarin, corchoroside, convallatoxin	Inflammation
Angelica sinensis	Dong quai	Chinese angelica	Ligustilide	Women's diseases, thrombophlebitis
Artemisia annua	Quing hao su	Sweet annie	Artemisinin	Malaria, lupus, diarrhea
Asarum sieboldi	Xi Xin	Azamaru, wild ginger	Asarinine	Pain, colds
Astragalus membranaceous	Huang Se	Milk vetch	Astragalosides	Infections, fatigue,aids, immunodeficiency
Atractylodes chinensis	Cang Zhu	Thistle	Atractylol	Digestive disorders, pain
Camellia sinensis	Cha i	Tea	Polyphenols, theophylline	Stress diseases, fatigue, dyspepsia
Chysanthemum indicum	Yao Jin Hua	Chyrsanthemum	Chrysanthinin	Headache, insomnia, dizziness
Cimicifuga foetida	Sheng Ma	Bugbane	Cimifugin	Infections, headache, fever, bronchitis, tonsillitis
Coptis sinensis	Huang Lian	Goldthread	Coptisine	Fever, diarrhea
Evodia rutaecarpa	Wu-chu-yu	Evodia	Rutaecarpine	Hypertension
Ganoderma lucidum	Ling Chi	Reishi mushroom	Ganoderic acids	Bronchitis, cancer, allergy, immunodeficiency
Ginkgo biloba	Bai Guo	Ginkgo	Ginkgolides	Circulatory diseases, dementia, asthma, cough
Gossypium hirsutum	Mian Hua Gan	Indian cotton	Gossypol	Fertility (prevention)

continued on page next page

Table 1
Examples of traditional Chinese herbal medicine (*continued*)

Latin name	Chinese name	English name	Main constituent(s)	Conditions frequently treated
Glycyrrhiza uralensis	Gan Cao	Liquorice	Glycyrrhizin	Peptic ulcers, hepatitis, eczema, cough
Gynostemma pentaphyllum	Jiao Chiu Lan	Sweet tea, vine, Southern ginseng	Gypenosides	Stress diseases, anxiety, hypertension, cancer
Ligusticum wallichii	Chuan xiong	Ligusticum	Alkaloids	Hypertension
Ligustrum lucidum	Nu Zhen Zi	Glossy privet	Ligustrin	Infection, immuno-deficiency
Lobelia chinensis	Ban Bian Lian	Lobelia	Lobeline	Hydro-retention
Lonicera japonica	Jin Yin Hua	Honeysuckle	Saponins	Fever, pharyngitis, diarrhea
Lycium chinense	Di Gu Pi	Wolfberry	Kukoamines	Diabetes mellitus
Magnolia liliflora	Xin Yi Hua	Magnolia	Citral	Nasal congestion, sinusitis
Momordica charantia	Ku Gua Zi	Bitter melon	Charantin	Diabetes, infections, aids
Momordica grosvernorii	Luo Han Guo	Monk fruit	Mognosides	Cough, dyspepsia
Morus alba	Sang Zhi	Mulberry	Morin	Rheumatic complaints, hypertension, hydro-retention
Nerium indicum	Jia Zhu Tao	Rose laurel	Oleandrin	Congestive heart failure
Ophiopogon japonicus	Mar Dong	Onion grass	Mucilage	Bronchitis, laryngitis, cough
Paeonia lactiflora	Bai Shao	Peony	Paeoniflorin	Dysmenorrhea, spasm
Panax ginseng	Ren shen	Ginseng	Ginsenosides	Stress diseases, diabetes, heart disease, cancer
Panax notoginseng	San Qi	Tienchi ginseng	Ginsenosides	Bleeding disorders, heart disease
Perilla frutescens	Zi Su Zi	Beefsteak plant	Perilla aldehyde	Colds, cough, fever
Periploca sepium	Xiang Jia Pi	Chinese silkvine	Periplocin	Rheumatic complaints
Phellodendron chinense	Huang Bai	Cork-tree	Isoquinolines	Diarrhea, vaginitis, inflammation
Picrorhiza kurroa	Hu Huang	Picrorhiza	Kutkin	Antipyretic, asthma, vitiligo
Pinellia ternata	Banxia	Pinellia	Coniine	Cough, bronchitis

continued on page next page

Table 1

Examples of traditional Chinese herbal medicine (*continued*)

Latin name	Chinese name	English name	Main constituent(s)	Conditions frequently treated
Platycodon grandiflorum	Jie Geng	Balloon flower	Playcodigenin	Bronchitis, tonsillitis, parasite infections
Polygala tenuifolia	Yuan Zhi	Chinese senega	Teneuifolin	Cough, bronchitis
Polygonum multiflorum	Ho Shou Wu	Knotweed, cornbind, fleece flower	Antraquinones	Bronchitis, infections, atherosclerosis, neurasthenia
Pueraria lobata	Geh Gen	Kudzu vine	Daidzen	Alcohol abuse, fever
Pulsatilla chinensis	Bai Tou Weng	Anemone Pasque flower	Anemonin	Fever, infections, dysentery, analgesia
Rauwolfia verticillata	Luo Fu Mu	Rauwolfia	Reserpine	Anxiety and insomnia, hypertension
Rehmania glutinosa	Di Huang	Chinese foxglove	Jionosides	Allergies, bleeding disorders, rheumatism
Rheum palmatum	Tai Huang	Rhubarb	Antraquinones	Constipation, fever
Rhododendron molle	Ba Li Ma	Chinese azalea	Rhomotoxin	Hypertention, anxiety
Salvia miltiorrhiza	Tan Seng	Red root sage	Tanshinones	Circulatory disease, hepatitis, menstrual disorders
Schizandra chinensis	Wu Wei Zi	Magnolia vine	Schizandrins	Liver disease, cough, stress states
Scutellaria baicalensis	Huang Qin	Skullcap, scute	Baicalin	Allergies, bronchitis, enteritis, hypertension, inflammation
Sophora japonica	Huai Hua Huai Mi	Pagoda tree	Sophoretin	Bleeding disorders, fever, hypertension
Stephania tetrandra	Fang Ji Han Fang Ji		Tetrandrine	Hydro-retention, rheumatic complaints, inflammation
Syzygium aromaticum	Ding Xiang	Clove	Eugenol	Emesis, dental pain, local anaesthesia

continued on page next page

Table 1
Examples of traditional Chinese herbal medicine (*continued*)

Latin name	Chinese name	English name	Main constituent(s)	Conditions frequently treated
Thevetia spp.	Huang Hua Jia Zhu Tao	Yellow oleander	Thevetin	Cardiac disease
Trichosanthes kirilowii	Gua Lou, Tian Hua Fen	Chinese cucumber	Tricosanthin	Cancer, AIDS, angina
Tripterygium wilfordii	Lei Gong Teng	Thunder God vine	Triptolides	Arthritis, inflammation, immune diseases (immunosuppressant)

(From Rotblatt and Ziment, modified)

control and the absence of scientific and clinical proof of their effectiveness. Serious consideration of Chinese herbal medicines as a form of medical treatment requires a thoughtful examination of certain fundamental issues such as source materials, standardization, biological assays and clinical studies.

Herbs in Ayurvedic Medicine

Ayurveda has been the main medical approach in India for more than six thousand years. "Ayurveda" means the "science of life and longevity": this practice combines diet, exercise, spiritual activities and medicinal herbs in a holistic healing system. For an Ayurvedic doctor the health is a state of balance of the body's systems (physical, emotional, spiritual), while the illness is a state of imbalance. Ayurvedic medicine treats the whole person, rather than the disease, and every therapeutic regime is highly individualized.

The use of herbs in traditional Indian medicine is based on experience, philosophy and some crude beliefs. Some herbs are considered of value in enhancing the physical and mental performance, many others work by improving the body's ability to fight disease without specific effect. Also, modern Ayurvedic books emphasize the use of herbal products in a number of specific diseases (Table 2).

As in the case of traditional Chinese Medicine, there is still insufficient clinical evidence to justify the use of Ayurvedic herbs. Other concerns include lack of standardization, contamination, paucity of toxicology studies and a dearth of critical evaluation.

Table 2
Examples of traditional Indian (Ayurvedic) herbal medicines

Latin name	Indian name (sanskrit)	English name	Major constituent(s)	Conditions frequently treated
Abies spectabilis	Talisapatra	Himalayan silver	Taxins	Pulmonary affections
Acorus calamus	Vacha	Sweet flag	Volatile oil (asaryl aldehyde)	Bronchitis, cough, spasms
Adhatoda vasica	Vasaka	Malabar nut	Vasicine	Asthma, bronchitis
Aegle marmelos	Bilva - Shriphala	Bael fruit	Marmelosin	Diarrhea, colitis, worms
Albizzia lebbek	Shirish	Siris	Echinocystic acid	Cancer, parasites infestation
Alpinia galanga	Malayavach	Java glangal	Galangol	Sexual disfunction, bronchitis, rheumatic disorders
Andrographis paniculata	Kirta	Andrographis	Andrographolides	Infections, liver disease, cardiovascular disease
Areca catechu	Pooga	Areca nut	Arecoline	Lack of stamina
Asparagus racemosus	Shatavari	Asparagus	Asparasaponin	Immunodeficiency, spasms, reduced milk secretion
Azadiracta indica	Aristha	Persian lilac	Azadiratin	Bacterial infections, skin diseases
Boswellia serrata	Shallaki	Indian olibaum	Boswellic acid	Arthritis, inflammation
Boerhaavia diffusa	Punarnava	Spreading	Punarnavine	Hydro-retention, bronchitis
Bacopa monniera	Brahmi	Bacopa	Bacosides	Dementia, epilepsy
Centella asiatica (*Hydrocotile asiatica*)	Mandukaparni	Hydrocotyle	Triterpenes	Reduced memory, lack of stamina, stress states
Commiphora mukul	Goggulu	Indian myrrh (guggul)	Myrcene	Hypercholesterolemia, menstrual disease
Datura metal	Datura	Thornapple	Hyoscine	Asthma, spasms, eye disease
Emblica officinalis	Amalik	Emblic myrobalan	Tannins phillemblic acid	Dyspepsia, diarrhea
Gymnema sylvestre	Meshasringi	Gymnema	Gymnemic acid	Diabetes, hypercholesterolemia

continued on page next page

Table 2
Examples of traditional Indian (Ayurvedic) herbal medicines (*continued*)

Latin name	Indian name (sanscrit)	English name	Major constituent(s)	Conditions frequently treated
Hemidesmus indicus	Sariva	Indian sarsaparilla	Coumarins	Skin disease, arthritis
Picrorhiza kurroa	Katula	Picrorhiza	Kutkin	Infections, hepatitis, immunodeficiency
Piper longum	Pipali	Long pepper	Piperine	Bronchitis, dyspepsia
Rauwolfia serpentina	Sarpagandha	Snakeroot	Reserpine	Hypertension, anxiety
Terminalia arjuna	Arjuna	Arjun tree	Arjungenin	Heart and circulatory diseases
Terminalia chebula	Haritaki	Chebulic myrobalan	Chebulinic acid	Bronchitis, dyspepsia, constipation
Tribulus terrestris	Gokshura	Small caltrops	Harmine	Genitourinary disorders, pain
Withania somnifera	Ashwagandha	Winter cherry	Withanolides	Stress states, lack of stamina, immunodeficiency

Further Reading

Chang Uang K (1999) The pharmacology of Chinese herbs. CRP Press LLC, Boca Raton

Chopra A, Doiphode VV (2002) Ayurvedic medicine. Core concept, therapeutic principles, and current relevance. Med Clin North Am 86:75-89

Khan S, Balick MJ (2001) Therapeutic plants of Ayurveda: a review of selected clinical and other studies for 166 species. J Altern Complement Med 7:405-415

Nestler G, Dovey M (2001) Traditional Chinese medicine. Clin Obstet Gynecol 44:801-13

Rotblatt M, Ziment I (2002) Herbal Medicine. Harley and Belfus Inc, Philadelphia

Tripathi YB (2000) Molecular approach to ayurveda. Indian J Exp Biol 38:409-414

Yuan R, Lin Y (2000) Traditional Chinese medicine: an approach to scientific proof and clinical validation. Pharmacol Ther 86:191-198

Appendix D

Summary of the Clinical Efficacy of Herbal Medicines

In view of the level of popularity of herbal medicine, it is desirable to have reliable information about their efficacy. This can be achieved by performing clinical trials, i.e. experiments carried out to assess the effectiveness in humans. In **controlled clinical trials**, volunteers are allocated to one of two groups, the treatment group or the control group. The treatment group receives the drug (e.g. herbal medicine) to be evaluated. The control group receives either a standard drug for the condition (generally a synthetic drug of proven effectiveness) or a **placebo** (an inactive material identical in appearance to a drug undergoing testing). Any placebo effects are assumed to be psychological, or suggested by the process of taking a medicine. Such effects are discounted from the real actions of the drug under study. **Randomisation** (random allocation of participants to the treatment and control groups) avoids any bias in selection. Whenever possible, it is preferable that neither the participant nor the investigator knows which treatment has been administered until after the end of the trial. This is called a **double-blind** design. A **single-blind** design is when the investigator, but not the participant, knows the treatment administered.

In evaluating a herbal medicine for a specific pathological state, different clinical trials could not always agree in their conclusion. Hence, only the totality of the available data will provide the most reliable evidence of effectiveness (or lack of effectiveness). The aim of summarizing research evidence can be achieved by conducting systematic reviews and meta-analysis. **Systematic reviews** take care to find all relevant studies published and unpublished, assess each study, synthesize the findings from individual studies in an unbiased way and present a balanced and impartial summary of the findings with due consideration of any flaws in the evidence. **Meta-analysis** represent a sub-species of systematic reviews, which pool data from individual trials and calculate a new overall effect size of a particular outcome measure. In herbal medicine, systematic reviews/meta-analysis are of particular importance because i) people often do not have objective views, ii) the literature is scarce and often published in journals which are not easily accessible, and iii) clinical trials of herbal medicine are often published in languages other than English (most are, in fact, published in German).

Clinical evidence of herbal medicines in a specific pathological state depends on three different factors: i) the type of trial (the highest level of evidence is given by systematic review/meta-analysis, followed by randomised clinical trials, controlled clinical trials and uncontrolled studies); ii) the methodological quality of the studies which can be judged, for example, by assessing methods of randomisation and blinding and the description of dropouts (subjects who withdraw from the trial); iii) the number of subjects participating in a single trial and the number of trials. Table 1 reports the clinical evidence of some herbal medicines in specific pathological states.

Table 1

Clinical efficacy of herbal medicines in specific pathological states. Reference of systematic reviews, meta-analyses and recent relevant papers are indicated by a superscript number in the column "source of evidence". Other references can be found in "The Desktop Guide to Complementary and Alternative Medicine – an Evidence-based Approach", edited by E. Ernst et al. (2001), Mosby – Harcourt Publishers Limited, London, UK

Pathological state	Herbal medicine Latin name	Herbal medicine Common name	Clinical evidence	Source of evidence
AIDS infection	*Buxus sempervirens*	Boxwood	Preliminarily positive	One RCT
Acne	*Melaleuca alternifolia*	Tea tree oil	Clearly positive	Systematic review one RCT (n=124)[1]
Alzheimer's disease	*Ginkgo biloba*	Ginkgo	Clearly positive (modest effect)	Meta-analysis (4 placebo-controlled, double-blind RCTs, n=424)[2]
Anxiety	*Piper methysticum*	Kava	Clearly positive	Systematic review (7 RCTs, n=377)[3]
Asthma	*Ginkgo biloba*	Ginkgo	Preliminarily positive	Systematic review (1 placebo-controlled study, n=61)[4]
	Ligusticum walichii	Sichuan lovage	Preliminarily positive	Systematic review (1 placebo-controlled RCT, n=150)[4]
	Tylophora indica	Indian ipecac	Tentatively negative	Systematic review (5 RCTs, n=583)
	Picrorhiza kurroa	Picrorhiza	Clearly negative	Systematic review (1 double-blind placebo-controlled RCT, n=72)[4]

continued on page next page

Table 1
Clinical efficacy of herbal medicines in specific pathological states (*continued*)

Pathological state	Herbal medicine Latin name	Herbal medicine Common name	Clinical evidence	Source of evidence
	Solanum spp.	Kantakari	Preliminary positive	Systemic review (1 RCT, n=60)[4]
	Boswellia serrata	Boswellia (Indian olibaum)	Preliminarily positive	Systematic review (1 double-blind placebo-controlled RCT, n=80)[4]
	*	Tsumura saiboku-to (TJ-96)	Preliminarily positive	Systematic review (1 double-blind placebo RCT)[4]
	Hedera helix	English ivy	Preliminarily positive	Systematic review (1 double-blind placebo-controlled RCT, n=24)[4]
Atopic eczema	*Borago officinalis*	Borage	Tentatively negative	Two double-blind RCTs (n=210)
	Oenothera biennis	Evening primrose	Tentatively negative	Four double blind RCTs (n=273)
	Matricaria recutita	German chamomile	Uncertain	One non-randomized trial (n=161)
Back pain	*Harpagophytum procumbens*	Devil's claw	Preliminarily positive	One placebo-controlled, double-blind RCT (n=118)
Benign prostatic hyperplasia	*Pygeum africanum*	Pigeum (African plum)	Clearly positive (modest effect)	Meta-analysis (18 RCTs) (n=1562)[5]
	Urtica dioica	Nettle	Tentatively positive	Four placebo-controlled, double-blind RCTs (n=210)
	Cucurbita pepo	Pumpkin	Clearly positive	One double-blind RCT in combination with saw palmetto
	Pollen of *Secale cereale*	Rye grass pollen	Clearly positive (modest effect)	Systematic review (4 RCTs, n=444)[6]
	Serenoa repens	Saw palmetto	Clearly positive	Meta-analysis (18 RCTs, n=2939) (16 double-blind)[7]
Cancer (prevention)	*Allium* spp	*Allium* vegetables such as garlic and onion	Preliminarily positive	Systematic review (20 epidemiological studies)[8]
	Thea sinensis	Green tea	Clearly positive	Systematic review (31 epidemiological studies)[9]

continued on page next page

Table 1

Clinical efficacy of herbal medicines in specific pathological states (*continued*)

Pathological state	Herbal medicine Latin name	Herbal medicine Common name	Clinical evidence	Source of evidence
	Panax ginseng	Ginseng	Tentatively positive	One epidemiological study (n=4634)
Cancer (treatment)	*Arctium lappa, Rheum palmatum, Rumex acetosella, Ulmus fulva*	Essiac (a combination of rhubarb, shepp sorrel, burdock and slippery elm)	Uncertain	Unpublished observation
	**	PC – SPES	Tentatively positive	Preclinical studies in humans
	Viscum album	Mistletoe	Uncertain	Small poor quality clinical trials
Chronic fatigue syndrome	*Oenothera biennis*	Evening primrose	Uncertain	Two placebo-controlled, double-blind (n=113)
Chronic venous insufficiency	*Fagopyrum esculentum*	Buckwheat	Preliminarily positive	One double-blind RCT (n=67)
	Ruscus aculeatus	Butcher's broom	Preliminarily positive	One placebo-controlled, double-blind RCT (n=166)[10]
	Centella asiatica	Gotu kola	Clearly positive	Three double-blind RCTs (two with placebo)
	Aesculus hippocastanum	Horse chestnut	Preliminarily positive	Systematic review (13 RCTs, n=1083) (7 with placebo)[11]
	Vitis vinifera	Grape leaves	Preliminarily positive	One placebo-controlled double-blind RCT (n=260)
	Pinus pinaster	French maritime pine	Clearly positive	Nine double-blind CCT (n=420) (6 placebo-controlled)[12]
Congestive heart failure	*Panax ginseng*	Ginseng	Preliminarily positive	One CCT (n=45)
	Crataegus laevigata	Hawthorn	Clearly positive	Several placebo-controlled RCTs
	Terminalia arjuna	Arjun tree	Preliminarily positive	One RCT (n=12)

continued on page next page

Table 1

Clinical efficacy of herbal medicines in specific pathological states (*continued*)

Pathological state	Herbal medicine Latin name	Herbal medicine Common name	Clinical evidence	Source of evidence
Constipation	*Plantago psyllium*	Psyllium positive	Tentatively placebo controlled	One double-blind, RCT (n=20)
	***	Misrakasneham	Preliminarily positive	One RCT (n=20)
Depression (mild to moderate)	*Hypericum perforatum*	St John's wort	Clearly positive	Meta-analysis (27 placebo-controlled RCTs, n=2291)[13]
Depression (major depression)	*Hypericum perforatum*	St John's wort	Preliminarily negative	One double-blind placebo controlled RCT (n=200)[14]
Diarrhea	*Musa sapientum*	Banana (unripe)	Preliminarily positive	One double-blind RCT (n=62)[15]
Dyspepsia	*Chelidonium majus*	Greater celandine	Preliminarily positive	One placebo-controlled double-blind RCT (n=60)[16]
	Curcuma longa	Turmeric	Preliminarily positive	One double-blind placebo-controlled RCT (n=116)[16]
	Capsicum annuum	Chili	Clearly positive	One double-blind placebo-controlled clinical trial (n=30)[17]
	Gentiana lutea	Gentian	Preliminarily positive	One RCT (n=359)[16]
	Musa sapientum	Banana	Preliminarily positive	One RCT (n=46)[16]
	Emblica officinalis	Emblic myrobalan	Preliminarily positive	One RCT (n=38)[16]
	Mentha piperita *Carum carvi*	Peppermint and Caraway	Clearly positive	Four RCTs (n=484)[16]
Drug/alcohol dependence	*Pueraria lobata*	Kudzu	Preliminarily negative	One RCT (n=38)
Erectile dysfunction	*Ginkgo biloba*	Ginkgo	Preliminarily positive	Uncontrolled study (n=73)
	Panax ginseng	Ginseng	Preliminarily positive	One placebo-controlled RCT (not double-blind) (n=90)

continued on page next page

Table 1
Clinical efficacy of herbal medicines in specific pathological states (*continued*)

Pathological state	Herbal medicine Latin name	Herbal medicine Common name	Clinical evidence	Source of evidence
	Mucuna pruriens, Withania somnifera	Mustang Ashwagandha	Preliminarily positive	One uncontrolled study (n=25)
Hay fever	*Urtica dioica*	Stinging nettle	Preliminarily positive	One double-blind RCT (n=69)
Headache	*Mentha piperita*	Peppermint oil (local application)	Clearly positive	One placebo-controlled RCT (n=205)
Hepatitis	*Glycyrrhiza glabra*	Liquorice	Preliminarily positive	One RCT (n=28) and a retrospective analysis (n=84)
	Silybum marianum	Milk thistle	Tentatively positive	Systematic review (4 RCTs)
	Phyllanthus spp. (e.g. P. Amarus, P. urinaria, niruri)	Black catnip	Tentatively positive	Systematic review (22 placebo-controlled RCTs, n=1947)[18]
Herpes simplex (prevention)	*Eleutherococcus senticosus*	Siberian ginseng	Preliminarily positive	One placebo-controlled RCT (n=93)
Herpes simplex (treatment)	*Melissa officinalis*	Lemon balm	Preliminarily positive	One placebo-controlled RCT (n=66)
Herpes (genital herpes)	****	Propolis	Preliminarily positive	Three controlled RCTs (n=30)
	Aloe spp.	Aloe gel	Preliminarily positive	Systematic review (2 RCTs (n=180)[19]
Herpes zoster	*Clinacanthus nutans*	Phaya Yo	Preliminarily positive	1 CCT (n=51) and 1 larger RCT
Hypercholesterolemia	*Trigonella foenum graecum*	Fenugreek	Clearly positive	Systematic review (6 RCTs)[20]
	Commiphora mukul	Gugulipid	Tentatively positive	Systematic review (5 RCTs)
	Cynara scolymus	Artichoke	Preliminarily positive	Systematic review (1 double-blind RCT, n=44)
	Plantago psyllium	Psyllium	Clearly positive (modest effect)	Meta-analysis (8 RCTs, n=384)[20]
	Allium sativum	Garlic	Clearly positive (modest effect)	Meta-analysis (13 double-blind, placebo-controlled RCTs, n=781)

continued on page next page

Table 1
Clinical efficacy of herbal medicines in specific pathological states (*continued*)

Pathological state	Herbal medicine Latin name	Herbal medicine Common name	Clinical evidence	Source of evidence
	Cyamopsis tetragonolobus	Guar gum	Preliminary positive	Systematic review (1 double blind, placebo-controlled RCT[20]
Insomnia	*Piper methysticum*	Kava	Preliminarily positive	One placebo-controlled trial (n=12)
	Valeriana officinalis	Valerian	Tentatively positive	Systematic review (9 placebo-controlled RCTs, n=390)[21]
Intermittent claudication	*Allium sativum*	Garlic	Preliminarily positive	One double-blind, placebo-controlled RCT (n=64)
	Ginkgo biloba	Ginkgo	Clearly positive	Meta-analysis (8 double-blind, placebo-controlled RCTs, n=415)[22]
Irritable bowel syndrome	*Plantago psyllium*	Isphagula	Tentatively positive	Three double-blind placebo-controlled RCTs (n=202)
	Mentha piperita	Peppermint oil	Tentatively positive	Meta-analysis (8 RCTs, n=295) (seven studies double-blind)[23]
Menopausal symptoms	*Cimicifuga racemosa*	Black cohosh	Preliminarily positive	Systematic review (4 RCTs, n=226)[24]
	Angelica sinensis	Dong quai	Preliminarily negative	One double-blind placebo-controlled RCT (n= 71)
	Oenothera biennis	Evening primrose oil	Preliminarily negative	One double-blind placebo-controlled RCT (n= 56)
	Panax ginseng	Ginseng	Preliminarily positive	One double-blind, placebo-controlled RCT (n=384)
	Piper methysticum	Kava	Preliminarily positive	Two double-blind, placebo-controlled RCTs (n=40)

continued on page next page

Table 1

Clinical efficacy of herbal medicines in specific pathological states (*continued*)

Pathological state	Herbal medicine Latin name	Herbal medicine Common name	Clinical evidence	Source of evidence
	Trifolium pratense	Red clover	Clearly negative	Systematic review (2 double-blind RCTs)[25]
	Hypericum perforatum	St John's wort	Preliminarily positive	One uncontrolled study and 1 RCT
Migraine	*Tanacetum parthenium*	Feverfew	Tentatively positive	Systematic review (4 placebo-controlled RCTs, n=196)[26]
	Petasites hybridus	Butterbur	Preliminarily positive	One double-blind CCT[27]
Nausea and vomiting	*Zingiber officinale*	Ginger	Clearly positive	Systematic review (6 placebo-controlled RCTs, n=480)[28]
Osteoarthritis	*Harpagophytum procumbens*	Devil's claw	Clearly positive	Systematic review (2 double-blind, placebo controlled RCTs, n=139)[29,30]
	Zingiber officinale	Ginger	Uncertain	Systematic review (one double-blind, placebo controlled RCTs, n=56)[29,30]
	Populus tremula *Fraxinus excelsior* *Solidago virgaurea*	Phytodolor®	Clearly positive	Systematic review (6 double blind RCTs, n=537)[29,30]
	Petiveria alliacea	Tipi	Preliminarily negative	One placebo-controlled RCT
	Urtica dioica	Stinging nettle (topical treatment)	Preliminarily positive	Systematic review (1 double-blind placebo-controlled RCT, n=27)[29,30]
	Salix spp .	Willow bark	Preliminarily positive	Systematic review (1 double-blind placebo-controlled RCT, n=78)[29,30]

continued on page next page

Table 1
Clinical efficacy of herbal medicines in specific pathological states (*continued*)

Pathological state	Herbal medicine Latin name	Herbal medicine Common name	Clinical evidence	Source of evidence
Obesity	*Cyamopsis tetragonolobus*	Guar gum	Clearly negative	Meta-analysis (20 double-blind, placebo-controlled RCTs, n=392)
	Garcinia cambogia	Malabar tamarind	Preliminarily negative	One double-blind placebo-controlled RCT (n=135)
	Rheum palmatum	Rhubarb	Preliminarily positive	Three RCTs (n=472)[32]
Premenstrual syndrome	*Vitex agnus castus*	Chasteberry	Tentatively positive	Several uncontrolled studies (n=1634) and three double-blind RCT (n=522)[33]
	Oenothera biennis	Evening primrose oil	Tentatively negative	Systematic review (11 clinical trials, n=455) (4 RCTs)[34]
	Ginkgo biloba	Ginkgo	Preliminarily negative	One double-blind placebo-controlled RCT (n=163)
	Hypericum perforatum	St John's wort	Preliminarily positive	One small pilot study (n= 19)
Psoriasis	*Aloe vera*	Aloe gel	Preliminarily positive	One RCT (n=60)[19]
Rheumatoid arthritis	*Ribes nigrum*	Blackcurrant	Tentatively negative	Systematic review (1 placebo-controlled RCT, n=34)[30]
	Borago officinalis	Borage	Clearly positive	Systematic review (2 placebo-controlled double-blind RCTs, n=93)[30]
	Boswellia serrata	Boswellia (Indian olibaum)	Preliminarily negative	One placebo-controlled RCT, n=37)[30]
	Oenothera biennis	Evening primrose oil	Tentatively positive	Systematic review (one placebo-controlled double-blind RCT, n=49)[30]

continued on page next page

Table 1
Clinical efficacy of herbal medicines in specific pathological states (*continued*)

Pathological state	Herbal medicine Latin name	Herbal medicine Common name	Clinical evidence	Source of evidence
	Tanacetum parthenium	Feverfew	Clearly negative	One placebo-controlled RCT, n=41)
	Allium sativum	Garlic	Preliminarily positive	One RCT (n=15)
	Zingiber officinale	Ginger	Preliminarily positive	One uncontrolled trial (n=28)
	Populus tremula *Fraxinus excelsior* *Solidago virgaurea*	Phytodolor®	Clearly positive	Systematic review (ten RCTs, 6 with placebo, 4 against reference medication, n=1035)[30]
	Tripterygium wilfordii	Thunder God vine	Preliminarily positive	Two RCTs
Rhinitis	*Petasites hybridus*	Butterbur	Preliminarily positive	One double-blind controlled RCT (n=256)[35]
Stroke	*Allium sativum*	Garlic	Preliminarily positive	One placebo-controlled RCT (n=60)
	Ginkgo biloba	Ginkgo	Preliminarily positive	One placebo-controlled RCT (n=50)
Tinnitus	*Ginkgo biloba*	Ginkgo	Tentatively positive	Systematic review (5 placebo-controlled RCTs, n=541)[36]
Upper respiratory tract infection	*Andrographis paniculata*	Andrographis	Preliminarily positive	Two double-blind RCTs (n=208)
	Echinacea spp.	Echinacea (prevention)	Tentatively negative	Systematic review (4 placebo-controlled RCTs (n=1152)[37]
	Echinacea spp .	Echinacea (treatment)	Tentatively positive	Systematic review (9 placebo-controlled, RCTs, n=1364)[37]
	Matricaria recutita	German chamomile	Preliminarily positive	One placebo-controlled RCT
	Panax ginseng	Ginseng	Preliminarily positive	One placebo-controlled RCT (n=227)

continued on page next page

Table 1
Clinical efficacy of herbal medicines in specific pathological states (*continued*)

Pathological state	Herbal medicine Latin name	Herbal medicine Common name	Clinical evidence	Source of evidence
Urinary tract infections	*Vaccinium macrocarpon*	Cranberry	Tentatively positive	Systematic review (4 placebo-controlled RCTs)[38]
Dermatological wounda	*Aloe vera*	Aloe gel	Preliminarily positive	Systematic review (2 RCTs,n=57)[19]

* Kampo (Japanese) formulation containing 10 herbs
** The herbal formula PC-SPES contains eight herbal medicines (see Appendix B)
*** Ayurvedic herbal preparation
**** Propolis is a resinous material which is collected by honey-bees from the buds of living plants mixed with bee wax and salivary secretions
Abbreviations: spp = species; CCT = controlled clinical trial; RCT = randomized clinical trial

References for Table 1

1. Ernst E, Huntley A (2000) Tea tree oil: a systematic review of randomized clinical trials. Forsch Komplementärmed 7:17–20
2. Meta-analysis Ginkgo for Alzheimer's disease. Arch Neurol 1998; 55:1409–1415
3. Pittler MH, Ernst E (2000) Efficacy of kava extract for treating anxiety: a systematic review and meta-analysis. J Clin Psychopharmacol 20:84–89
4. Ernst E, Huntley A (2000) Herbal medicine for asthma: a systematic review. Thorax 55:925–929
5. Ishani A, MacDonald R, Nelson D, Rutks I, Wilt TJ (2000) *Pygeum africanum* for the treatment of patient with benign prostatic hyperplasia: Systematic review and quantitative meta-analysis. Am J Med 1:654–664
6. Wilt TJ, MacDonald R, Ishani A, Rutks I, Stark G (2000) Cemilton for benign prostatic hyperplasia. Cochrane Database Syst Rev 2:CD001042
7. Wilt TJ, Ishani A, Stark G, MacDonald R, Lau J, Murlow C (1998) Saw palmetto extract for treatment of benign prostatic hyperplasia. JAMA. 280:1604–1609
8. Ernst E (1997) Can Allium vegetables prevent cancer? Phytomedicine 4:79–83
9. Kaegi E. (1998) Unconventional therapies for cancer: 2 Green tea. Can Med Assoc J, 158:1621–1624
10. Vanscheidt W, Jost V, Wolna P *et al.* (2002) Beneficial effects of *Ruscus aculeatus* L. for chronic venous insufficiency. Arzneim-Forsch/Drug Res 52:243–50
11. Pittler MH, Ernst E (1998) Horse-Chestnut seed extract for chronic venous insufficiency. Arch Dermatol 134:1356–1360
12. Rohdewald P (2002) A review of the French maritime pine bark extract (Pycnegol®), a herbal medication with a diverse clinical pharmacology. Inter J Clin Pharm Ther 40:158–168

13. Linde K, Mulrow CD (2000) St John's wort for depression. In The Cochrane Library (Issue 3), Oxford, Update Software
14. Shelton RC, Keller MB, Gelenberg A *et al.* (2001) Effectiveness of St John's Wort in major depression, a randomized controlled trial. JAMA, April 18, 285:1978–1986
15. Rabbani GH, Teka T, Zaman B *et al.* (2001) Clinical studies in persistent diarrhea: dietary management with green banana or pectin in Bangladeshi children. Gastroenterology, 121:554–560
16. Coon JT, Ernst E (2002) Systematic review: herbal medicinal products for non-ulcer dyspepsia. Aliment Pharmacol Ther 16:1689–1699
17. Bortolotti M, Coccia G, Grossi G, Miglioli M (2002) The treatment of functional dyspepsia with red pepper. Aliment Pharmacol Ther 16:1075–1082
18. Liu J, Lin H, McIntosh H (2001) Genus *Phyllantus* for chronic hepatitis B virus infection a systematic review. J Viral Hepatitis 8:358–366
19. Vogler BK, Ernst E (1999) *Aloe vera*: a systematic review of its clinical effectiveness. Br J Gen Pract 49:823–828
20. Thomson Coon J, Ernst E (2003) Herbal medicinal products for the treatment of hypercholesterolemia: a systematic review. Perfusion 16:40–55
21. Stevinson C, Ernst E (2000) Valerian for insomnia: a systematic review of randomised clinical trials. Sleep Medicine 2000; 1:91–99
22. Pittler M, Ernst E (2000) Ginkgo biloba extract for the treatment of intermittent claudication: a meta-analysis of randomized trials. Am J Med 108:276–280
23. Pittler M, Ernst E. (1998) Peppermint oil for irritable bowel syndrome: a critical review and meta-analysis. Am J Gastroenterol 93:1131–1135
24. Borrelli F, Ernst E (2002) *Cimicifuga racemosa*: a systematic review of its clinical efficacy. Eur J Clinical Pharmacol 58 (4):235–243
25. Fugh-Berman A, Kronenberg F (2001) Red clover (Trifolium pratense) for menopausal women: Current state of knowledge. Menopause 8:333–337
26. Pittler MH, Vogler BK, Ernst E (2000) Feverfew for preventing migraine. The Cochrane Library 3:1–10
27. Grossman M, Schmidramsl H (2000) *Petasites* extract effective for short-term migraine prophylaxis. Int J Clin Pharmacol Ther 38:430–435
28. Ernst E, Pittler MH (2000) Efficacy of ginger for nausea and vomiting: a systematic review of randomised clinical trials. Br J Anaesth 84:367–371
29. Ernst E, Chrubasik S (2000) Phyto-anti-inflammatories. a systematic review of randomised, placebo-controlled, double-blind trials. Rheumatic Disease Clinics of North America 26:13–27
30. Long L, Soaeken K, Ernst E (2001) Herbal medicines for the treatment of osteoarthritis: a systematic review. Rheumatology 40:779–793
31. Pittler MH, Ernst E (2001) Guar gum for body weight reduction: meta-analysis of randomized trials. Am J Med 110:724–730
32. Jiao DH, Shen XM, Gao YP, Chen MX, Wang ML (2001) Rhubarb extract – helpful in treating obesity? Chin J Integr Tradit West Med 7:33–35
33. Schellenberg R (2001) Treatment for the premenstrual syndrome with agnus castus fruit extract: prospective, randomized, placebo controlled study. Br Med J 322:134–137

34. Budeiri D, Li Wan Po A, Doman JC (1996) Is evening primrose oil of value in the treatment of premenstrual syndrome? Controlled Clin Trials, 17: 60–68
35. Schapowal A (2002) Randomized controlled trial of butterbur and cetirizine for treating seasonal allergic rhinitis. Br Med J 324:1–4
36. Ernst E, Stevinson C (1999) Ginkgo biloba for tinnitus: a review. Clin Otoryngol 24:164–167
37. Barrett B, Vohmann M, Calabrese C (1999) Echinacea for upper respiratory tract infection. J Fam Pract 48:628–635
38. Jepson RG, Mihaljevic L, Craig J (2000) Cranberry for treating urinary tract infections. Cochrane Database Syst Rev 2:CD001322

Glossary of Botanical Terms

Acuminate	Terminating very gradually in a point (apex) (refers to leaves)
Adventitious	Refers to an organ (root) that arises from an unusual position
Berry	Fleshy fruit containing many seeds
Biennial	A herb that normally requires two years to complete its life cycle
Bush	Clump of shrubs
Capitulum	An inflorescence consisting of sessile or subsessile flowers borne by the enlarged top of the peduncle (receptacle)
Caulescent	A herb whose stem bears leaves separated by visible elongated internodes, as opposed to a rosette plant
Coriaceous	Having the consistency of leather (refers to leaves)
Corymb	Indefinite inflorescence. The insertion points of the peduncles are spread along the axis and the peduncles are of uneven length, so that all of the flowers are approximately at the same level
Deciduous	Refers to leaves which fall off during the year
Decussate	With successive pairs at right angles to one another (refers to leaves)
Endosperm	A triploid (3n) nutritive tissue, formed within the embryonic sac from the union of a male nucleus and the polar nuclei of the central cell; it is consumed by the growing sporophyte either before or after the maturation of the seed; found only in Angiosperms
Floret	One of the flowers that make up a capitulum
Flower-head	An inflorescence, typical of the composite family, in which flowers are grouped closely on a receptacle
Herb	A non-woody seed plant with a relatively short-lived aerial portion.
Lamina	Flat and enlarged part of a leaf

Paripinnatus	When the petiole is terminated by neither leaflet nor tendril (e.g. senna leaves)
Perennial	A herb that lives from year to year
Pericarp	Wall of the fruit (pericarp + mesocarp + endocarp)
Periderm	Outer protective tissue that replaces epidermis after secondary growth is initiated; consists of cork, cork cambium, and phelloderm (refers to rhizome)
Pubescent	Covered with trichomes
Raceme	An inflorescence in which the main axis is elongated but the flowers are borne on pedicles that are about equal in length
Scarious	Membranous, thin, and transparent
Schizocarp	Dry fruit with two or more united carpels that split apart at maturity
Sessile	Inserted directly on the axis (with no peduncle or petiole) (generally refers to leaves)
Shoot (flowering)	A young branch that shoots out from the main stock of a tree, or the young main portion of a plant growing above ground
Shrub	A perennial woody plant of relatively low stature, typically with several stems arising from or near the ground
Spike	Indefinite inflorescence consisting of an axis bearing sessile flowers or groups of flowers (spikelet) spread along the axis
Squamous	Covered with minute scales, fixed by one end
Stolon	A stem that grows horizontally along the ground surface and may form adventitious roots
Strobilus	A reproductive structure consisting of a number of modified leaves (sporophylls) or ovule bearing scales grouped together or an axis, a cone. Strobili occur in many kinds of sphenophytes, lycophytes, and gymnosperms
Style	Narrow part between the ovary and the stigma
Succulent	A plant with fleshy, water-storing stems or leaves
Tap-root	The primary root of a plant that develops directly from the embryonic radicle; forms a stout, tapering main root from which arise smaller, lateral roots
Thallus	A plant body without true roots, stems, or leaves; the word thallus was commonly used when fungi and algae were considered to be plants, to distinguish their simple construction from the differentiated bodies of plant sporophytes

Tuberous Refers to a subterraneous organ, much-enlarged, in which reserves are stored

Weed Generally a herbaceous plant or shrub not valued for use or beauty, growing where unwanted, and regarded as using ground or hindering the growth of useful vegetation

Subject Index

A

D

E

G

M

N

O

S